PREFRONTAL CORTEX: ROLES, INTERVENTIONS AND TRAUMAS

PREFRONTAL CORTEX: ROLES, INTERVENTIONS AND TRAUMAS

LORENZO LOGRASSO
AND
GIOVANNI MORRETTI
EDITORS

Nova Biomedical Books
New York

For permission to use material from this book please contact us:
Telephone 631-231-7269; Fax 631-231-8175
Web Site: http://www.novapublishers.com

Library of Congress Cataloging-in-Publication Data

Prefrontal cortex : roles, interventions & traumas / [edited by] Lorenzo LoGrasso & Giovanni Morretti.
p. ; cm.
Includes bibliographical references and index.
ISBN 978-1-60692-415-0 (hardcover)
1. Prefrontal cortex. 2. Prefrontal cortex--Pathophysiology. 3. Schizophrenia. I. LoGrasso, Lorenzo. II. Morretti, Giovanni.
[DNLM: 1. Prefrontal Cortex. 2. Mental Processes--physiology. 3. Schizophrenia--physiopathology. WL 307 P9236 2009]
QP383.17.P746 2009
612.8'25--dc22

2008047557

Published by Nova Science Publishers, Inc. ✝ New York

Contents

Preface

Intellectual disabilities have been related to the dysfunction of the prefrontal cortex. The prefrontal cortex is located on the anterior part of the frontal lobes of the brain, lying in front of the motor and premotor areas. This brain region has been implicated in planning complex cognitive behaviors, personality expression, and moderating correct social behavior.This book presents a review of present day evidence of the reduction of the prefrontal cortex; links between abnormalities and functional or clinical features of intellectual disabilities such as schizophrenia. The book presents the latest research from around the world in this field.

Chapter 1 - Dysfunction of the prefrontal cortex is a hallmark of schizophrenia. This dysfunction can be demonstrated using many approaches, including functional neuroimaging techniques, neuropsychological tests focused on working and verbal memory, problem solving, or verbal fluency. Histopathological studies demonstrate the presence of cortical thickness reduction (layers II and III in particular) that is due to the neuropil loss with reduction of pyramidal neuronal size. These neuropathological changes are reflected in neuroimaging studies (volumetric studies and voxel-based studies) with findings of cortical gray matter shrinkage. All of these changes can be viewed in the context of the prefrontal disconnection that is behind many signs and symptoms of the disease, including dopamine system dysregulation and cognitive abnormalities. This chapter reviews the present-day evidence for the reduction of the prefrontal cortex and then focuses on the links between this abnormality and the functional and clinical features of schizophrenia.

Chapter 2 - There is a growing body of evidence to suggest that alterations in the cholinergic systems of the central nervous system are important in the pathology of schizophrenia. This data has arisen from studies into preclinical and clinical pharmacology, patient treatment, post-mortem neurochemistry and neuroimaging of patients with the disorder. The neuropharmacology of antipsychotics used to treat the disorder first led scientists to investigate changes in both the neurotransmitters and their receptors that are targeted by these therapeutic agents. These investigations have revealed that some atypical antipsychotics increase acetylcholine release in the prefrontal cortex, possibly contributing to improvements seen in some of the cognitive dysfunction for these drugs. Whilst there are data that show that some current atypical antipsychotic drugs have some impact on negative symptoms and cognitive deficits, none of these drugs are truly effective in treating these symptoms. Thus, in schizophrenia, various components within the cholinergic system are being investigated as potential targets for drugs that might effectively reverse these symptoms that are currently treatment-resistant. In this regard, post-mortem studies have revealed that patients with schizophrenia have low levels of cholinergic muscarinic receptors (CHRMs) in the CNS, and it is now well established that CHRM1 is decreased in the dorsolateral prefrontal cortex from subjects with the disorder; this receptor deficit is believed to play an important role in the cognitive dysfunctions associated with the disease. Recent information from basic research, in particular from studies using $CHRM^{-/-}$ mice, has enabled us to develop hypotheses as to what the functional consequences of deficits in CHRMs might be. Several lines of evidence also suggest a pathophysiological function for nicotinic acetylcholine receptors in schizophrenia. Nicotine administration has been shown to improve cognition in patients with schizophrenia. In the prefrontal cortex this receptor is thought to affect cognition through its activation-dependent effects on dopamine D_1 receptor mediated neurotransmission. Thus, both muscarinic and nicotinic receptors are viable drug targets with respect to cognitive deficits in schizophrenia. Using previous findings, in combination with data, it is possible to understand the specific changes in the various neurotransmitter receptors in the brains of schizophrenic patients, the functional effects of these changes and the roles the receptors may play in the pathology of the disorder.

Chapter 3 - Sexual and maternal behaviors constitute motivated behaviors, the adequate manifestation of which requires an appropriate integration of external stimuli and internal states. In both is required the perception of an appropriate stimulus. For a male rat, one appropriate sexual incentive stimulus could be a receptive female, while for a female mother rat the appropriate maternal incentive could be a pup rat. The sensory clues emitted by either the potential sexual partner or the pups must be first detected and then processed in order to be perceived as incentives and as potentially rewarding. The prefrontal cortex (PFC) plays an important role both in mediating the assignation of the incentive value and in information processing. Thus, using electroencephalographic (EEG) recordings,this book characterizes the prefrontal functioning during motivational states of sexual and maternal behavior in rats. In a first study, it was observed that the EEG activity of the medial (mPFC) and orbital prefrontal cortices (oPFC) was modified during the performance of male rats in a T-maze under two different conditions: sexually-motivated (with previous intromission and one receptive and one non-receptive female placed in the goal boxes of the lateral arms); and not sexually-motivated (no previous intromission and empty goal boxes). Only the sexually-motivated males showed a higher proportion in the 6-7 Hz band and a lower proportion in the 8-11 Hz band during the awake-quiet state and while walking in the maze stem. In addition, they showed an increased correlation of the 6-7 Hz band while walking in the maze stem and when remaining close to a receptive female. Similar EEG changes were obtained in estrous female rats that were subjected to a sexually-motivated task using the same paradigm of the T-maze. In the oPFC of the sexually-motivated females and males, different EEG patterns were observed, results that suggest a different functionality of the mPFC and oPFC, which may work together in the processing of sexual incentive stimuli. Another study explored whether the mPFC of female rats shows characteristic EEG patterns during the presentation of olfactory stimuli, when (1) associated with pups (nest-bedding); and, (2) not-associated, with pups (female bedding), during the following distinct reproductive states: proestrus-estrus (P-E), diestrus (D) and lactation (L). During the smelling of nest-bedding, only the L rats showed a higher proportion in the 8-11 Hz band. This finding may represent a characteristic processing of the olfactory stimuli related to pups in the mPFC of L rats. Taken together, these data allow suggest that in rats the prefrontal cortex participates in identifying and processing sexual and maternal incentives.

Chapter 4 – This chapter shows the way in which animals acquire problem-solving behavioral strategies. The focus was on the search for sequential feedback rules that guide an individual along the stepwise learning process from the initial conflict generated by a novel situation to the context-adequate, problem-solving and, therewith, successful behavioral strategy.

The medial prefrontal cortex plays a complex role in acquisition and storage of behavioral strategies. It is an important part of the internal reward system, inducing a motivational drive for the development of a memory-guided, goal-directed behavioral strategy. This view is also strongly supported by work on the learning-related dynamics of prefrontal dopamine release.

Using Mongolian gerbils (Meriones unguiculatus) as an animal model, this chapter shows the formation of an avoidance strategy in a shuttle-box during the stage of avoidance learning is accompanied by a strong increase of the activity in the prefrontal dopamine system. Cortical theta activation was found to be, overall, negatively correlated with the formation of avoidance strategy during learning. In learning stages preceding the stage of avoidance learning there are different decreases of theta activity. However, when the animals entered the stage of avoidance learning, i.e., the phase when prefrontal dopamine release increases, theta activity increased again as well. A detailed analysis of theta activation revealed unique events in single trials marking the transition between behaviorally-defined learning stages and reflecting the actual change of the task-context for the animal.

Based on the correlation between behavioral data and data of learning-relevant physiological parameters, i.e., prefrontal dopamine and theta activation, cognitive processes like feedback learning, error processing, planning, decision making, and short-term memory as components of working memory functions during stepwise learning are discussed. The detailed analysis of learning processes in simple avoidance conditioning paradigms is a prerequisite for a deeper understanding of information processing during the goal-directed formation of behavioral strategies.

Chapter 5 - The orbital part of the prefrontal cortex is known to be crucially involved in emotional decision-making. Its function seems to be, first, to associate affective value with behavioral bias (i.e., approach or withdrawal) in complex choice situations, and secondly, to flexibly control and transiently inhibit affective and behavioral impulses. Dysfunction of this region due to damage or immaturity of OFC cells leads to impulsiveness, behavioral perseveration, and reduced sensitivity for risk, as observed in children as well as various patients groups. The evidence is reviewed with a focus on the much less investigated question of whether and how *hyper*activation (or hyperfunctioning of modules and processes) involving OFC leads to the opposite behavioral tendencies, namely risk-aversion, enhanced inhibition, undecidedness and higher risk sensitivity including heightened anxiety. Two perspectives with opposing views onto this issue, some unpublished studies of populations with children and patients with anxiety disorders using the Iowa gambling task, a task that is presumed to be sensitive to OFC function are discussed. Reports find that, if anything, anxiety has the same beneficial effects onto performance as cortical maturation. Although effects of anxiety are much weaker and less conclusive than those of age during childhood, it seems that there are situations in which enhanced anxiety can support advantageous decision-making. Results highlight the important role of orbitofrontal cortex in integrating approach- and withdrawal-tendencies mediated by mesolimbic and mesostriatal structures on the one hand and higher cognitive centres on the other, with the latter ones recruiting more dorsal parts of the prefrontal cortex and allowing for conscious thinking, reasoning, and problem-solving. Behavioral interventions as in education, cognitive training, and psychotherapy are most effective when they take into account the motivational and evaluative function of this region.

Chapter 6 - In macaque monkeys, area 8B may be considered cytoarchitectonically as a transitional area between the granular area 9, rostrally, and the rostral part of the dorsal agranular area 6 (FC or F7), caudally. This area is anatomically connected with auditory cortical areas, cerebellum and superior colliculus. Microstimulation of area 8B evokes ear movements or eye movements in some sites; in other sites, it evokes both ear and eye movements by varying the intensity of electric stimulation. Unit activity recording shows that neurons in area 8B have a role in encoding different auditory environmental stimuli and movements of the ear and eye. In addition, fixation of a visual stimulus, when attention is engaged, modulates the discharge of auditory environmental neurons, and sensory-motor neurons.

Current functional and anatomical evidences strongly support the proposal that area 8B is a specific Premotor Ear-Eye Field (PEEF) involved in the recognition of auditory stimuli and in orienting processes. Moreover, activation by specific environmental auditory stimuli, suggests that PEEF is an important node in the hierarchical organisation of the auditory network. The inhibitory effects on neural discharge of auditory and auditory-motor cells might be a consequence of the engagement of attention during visual fixation. This phenomenon may be the expression of a combination of a covert orienting of attention relative to eye effectors, and an overt orienting of attention relative to ear effectors. It seems that attention may affect more than one channel at the same time during a conditioned task or during natural behaviour. Then the PEEF, based on its connections and functional characteristics may be involved in three circuits: 1) an auditory circuit, 2) an oculomotor circuit, 3) and a fronto-cerebellar circuit.

Expert Communication A - Parkinson's disease (PD) is a neurodegenerative disorder, classically characterized by the chronic loss of dopaminergic neurons primarily in substantia nigra pars compacta, which leads to a reduction of dopamine levels in the striatum. The motor symptoms do not become obvious until at least an 80% reduction in striatal dopamine levels. Recent works have demonstrated that cognitive impairment occurs even in the early course of PD which is correlated with dopaminergic dysfunctions in the prefrontal cortex (Brück, 2005b; Chudasama and Robbins, 2006) and not necessarily related to motor disorders. This commentary will discuss the current knowledge of the prefrontal cortex and its association with cognitive deficits in PD.

Expert Communication B - This chapter reviews the important role of prefrontal cortex (PFC) in the regulation of behavior and attention, and evidence that these processes are weakened in Attention-Deficit/Hyperactivity Disorder (AD/HD). Norepinephrine (NE) has been found to have a critical beneficial effect on PFC function through actions at post-synaptic, α2A-adrenoceptors, while high levels of NE release during stress impair PFC regulation of behavior through actions at α1 adrenoceptors. The PFC regulates its own NE input through projections to NE-containing locus coeruleus (LC) neurons. The LC fires according to arousal state and attentional demands. Most medications effective for the treatment of AD/HD powerfully influence NE transmission, either by blocking reuptake or mimicking its actions at α2A-adrenoceptors. The importance of NE to AD/HD is increasingly appreciated.

Short Communication A - Modern imaging techniques allow the mapping of gross brain structure to an exacting standard; however, these methodologies have been applied inappropriately in recent times to the study of the prefrontal cortex – the structure identified by Brodmann as being central to intelligence. Currently, these methodologies cannot detect prefrontal cortex, nor be used to quantify it. Here Brodmann's data on comparative aspects of the gross structure of the cerebral cortex, some of which have been largely ignored in recent times, is reviewed. This still remains the definitive data set for prefrontal cortex. In addition, Brodmann's observations are compared with those of his contemporary Santiago Ramon Cajal. Cajal's studies of the fine structure of the cerebral cortex led him to the conclusion that human intelligence is largely attributable to the complexity of the pyramidal (psychic) cell. These observations are compared and contrasted with modern data on prefrontal cortex, essentially substantiating the conclusions of these two great founding fathers of modern neuroscience.

Short Communication B - The developmental characteristics of semantic category generation were studied in a sample of 200 neurologically intact subjects from 6 to 30 years old. Results indicate that diverse brain areas support different the category criteria used: subjects in the 6-8 age range used a concrete criteria (posterior brain areas), in the 9-11 age range a functional criteria is dominant (dorsolateral prefrontal cortex), while abstract criteria becomes dominant in the 12-14 age-range (anterior prefrontal cortex) and continuous to develop in the 16 to 30 age range. It is proposed that different prefrontal areas participate during development, shaping cognitive approach to categorisation during childhood and adolescence.

In: Prefrontal Cortex: Roles, Interventions and Traumas
Editors: Lorenzo LoGrasso and Giovanni Morretti
ISBN 978-1-60692-415-0

Chapter 1

Prefrontal Morphology, Neurobiology and Clinical Manifestations of Schizophrenia

Tomáš Kašpárek*
Department of Psychiatry,
Masaryk University and Faculty Hospital Brno
Jihlavska 20, 625 00, Brno, Czech Republic

Abstract

Dysfunction of the prefrontal cortex is a hallmark of schizophrenia. This dysfunction can be demonstrated using many approaches, including functional neuroimaging techniques, neuropsychological tests focused on working and verbal memory, problem solving, or verbal fluency. Histopathological studies demonstrate the presence of cortical thickness reduction (layers II and III in particular) that is due to the neuropil loss with reduction of pyramidal neuronal size. These neuropathological changes are reflected in neuroimaging studies (volumetric studies and voxel-based studies) with findings of cortical gray matter shrinkage. All of these changes can be viewed in the context of the prefrontal disconnection that is behind many signs and symptoms of the disease, including dopamine system dysregulation and cognitive abnormalities. We review the present-day evidence for the reduction of the prefrontal cortex and then focus on the links between this abnormality and the functional and clinical features of schizophrenia.

A. Introduction

Schizophrenia is a heterogeneous condition with highly variable clinical manifestation, time-course, and response to various treatment approaches. During the course of the illness, subjects with schizophrenia experience periods of psychosis with symptoms such as

* Tel.: +420 53223 2560; Fax: +420 53223 3706; E-mail: tomas.kasparek@centrum.cz

hallucinations, delusions or disorganization of thoughts and behavior. Simultaneously as well as after the psychosis alleviation, they may experience so-called negative symptoms such as emotional withdrawal, apathy, anhedonia, lack of initiative, etc. and a varying degree of cognitive dysfunction, with working memory, verbal learning and memory, sustained attention or executive functions being affected the most (Nuechterlein et al., 2004). One of the cardinal features of schizophrenia is its typical time window of onset: although there are exceptions, the illness manifests during late adolescence or early adulthood in most cases. The outcome of the illness is inherently variable in the sense of the expression of symptoms and functional impairment. Unfortunately, it is very hard to predict the probable course of the illness in individual patients (Bromet et al., 2005; Fleischaker et al., 2005; Jobe and Harrow, 2005). The failure of current operationally-based diagnostic approaches to provide homogenous subgroups of patients with similar outcomes and responses to treatment led to a search for distinct neurobiologically-defined syndromes that may share clinical manifestations (Braf et al., 2007). Studies of brain morphology may help in this effort.

Schizophrenia was considered a functional condition for a significant period of time. This view stemmed from the inability to find any specific morphological correlates of the disease during the period of the neuropathological era in neuropsychiatry in the late nineteenth and early twentieth century. From the late 1970s when the first CT studies of chronic schizophrenia patients were published (Johnstone et al., 1976), it is more and more obvious that morphological abnormalities play a considerable role in the neurobiology of schizophrenia. Until today, brain morphology is in principle studied by two approaches: histopathology and neuroimaging.

B. Neuropathological Findings in the Prefrontal Cortex in Schizophrenia

Contrary to the expectations in the golden era of neuropathological studies in neuropsychiatry, in the age of Kraepelin and Alzheimer, the structural correlate of schizophrenia remained uncovered for a long time, and the phrase "schizophrenia as a graveyard of neuropathologists" emerged. Despite recent advances, the definite pattern of neuropathological abnormalities in schizophrenia is still missing. Many older studies yielded inconsistent or contradictory findings. As in other areas of schizophrenia research, consistency was complicated by the lack of diagnostic validity and reliability, clinical heterogeneity of the illness, or lack of information from other methodologies for identification of regions of interest in older studies (Powers, 1999).

As recently as the last two decades, with the improvements in both diagnostic and neuropathological methodologies, a much clearer picture has emerged. There seem to be several cortical as well as subcortical morphological changes in schizophrenia. Morphological studies of cortical structures focus mainly on prefrontal cortex, anterior cingulate, and temporal lobe regions such as superior temporal gyrus and medial temporal structures. In general, the changes are relatively inhomogeneous in individual patients, both in type and localization; there is a considerable overlap between the patients and healthy controls with no pathognomic features useful for differential diagnosis (Bogerts, 1999).

Furthermore, imaging studies suggest that the neuropathological changes are more widespread than recent neuropathological studies demonstrate – simply because the neuropathological examinations have not yet focused attention on these regions.

Pattern of Neupathological Neocortical Changes

In schizophrenia, a smaller volume of frontal, parietal, and termporal cortices were shown (Pakkenberg et al., 1993; Selemon et al., 2002).

Dorsolateral prefrontal cortex (DLPFC, area 9, 46): Changes of the dorsolateral prefrontal cortex are the most studied and the findings form the most established neuropathological evidence in schizophrenia. In the prefrontal cortex *increased neuronal density* was observed in the dorsolateral prefrontal cortex, - by 17% in area 9 and 21% in area 46 across layers III–VI (Selemon, 1995, 1998), with some data suggesting a similar pattern in the whole frontal lobe or even cortex as a whole (Pakkenberg, 1993). The increased density was observed for pyramidal as well as non-pyramidal neurons (Selemon, 1998). No significant changes of glial density were observed (Selemon et al., 1995; Selemon et al., 1998). The *cortical thickness is reduced*, especially in layers II and III, probably as a consequence of increased neuronal density (Pakkenberg, 1987; Selemon 1998; Woo, 1998). The total *number of neurons* in the frontal cortex seems to be preserved (Pakkenberg, 1993; Thune et al., 2001). Furthermore, the *neuronal size* of pyramidal neurons is reduced, especially in the deep layer III of BA 9, but not in layer V (Rajkowska 1998; Pierri et al., 2001). Reduction of the neuronal size and increased neuronal density are in accord with or are consequences of the *decreased neuropil density* as demonstrated by the findings of reduced presynaptic terminals as inferred from *synaptophysin* levels, which is a protein associated with synaptic vesicles (Glantz and Lewis, 1997) and by lower density of *dendritic spines:* on layer III (Garey, 1998; Glantz and Lewis, 2000) but not on layer V and VI (Kolluri et al., 2005) pyramidal neurons in dorsolateral prefrontal area 46 and on layer V in area 9 (Jones et al., 2002). The magnitude of the reduction was determined to be almost 50 % of the spine density in healthy controls. Changes in the deep cortical layers might be a consequence of exposure to antipsychotics – see below – and thus they should be considered with caution. Reduction of glial cells was also observed (Hof et al., 2003).

Other prefrontal areas: In the *frontopolar cortex* (area 10), increased density of pyramidal neurons with decreased density of interneurons was observed in layer V (Benes et al., 1991), and lower density of dendritic spines (Garey et al., 1998). Lower levels of synaptophysin (Perrone-Bizzozero et al., 1996) were observed. Changes of neuronal cell size or glial density were not seen (Benes et al., 1991). In *Broca's area* (area 44) not significant changes of cell density were observed in the same subjects in whom the increase was found in the DLPFC (Selemon et al., 2003). *Anterior cingulate* seems to be morphologically distinct from lateral and rostral parts of the frontal cortex. In contrast to findings in the DLPFC, no changes in neuronal density in the cingulate cortex were reported (Benes et al., 1991; Kalus et al., 1997). A decrease in the number of dendrites in layer V in medial prefrontal area 32 was reported (Broadbelt et al., 2002), however, with findings of preserved levels of synaptophysin (Honer et al., 1997; Eastwood et al., 2000). Moreover, an increase of certain

GABA-ergic parameters was observed, whereas decrease was observed in dorsolateral prefrontal cortex: Kalus et al. (1997) found an increase of parvalbumin-immunoreactive neurons and similar increase of chandelier axonal cartridges. No changes of glia cells were observed in some studies (Benes et al., 1991; Radewicz et al., 2000), although newer study found significant reduction of glial cells in area 24 (Hof et al., 2003).

Table 1. Neuropathology of dorsolateral prefrontal cortex in schizophrenia

LAYER II, III
Decreased dendritic density, loss of dendritic spines
Decreased neuronal cell bodies of pyramidal and GABA neurons
Increased neuronal density
Reduced cortical thickness
NO GLIOSIS
NO NEURONAL LOSS
LOSS OF DENDRITIC SPINES IN LAYER V???

The findings in all these prefrontal areas are less extensive than the changes in dorsolateral prefrontal cortex suggesting that although not uniquely, DLPFC is affected prominently. It is not known If the changes are present also in other frontal areas since they have not been systematically studied. Overall, the pattern of changes in the prefrontal cortex in schizophrenia subjects suggests abnormalities of cortical connectivity, or, in other words, disease of the cortical microcircuitry.

Changes of Cortical Microcircuitry in Schizophrenia

It is possible to look at the changes in much greater detail: several lines of evidence point to layer III pyramidal neurons, parvalbumin-immunoreactive GABA-ergic interneurons and cortical dopaminergic projections.

From the point of view of layer III pyramidal neuronal inputs, reduction of dendritic spines, which is the hallmark of the neuropathology of schizophrenia, may reflect the impairment of connections from other cortical areas (association fibers), nearby PN of the same layer (intrinsic connections), mediodorsal thalamus (thalamocortical projections) and dopaminergic projections. Dendritic spines of layer III pyramidal neurons are the target of these excitatory inputs (DeFelipe and Farinas, 1992), thus the reduction of the spines seems to reflect a reduction of such inputs. Alternatively, the reduction of the dendritic arbor may result from altered capacity of pyramidal neurons to support it, perhaps due to cytoskeleton regulation abnormalities, and consequently, the number of excitatory synapses is diminished.

As there is a reduction of *mediodorsal thalamus* volume in schizophrenia, a deficit of thalamo-cortical connections may contribute to the overall pattern of the cortical microcircuitry changes. The projections from MD thalamus terminate in deep layer III on basal dendritic spines of layer III PN (Erickson adn Lewis, 2004). The reduction of neurons in mediodorsal nucleus, as well as changes of thalamo-cortical afferent fiber bundles were described (Pakkenberg 1990; Dorph-Petersen et al., 2004). However, as the thalamocortical afferents appear to compose a small proportion (< 10 %) of the total cortical excitatory inputs - as demonstrated in visual cortex of cats (Ahmed et al., 1994) – and lesions of mediodorsal thalamus produce no changes in GAD67 mRNA expression (Volk and Lewis, 2003; see below) it is clear that other inputs should contribute to the pattern of changes.

Cortical architecture, connectivity as well as performance of the dorsolateral prefrontal cortex mature during adolescence, which is the time of typical onset of schizophrenia. During that time the prefrontal cortex starts to augment the activity of other neural circuits during the performance of tasks such as delayed action, working memory paradigms (Alexander and Goldman 1978). This increase of the prefrontal cortex involvement correlates with interrelated changes of *connectivity of layer III pyramidal neurons*, parvalbumin-immunoreactive wide-arbor GABA-ergic interneurons and dopaminergic projections, as emerges from primate studies (Lewis 1997): Layer III pyramidal neurons send axonal associational projections to other cortical regions as well as intrinsic axonal collaterals that run horizontally through gray matter to superficial cortical layers where they terminate on dendritic spines of neighboring pyramidal cells thus giving rise to functionally interconnected clusters of pyramidal neurons (Levitt et al., 1993). During adolescence the dendritic spines of layer III pyramidal neurons are extensively pruned (Bourgeois et al., 1994). Changes in dendritic spine density reflect parallel changes in excitatory inputs formed by intrinsic, and not associational, projections to these neurons (Lund and Holbach, 1991; Woo et al., 1997).

The layer III PN also send collateral connections to the dendrites of *GABA-ergic parvalbumin-immunoreactive (wide arbor and chandelier) interneurons* (Levitt et al., 1993; Lund et al., 1993; Melchitzky et al., 1995). Interestingly, the maturation changes of dendritic spines on pyramidal neurons are accompanied by the changes of PV-interneurons that may be a kind of compensatory mechanism of the changes of excitatory inputs to pyramidal neurons (Lewis 1997). There is a growing evidence of the involvement of GABA dysfunction in schizophrenia (Lewis et al., 2005). In schizophrenia decrease of *GAD67* mRNA encoding GABA synthesizing enzyme glutamic acid decarboxylase in the prefrontal cortex was replicated several times (Akbarian et al., 1995; Volk et al., 2000; Guidotti et al., 2000), with a consequent reduction of the protein levels (Guidotti et al., 2000). GAD67 positive neurons density was decreased in layer III-V, but not VI in DLPFC in schizophrenia (Akbarian et al., 1995; Volk et al., 2000) with no changes of the GAD67 mRNA level in individual neurons (Volk et al., 2000). However, *a proportion of GABA neurons did not express detectable levels of GAD67 mRNA*, together with reduced levels of GABA transporter *GAT1* (Volk et al., 2001). These changes seem to be specific to parvalbumin-immunoreactive cells (Beasley and Reynolds 1997; Hashimoto et al., 2003). *PV levels* were reduced in the layer III and IV neurons in the DLPFC (Hashimoto et al., 2003). There is not a loss of PV positive neurons in DLPFC, rather normal numbers of neurons express lower levels of PV. PV positive neurons are of two types: chandelier and wide-arbor basket cells. *Chandelier cells* project axons to initial axonal segments of pyramidal neurons and form there multiple synaptic connections called *"cartridges"*, carrying GAT1 transporters. The density of these GAT1 immunoreactive cartridges was reduced in middle cortical layers of DLPFC in schizophrenia (Woo et al., 1998). On the postsynaptic side up-regulation of *alpha2 subunit containing GABA-A receptors* was seen (Volk et al., 2002). Similar pattern of synaptic changes is present in the case of *wide-arbor basket cells* (Lewis et al., 2001; Benes et al., 1996). These cells send axons that form synpases on the cell bodies of pyramidal neurons. Possible unifying mechanism of the PV associated pattern of changes was proposed: *BDNF receptor TrkB* dysfunction – expressing regional specificity to PV cells – with consequent changes of GAD67 expression and reduction of GABA synthesis and compensatory decrease of parvalbumin levels leading to higher levels of free calcium, decreased GABA re-uptake through down-regulated GAT1 – both leading to increase GABA synaptic levels - and increase of postsynaptic GABA receptors (Hashimoto et al., 2005; Lewis et al., 2005). Although the changes were not seen for calretinin-immunoreactive cells (Hashimoto et al., 2003), there seem to be changes in other GABA cells, such as somatostatin-positive cells (Morris et al., 2008) since PV interneurons cannot explain the changes in layers I and II. PV interneurons inhibit the somata and initial axonal segments of several pyramidal neurons and they share excitatory inputs from mediodorsal thalamus and other pyramidal neurons with local pyramidal neurons (Melchitzky et al., 1999; Melchitzky et al., 2001; Melchitzky and Lewis, 2003), thus enabling their coordinated and timed activity. Functional consequences of this action are synchronized neuronal oscilations in several discrete frequency bands (Cobb et al., 1995; Tamás et al., 2000; Szabadics et al., 2001; Blatow et al., 2003), such as gamma band oscillations, electrophysiological activity linked to many higher order cognitive operations. Several studies reported abnormalities of gamma band oscillations in schizophrenia (Spencer et al., 2003; Cho et al., 2006). Superficial GABA PV and CB positive interneurons give rise to theta band oscillations (Blatow et al., 2003), another band of interest in schizophrenia.

Furthermore, it was shown that also *dopaminergic projections* to the dorsolateral prefrontal cortex undergo substantial changes during adolescence. They form connections with dendritic spines of pyramidal neurons (Goldman-Rakic et al., 1989; Smiley et al., 1992) as well as with dendrites of PV-interneurons (and not with calretinin-immunoreactive GABA interneurons; Sesack et al., 1995a,b). The maturation changes of DA projections just precede the changes of PN a PV cells and it is speculated that the neuromodulatory effect exerted by dopamine may influence the refinement of cortical architecture (Lewis et al., 1997). In accord with these effects of dopaminergic projections are the findings of dopamine neurotrophic effect: its depletion affects dendritic spine and synapse density (Deutch and Jing, 2003; Deutch, 2005). Amphetamine sensitisation, leading to a chronic dopamine dysregulation, is also linked with dendritic spine reduction on layer III pyramidal neurons in primates (Selemon et al., 2007). Thus, monoamine abnormalities may contribute to the structural abnormalities in schizophrenia. It was also demonstrated that dopaminergic signaling has a key functional role in the prefrontal cortex (Williams and Goldman-Rakic, 1995; Arnsten et al., 1994). Reduction of DA connection may be a correlate of both morphological and functional impairments seen in schizophrenia. Benes suggested a model of neuropathology of schizophrenia where abnormal connectivity of local neuronal circuits is caused by rearrangement of dopaminergic connections, which are supposed to shift from PN to nonpyramidal neurons, possibly as a way of compensation of the loss of their pyramidal targets (Benes et al., 1995; Benes 1997).

These data obtained mostly from animal studies seem to be parallel to the neuropathological changes seen in human subjects with schizophrenia: neuropil reduction of layer III pyramidal neurons, decreased cell size of pyramidal neurons as well as PV-interneurons – see above. In the light of animal as well as human neuropathological data we may view the pathology of schizophrenia as pathology of prefrontal cortical microcircuitry connectivity. Because of the developmental changes are prominent for the intrinsic connections between the clusters of pyramidal and PV-cells, with the tuning connections from dopaminergic centers, the basic pathology concerns local circuitry connectivity. These local circuitry abnormalities of prefrontal cortex may lead to difficulties in coordination of action of large populations of neurons with consequent discoordination or disconnection of neuronal nets subserving top-level information processing – leading to either overall impairment of cortical connectivity or rather specific disconnection of fronto-temporal areas (Friston and Frith, 1995). These ideas were formulated explicitly by Selemon and Goldman-Rakic who view the reduced neuropil as a cardinal feature of schizophrenia: The reduced neuropil hypothesis. In short they state that "disturbances in prefrontal cognitive functioning in schizophrenia may be mediated by a process which involves atrophy of neuronal processes but stops short of actual neuronal loss" (Selemon 1995, Selemon and Goldman-Rakic, 1999a). As shown below, several processes that may selectively afflict the neuropil without the induction of cell death exist. The reduced neuropil hypothesis receives support from an elegant computational simulation: Hoffman and Dobscha (1989) presented a model, where reduction of elements of a neuronal network led to the improvement of performance. However, when a certain threshold was crossed, the network produced outputs even without any inputs, which was interpreted as a correlate of autonomic behavior of cortex as a cause of hallucinations.

Dendritic arbor of layer V and VI PN seems to be relatively spared. These cells are the origin of cortico-striatal and cortico-thalamic projections, which seem to be intact in schizophrenia. Similarly, these cells receive very little inputs from mediodorsal thalamus (Erickson and Lewis, 2004), further supporting the view of layer III specific abnormality in schizophrenia.

Table 2. Cortical neurocircuitry changes in dorsolateral prefrontal cortex in schizophrenia

ABNORMALITIES OF EXCITATORY INPUTS ON DENDRITIC ARBOR OF PYRAMIDAL NEURONS
Reduction of intrinsic and cortico-cortical connections between pyramidal neurons
Reduction of dopaminergic projections
Reduction of thalamocortical projections from mediodorsal thalamus
ABNORMALITIES OF PERISOMATIC AND AXONAL INHIBITION OF PYRAMIDAL NEURONS
Reduction of chandelier cells synaptic cartridges on initial axonal segment of pyramidal neurons
Reduction of wide-arbor cells perisomatic inhibition
Up-reglation of GABA-A alpha 2 subunit postsynatptically on pyramidal neurons
= LOSS OF COORDINATION BETWEEN CORTICAL PYRAMIDAL NEURONS

Regional Specificity of the Changes Seen in Prefrontal Cortex

Are the above described changes specific for the prefrontal cortex? There is evidence of changes in many other areas, where similar as well as distinct neuropathological changes were described: disarray of hippocampal pyramidal neurons, reduction of their size, decrease of synaptic markers in hippocampus (Harrison, 2004); reduction of neurons in the mediodorsal nucleus and pulvinar of the thalamus (Pakkenberg et al., 1990; Popken et al., 2000); reduction of normal cortical asymmetry with some reports suggesting pronounced abnormalities in the left hemisphere (Crow et al., 1989); reduction of dendritic spine density in temporal neocortex (BA 20, 21, 22, and 38; Garey et al., 1993), reduction of dendritic spines, neuronal size of layer III PN and axonal terminals in primary – BA 41 – and association auditory cortex - BA 42 (Sweet et al., 2003; Sweet et al., 2008); or neuropil reduction in occipital cortex (Selemon et al., 1995).

C. Etiology

The origin of structural changes is still elusive as well. However, it is probable that there is not just one unique mechanism responsible for the changes. Intrauterine or neonatal lesions, genetic diathesis, oxidative stress, nutritional factors, infectious agents etc. are all mentioned in the etiopathogenetic frameworks of schizophrenia.

Neurodevelopment

From the first studies in the late 19th century it is known that changes in schizophrenia are not followed by gliosis, suggesting the lack of neurodegenerative processes in schizophrenia. Other features, such as frequent occurrence of cavum septi pellucidi in the adult age, cytoarchitectural changes, or reduction of brain asymmetry point to some abnormality in the development of the brain. There is not just one comprehensive developmental theory of schizophrenia, rather, several of them emerged with some of them being refined, some abandoned (de Haan and Bakker, 2004).

Some theories emphasize the involvement of *early developmental abnormalities,* possibly during the pre/perinatal period (Weinberger 1987; Murray and Lewis 1987; Roberts 1991; Benes 1997). The evidence for this view comes from the findings of absence of brain asymmetry, higher prevalence of schizophrenia in subjects born in winter, with obstetric complications, whose mothers had influenza during the 2nd trimester of pregnancy or first-trimester malnutrition, with some motor and language skills abnormalities or social skills impairments during childhood (for review see Murray 1994; Weinberger 1995, Harrison 1999, Maynard et al., 2001).

Neonatal hippocampal lesions: neonatal ventral hippocampal lesions as a model of the pathophysiology of schizophrenia is one of the most elaborated theories (Lipska et al., 1995; Lipska and Weinberger 1995; Sams-Dodd et al., 1997); it is one of the theories of early developmental lesions that can explain long latency between the lesion and clinical manifestation - early developmental lesions exert adverse influence on the consequent development of the brain leading to abnormal maturation of interconnected prefrontal areas. In particular, after neonatal hippocampal lesions in rats reduction of dendritic spines of layer III PN in the DLPFC (Flores et al., 2005), GAD67 mRNA reduction in the prefrontal cortex (Lipska et al., 2003), decrease of NAA levels in prefrontal cortex (Bertolino et al., 1997), postpubertal vulnerability to stress or dopaminergic challenge (Saunders et al., 1998), behavior in adulthood interpreted as a correlate of schizophrenia phenotype (Lipska et al., 1993) was observed. Findings in humans such as reduced hippocampal volume correlated with prefrontal activity (Weinberger et al., 1992), and poorer performance in neuropsychological tests focused on prefrontal cortex (Bilder et al., 1995; Szeszko et al., 2002), abnormal EEG coherence between prefrontal cortex and hippocampus (Ford et al., 2002), and correlation between lower level on prefrontal NAA and abnormal mesolimbic dopaminergic activity (Bertolino et al., 1999; Bertolino et al., 2000) are data that conform with the hypothesis. The chain of neuropathological changes begins with neonatal or perinatal hippocampal lesion leading to impairment of development of fronto-temporal connections with consequent morphological and functional changes of prefrontal cortex (which is a correlate of cognitive and negative symptoms of schizophrenia), loss of prefrontal regulation of dopaminergic system with consequent mesolimbic dopaminergic dysregulation, mechanism that lays behind psychosis.

Others argue against the idea that early affections of the brain can have such an effect in the adulthood and emphasize abnormalities of *late development.* The main arguments are the pattern of morphological changes – total brain volume reduction without the changes in the intracranial volume – and several lines of evidence suggesting the progression of the changes during certain phases during the course of schizophrenia.

These features seem to be in accord with abnormalities of synaptic pruning (Feinberg 1982; Keshavan 1994, Lewis 1997, Woods 1998), possibly via abnormalities of synaptic apoptosis (see below) as a way of the refinement of heteromodal cortical mircrocircuits during the late adolescence (Lewis 1997). On the other hand, the presence of (albeit non-specific) symptoms early in the childhood speaks in support of the early developmental theories.

Contemporary *syntheses* understand the importance of the late processes and remain open to the possibility of early developmental lesions: *a two-hit hypothesis* (Bayer et al., 1999; Maynard et al., 2001). In this view the disruption of some early maturation process changes the way the brain develops and causes a vulnerability to the consequent negative effect. Neither the first nor the second hit alone can cause schizophrenia, the key is their combination. *Cell-cell signaling* was proposed as a potential process that might be affected both during the early development and later maturation processes (Maynard et al., 2001).

Another mechanism was proposed in the *"sensitization model"* where the early lesion leads to reduced inhibition of the cortex with subsequent increase of reaction to stressful stimuli occurring during adolescence with neurotoxic and apoptotic consequences (Lieberman at al., 1997). Another view is the concept of schizophrenia as a *progressive developmental disorder* due to a disruption of late developmental processes leading to a progression after the illness onset (Woods, 1998).

Apoptosis

It was argued that in schizophrenia there is (at least transiently during critical periods of the disease) an increased likelihood of a certain apoptotic mechanism, *"synaptic apoptosis"* (Mattson et al., 1998) that could explain the loss of dendritic spines without complete neuronal death (Glantz et al., 2006). Synaptic apoptosis seems to be the mechanism underlying synaptic remodeling and elimination – the key processes in the physiological plasticity of the brain as well as in many pathological states (Gilman and Mattson, 2002; Garden at al., 2002); in schizophrenia it might be the mechanism of the accelerated synaptic pruning and other late neurodevelopmental changes (Feinberg, 1982; Weinberger, 1987). Apoptotic activity can be triggered by many stimuli, such as oxidative stress, inflamation, excitotoxicity, neurotrophins withdrawal, mitochondrial dysfunction (Sastry and Rao, 2000). On the other hand, neurotrophic activity can reverse or prevent the apoptosis (Guo and Mattson, 2000). In schizophrenia mitochondrial dysfunction, decreased capacity to deal with oxidative stress, glutamatergic abnormalities as well as decrease of neurotrophins was demonstrated, making the involvement of apoptotic mechanisms in the pathogenesis of schizophrenia probable (Glantz et al., 2006). Apoptosis was also implied as a potential mechanism underlying progressive gray matter volume loss around the onset of schizophrenia (Berger et al., 2003; Jarskog et al., 2005).

Genetics of Cortical Microcircuits

It is also apparent that at least some genes linked with schizophrenia play a role in the development, maintaining or plasticity of the brain structure and synapse formation. This is the case for BDNF, DISC1, dysbindin, neuregulin 1 etc. Other genes code proteins involved in receptor formation and signal transduction: COMT, CHRNA7, G72, RSG4 (Perlman et al., 2004; Harrison and Weinberger 2005; Iritani 2007). In accord with the pattern of neuropathological changes it seems that the genetic susceptibility is not expressed on the level of a certain type of the synapse, rather, on the level of a cortical microcircuitry underlying core cognitive functions impaired in schizophrenia. Reduced signal-to-noise ratio, impaired synchronization and other dysfunctions were demonstrated as features of cortical circuit abnormalities in schizophrenia and these might be the consequence of genetic variations of the above mentioned genes. We may view the morphological changes as a consequence of the abnormalities of the synapse formation and activity within these circuitries.

Direct evidence connecting genetic polymorphisms implied in schizophrenia with brain structure emerges. The *BDNF* 11757 G/C polymorphism was significantly associated with frontal gray matter in patients with schizophrenia as well as in healthy controls (Agartz 2006). Similarly, the BDNF Val66Met polymorphism was linked with regional gray matter volume in prefrontal, parietal, temporal as well as occipital areas, where the Val-alele carriers showed larger volume (Ho et al., 2006). Pericentriolar Material 1 (*PCM1*) gene located on chromosome 8p22, involved in the maintenance of centromere integrity and regulation of microtubule cytoskeleton important for synaptogenesis and intracellular transport along axons and dendrites, was identified as susceptible gene for schizophrenia; schizophrenia subjects who were carriers of the susceptible allele demonstrated gray matter reduction in bilateral medial orbitofrontal cortex when contrasted with schizophrenia subjects without susceptible allele (Gurling et al., 2008). In similar manner, schizophrenia-associated haplotypes of *DISC1* were associated with gray matter density reduction in prefrontal areas as well as with cognitive abilities linked with prefrontal functions (Cannon et al., 2005). As stated earlier, not only genes coding proteins involved in the brain development show association with the changes of the brain morphology. For example schizophrenia subjects homozygous for *Val-COMT* (Val158Met polymorphism) differ significantly from the Met-COMT carriers in the gray matter morphology in anterior cingulate, temporal cortex and thalamus (Ohnishi et al., 2006).

Environment

The neuropil abundance and condition is sensitive to many environmental influences. It was demonstrated that neuropil density changes physiologicaly (Wooley et al., 1990), as a correlate of learning associated plasticity (Moser et al., 1994). Many adverse events may change the neuropil density as well. Repeated exposure to *stress* was linked with a substantial reduction of dendritic spines of layer III pyramidal neurons in medial temporal cortex

(Radley et al., 2006) or apical dendritic arbor of layer II, III neurons in anterior cingulate, but not in lateral orbitofrontal cortex (Liston et al., 2006) of rats; adverse effect of *alcohol* (Ferrer et al., 1986), *social isolation* (Connor and Diamond, 19982; Glantz and Lewis, 2000), *protein malnutrition* (Brock and Prasad, 1992), or *sensory deprivation* (Bryan and Riesen, 1989; Valverde, 1967) were all shown to lead to neuropil reduction.

D. Brain Imaging Methods in Schizophrenia

Methods: Pros and Cons

The advent of MRI brought sufficient image resolution enabling in vivo morphological assessment. It also allows for clear delineation of gray, white matter and liquor compartments, i.e. segmentation, and their separate analysis. Since gray matter is composed primarily of neuropil and cell bodies, imaging of the gray matter in schizophrenia reflects the reduction of neuropil as described by neuropathological studies. However, the changes are not visible for the "naked eye". It is necessary to process the images, extract the relevant information and describe the changes using statistical apparatus. In general, there are two approaches: *region of interest- and voxel-based methods.*

Which method seems to be the best suitable for the detection of morphological abnormalities in schizophrenia? It is evident that the morphological changes do not respect the macroscopic brain structures; rather they stretch across gyri, sulci and even lobes. The substantially high variability of the macroscopic as well as microscopic structures – such as the course or shape of individual sulci or gyri, Brodmann areas locations and extents – complicates the situation even further. This variability is especially pronounced in the prefrontal cortex and in schizophrenia even more than in healthy subjects. Due to these attributes of the brain morphology it seems that region-of-interest (ROI) based approaches (formerly considered as a gold standard in the field of brain morphology research) are not adequate methods to characterize the pattern of prefrontal morphology in schizophrenia. Among the disadvantages of ROI approaches belong the need to define a macroscopic brain structure to be studied; to label the structure with a sufficient validity and reliability, with inherent trade-off between these parameters, and the necessity to introduce arbitrary borders; the ability to study limited number of structures; the implicit investigation of the structure as a whole.

The *voxel-based methods* (VBM) seem to have several advantages over the ROI-methods. They enable assessment of local features of brain morphology within the whole brain, without the necessity to define a priori the regions of interest. They use the computational resources thus limiting the subjective influence on the results as well as labor intensity. On the other hand, they may have lesser statistical power and not as a last point some still find the digital preprocessing of the images too complicated, elusive and prone to unwanted bias. However, these methods were validated several times, both in terms of direct comparison with ROI-approaches (Giuliani et al., 2005; Saze et al., 2007), or in their ability to detect apparent pathology in the brain, such as mesiotemporal sclerosis in temporal epilepsy (Keller et al., 2004). There are several modification of voxel-based morphometry;

generally two approaches can be identified – studies of regional gray matter concentration/density and volume. Both approaches are usually pooled together in systematic reviews; however, it should be beard in mind that they may provide quite different results. It is not clear what approach should be preferred - volume studies are used more frequently nowadays, since they allow better understanding of the units measured and easier interpretation. Keller et al. (2004) found the gray matter volume analysis was able to find more regional changes in temporal lobe epilepsy than did the gray matter concentration approach. On the other hand, Meda et al. (2008) found just the opposite: gray matter concentration analysis yielded much better results in a large sample of schizophrenia subjects than the gray matter volume approach; the reason was that modulation, step necessary to obtain volume information, resulted in higher variability with consequent decrease of statistical power.

In the context of schizophrenia, the VBM studies seem to provide neuropathologically meaningful information about cortical gray matter. It was demonstrated that VBM studying gray matter concentration detect analogues pathology as cortical thickness measurement (Narr et al., 2005). We may view the VBM studies of cortical structures in schizophrenia as a measure of regional cortical thickness and consequently of local abundance of neuropil or structural connectivity.

What follows is a review of the present day evidence concerning the brain morphology in schizophrenia with a focus on the prefrontal cortex and clinical features of the illness.

The Pattern of Morphological Changes

ROI-Based Approaches

There are innumerous volumetric studies in schizophrenia. The advantage of the volumetric studies is they may be relatively easily pooled together for meta-analysis. Such statistical re-assessment is available for several regions. Wright at al., (2000) performed a meta-analysis of most of the regions studied by ROI approaches between the years 1980 and 1998. They pooled studies of whole brain, gray matter, white matter volume, ventricular synstem volume, frontal and temporal lobe, temporal lobe areas: amygdala, hippocampus, superior temporal gyrus, subcortical areas: caudate nucleus, putamen, pallidum, and thalamus. Together they analyzed data from 1588 patients with schizophrenia. They expressed the volume of corresponding structures in healthy controls as 100%, and the volumes in schizophrenia as fractions of that value. Whole brain volume in schizophrenia represented 98% of healthy controls, frontal lobe 95% on both sides, temporal lobe 98% on left and 97% on right side, superior temporal gyrus 97% on both sides, amygdala 91% on both sides, hippocampus 93% on left and 94% on right side, parahippocampal gyrus 89% on left and 92% on right side, lateral ventricles 130% on left and 120% on right side, thalamus 96% on both sides, caudate 101% on left and 99% on right side, putamen 104% on both sides, and pallidum 118% on left and 121% on right side. Studies of both first-episode and chronic schizophrenia subjects, medicated and drug naive patients were included. Thus the pattern of changes may be biased by many confounding factors such as long-term exposure to antipsychotics, progression of the chronic illness, life-style changes as a consequence of severe mental condition, substance abuse etc. To rule out such factors it is advantageous to study first-episode, and if possible antipsychotic-naive schizophrenia patients. From the regions included in the meta-analysis it is also obvious that ROI studies focused mainly on regions where relatively easy delineation is possible, such as hippocampus, superior temporal gyrus or subcortical structures. Frontal regions are studied by a limited number of ROI studies and VBM techniques may be superior in these areas.

VBM Approaches

Honea et al., (2005) published a comprehensive review of 15 voxel-based studies in schizophrenia published through May 2004. Together they included 290 patients and 364 healthy controls. The aim was to specify the overlap of individual studies, which was expressed as a percentage of the studies that found reduction in a given structure. Individual studies found reduction in 50 regions. In more than 50% of studies the reduction was reported for left medial temporal lobe and left superior temporal gyrus. In 50% studies the reduction was seen in the left inferior frontal gyrus, left medial frontal gyrus, right superior frontal gyrus, and left parahippocampal gyrus. However, the changes were reported also in the precentral and postcentral gyrus, in insular, parietal and occipital cortex, in caudate nucleus, thalamus and cerebellum. The analysis included studies of both first-episode and chronic schizophrenia subjects. The authors also analyzed the methodological issues of individual studies and found a significant effect: studies that used smaller smoothing kernel tend to find reductions in more areas and more frequently in small structures such as medial temporal lobe structures or cingulate gyrus.

Similar summary is provided for 5 studies with first episode schizophrenia subjects published till the end of 2005 (Kasparek et al., 2007): all 5 studies found gray matter reduction in anterior cingulate gyrus, 4 in inferior frontal gyrus, 3 in superior temporal gyrus, hippocampus, and cerebellum.

Recent study used activation likelihood estimation (ALE), a statistical approach for meta-analytical analysis of neuroimaging data (Laird et al., 2005), to find a statistically consistent pattern of changes across published VBM studies with first-episode and chronic schizophrenia patients (Ellison-Wright et al., 2008). Data from seven VBM studies in first episode found gray matter reduction in inferior frontal gyrus (BA 47), cingulate gyrus (BA 32), precentral gyrus (BA 6), insula (BA 13), uncus, postcentral gyrus (BA 40), mediodorsal thalamus, caudate nucleus, and cerebellum, as well as gray matter increase in superior frontal gyrus (BA 6, 8), middle frontal gyrus (BA 9), precentral gyrus (BA 4), insula, superior temporal gyrus (BA 22), fussiform gyrus (BA 18), inferior parietal lobule (BA 40), lingual gyrus (BA 17), putamen, and cerebellum relative to healthy controls. Comparison of first-episode studies with studies with chronic schizophrenia patients showed greater decrease in the prefrontal cortex, specifically in the dorsolateral prefrontal cortex and medial frontal gyrus. The extent of decrease in cortical areas was greater in the chronic studies as well.

However, the results of the ALE analysis of VBM studies should be considered with caution. There are several issues that should be bear in mind: 1) no influence of negative studies on ALE results, 2) different methodology of pooled studies: concentration vs. volume, 3) different statistics of pooled studies: corrected, uncorrected, voxel-level, cluster-level etc. All these methodological factors may influence the results of a study and it may be inappropriate to pool studies with different methodologies together. It is especially important in the light of the Ellison-Wright meta-analysis results: many cortical areas were reported to have increased, and more importantly, simultaneously both decreased and increased gray matter. However, only two individual studies reported such substantial increase of gray matter (Salgado-Pineda et al., 2003; Whitford et al., 2006). Whitford et al. (2006) found gray matter volume increases in cortical areas BA 6, 8, 9, 10, 17, 18, 46, and in subcortical claustrum in a sample of first-episode schizophrenia subjects; however, two studies from the same center with the similar methodology and similar study samples did not find them (Farrow et al., 2005; Whitford et al., 2005). Of special interest is the report of increased gray matter in area 9, where a substantial body of evidence shows just the opposite: gray matter volume reduction, with a consistent pattern of findings in the neuropathological literature. Moreover the second study that reported gray matter increase did not find it in the prefrontal cortex; the changes were in areas 13, 22, 40, in the cerebellum, and in subcortical putamen. Thus, we have to understand the results of Ellison-Wright study in a following way: only two from seven studies found gray matter increases, and although the pattern of the two studies did not overlap, the ALE meta-analysis indicates that reported subset of foci of changes is distributed within the brain non-randomly. Apparently, the results of prefrontal gray matter increase lack replication in an independent observation.

However, recently published large scale study, that could not be included in the Ellison-Wright meta-analysis, brought some support for gray matter increase in schizophrenia: it was observed in bilateral orbitofrontal cortex (BA 10, 11), anterior cingulate (BA 24), left precentral gyrus (BA 6), left inferior temporal gyrus, right middle temporal gyrus, bilateral globus pallidus, and right medial cerebellum (Honea et al., 2008). All these findings survived quite stringent correction of multiple comparisons for VBM data: family wise errors with significance set to $p<0.05$ FWE corrected. However, the schizophrenia subjects included in this study were not the first episode cases and were exposed to antipsychotics for a substantial period of time. Of importance, in healthy siblings of the subjects, no gray matter volume increases were found, suggesting that the finding of prefrontal gray matter increases in schizophrenia does not reflect primary neurobiology – or endophenotype - of the illness. Moreover, the other recent study with similarly large samples found no gray matter increase (Meda et al., 2008) and the meaning of the findings of gray matter volume increase remain unclear.

The Meda ′s et al. (2008) study included 200 schizophrenia subjects and 200 healthy controls. It is a study with the biggest and sufficient statistical power from studies published till today to study gray matter morphology with sufficient correction of false positives without critical rise of false negative results. The study identified a reduction of gray matter concentration in many cortical and subcortical areas: in frontal lobe in both medial and lateral parts - in dorsolateral prefrontal cortex (BA 9, 46), orbitofrontal cortex (BA 10, 11, 47), pars opercularis and triangularis of inferior frontal gyrus (BA 44, 45), premotor and motor areas (BA 6, 8), cingulate cortex (BA 23, 24, 25, 32, 42); in insular cortex (BA 13); in temporal lobe in superior temporal gyrus (BA 22, 38, 41, 43), middle temporal gyrus (BA 21), inferior temporal gyrus (BA 19), uncus (BA 28); in parietal lobe in postcentral gyrus (BA 3, 1, 2, 40, 43), inferior parietal lobule (39); in occipital lobe in middle occipital gyrus (BA 19); and in mediodorsal thalamus, pulvinar and mammillary bodies, and caudate head. It is important to note that analysis of the gray matter volume showed similar pattern of changes, however on a lower, non-significant statistical threshold – which was due to the higher variability of volume data. This study also included chronic patients and such large scale and powerful study in first episode schizophrenia subgroup is still missing.

Dynamics of the Changes

Neuroimaging studies also observed progressive reduction of gray matter. Progressive gray matter loss in temporal, inferior frontal and cingulate cortex was seen in high-risk subjects who developed psychosis, i.e. the *conversion to psychosis* is linked with gray matter loss in heteromodal associative cortex (Pantelis et al., 2003; Wood et al., 2008). After the first episode of schizophrenia, *further reduction* of gray matter was demonstrated. Cahn et al. (2002) reported progressive loss of total gray matter, others observed progression in frontal (Farrow et al., 2005; Reig et al., 2008), temporal (Kasai et al., 2003; Farrow et al., 2005), or parietal (Farrow et al., 2005) cortex. No progression was observed in hippocampus (Lieberman et al., 2001). Some VBM studies observed dynamic spreading of the progressive loss of gray matter across several areas including prefrontal (inferior frontal gyrus), cingulate (posterior cingulate) temporal (superior temporal gyrus, parahippocampal gyrus), parietal (precuneus, postcentral gyrus, inferior parietal lobule), and occipital (lingual gyrus) cortices, and cerebellum (Thompson et al., 2001; Whitford et al., 2006). Progressive loss of gray matter in dorsolateral prefrontal cortex, superior temporal gyrus, thalamus, and caudate nucleus was observed also in chronically ill patients (van Haaren et al., 2007). For the interpretation of the findings of progressive gray matter loss a report of simultaneous worsening of functional impairment is of great value (Salisbury et al., 2007), i.e. the progression seen in imaging methods is not an epiphenomenon, rather it reflects certain neurobiological process with functional consequences.

This progressive loss of gray matter was interpreted in a *context of clinical progression*, or deterioration, through the first several years of the illness (Davidson and McGlashan, 1997). If there is a kind of ongoing pathogenetic process, at least in a certain subgroup of patients, the question arises if the treatment may stop or revert the changes and, subsequently, if such prevention of neuropathological progression leads to better outcome of the schizophrenia patients. Some data seem to support this possibility (Lieberman et al., 2005). However, it was speculated that the progression of the morphological changes reflect reversible processes of neuropil remodeling and that medication is just one of many factors that influence this plasticity (Weinberger and McClure, 2002). Several mechanisms that affect the plasticity and may lead to progression were proposed: dopaminergic overstimulation with consequent apoptosis (Ben-Schachar et al., 2004), glutamate excitotoxicity (Deutsch et al., 2001), GABA dysfunction (Farber et al., 2003), impaired apoptotic mechanisms (Luo et al., 1998; Datta et al., 1999), mitochondrial dysfunction (Beal et al., 1993; Ben-Schachar et al., 2004), decreased nitric oxid synthesis (Fiscus, 2002), oxidative stress (Mahadik et al., 2001).

In summary the neuroimaging studies provide quite widespread pattern of gray matter reduction, affecting not only dorsolateral prefrontal cortex, which is according to the neuropathological studies affected the most, and not even only heteromodal associative cortex, but also many primary and secondary sensory areas, as well as motor and premotor areas – see table 3. In some of these areas, fronto-temporal in particular, further gray matter loss was demonstrated. However, it seems that such widespread reduction and further progression is not present in all subjects, or subgroups, and substantial variability exists. How such variability can manifest itself on the clinical level is a topic of following sections of this chapter.

Table 3. Pattern of regional gray matter reduction in schizophrenia: neuroimaging data

FRONTAL LOBE
Motor and premotor cortex
Dorsolateral prefrontal cortex
Orbitofronal cortex
Ventrolateral prefrontal cortex
Medial frontal cortex
INSULA
TEMPORAL LOBE
Heteromodal neocortex
Primary and secondary auditory cortex
Mediotemporal structures (hippocampus, parahippocampal gyrus, amygdala)
PARIETAL LOBE
Somatosensory cortex
Heteromodal cortex
OCCIPITAL LOBE
Primary and higher order visual cortex
SUBCORTICAL REGIONS
Thalamus – mediodorsal nucleus, pulvinar
Caudate head

E. Clinical Correlates of Prefrontal Morphological Changes

Cognitive Functions

As schizophrenia is linked with cognitive dysfunction suggesting the involvement of dorsolateral prefrontal cortex, it is of importance to study if the above described morphological abnormality expresses itself as a functional impairment. Review of volumetric studies (Antonova et al., 2004) demonstrated that total frontal lobe volume is associated with executive functioning, working memory, verbal fluency, and immediate memory in schizophrenia. Dorsolateral prefrontal cortex volume was correlated with executive functions, attention, and verbal and visual memory, left DLPFC was associated with abstraction, flexibility, categorization and non-verbal immediate memory, right DLPFC with sustained attention. Orbitofrontal cortex had a complex relationship with many cognitive domains.

There were differences in the pattern of structure/function relationship between patients and healthy subjects which may reflect different variability in performance depending on the relative difficulty of the task (Baare et al., 1999) or different variability of brain morphology features. Another explanation was presented with the note that similar brain volume in schizophrenia patients may not predict the same performance as in healthy controls, possibly due to the abnormalities of brain connectivity.

Several voxel-based morphometric studies tried to refine the spatial pattern of the structure/function relationship and focused on the association between dorsolateral prefrontal gray matter volume and *executive functions*. There are reports demonstrating that this assumption holds true: significant correlation was found with the performance in Wisconsin Card Sorting Task (WCST) or Trial Making Test and dorsolateral prefrontal cortical gray matter (BA 9) (Bonilha et al., 2008), direct comparison of schizophrenia subjects with poor and good ability to solve WCST showed reduction in dorsolateral prefrontal cortex and anterior cingulate in poor realtive to good solvers (Rusch et al., 2007).

However, there are also negative reports: Antonova et al. (2005) performed voxel-based morphometry analysis of associations between gray matter and cognitive functions in 45 schizophrenia patients and 43 healthy subjects. The patients had smaller total gray matter volume by 9%, the whole brain volume by 9,5%, regional gray matter reduction in left inferior frontal gyrus (BA 45, 47), left lingual gyrus (BA 17) and gray matter increase in left precuneus (BA 7) and left putamen. Premorbid intelligence quotient (IQ) and actual performance in IQ tests were associated with total gray matter volume, verbal memory with precuneus in patients. In healthy controls inferior frontal gyrus volume was associated with both verbal and non-verbal memory, whereas in patients no such relationship was found. No association with executive functions as measured by Wisconsin card sorting test or Trial making test was observed. However, in contrast to Bonilha et al. (2008) study - which found quite widespread gray matter reduction, particularly in left supplementary motor area (BA 6), bilateral superior frontal gyrus (BA 6, 8), left middle frontal gyrus (BA 9), right opercular area (BA 44), left angular gyrus (BA 39), left superior temporal gyrus (BA 22) and left cerebellar hemisphere – Antonova et al. did not found changes in the dorsolateral prefrontal cortex in the strict sense (BA 9 and 46). Thus the inconsistency of the results may be a consequnece of neurobiological heterogeneity of the samples studied.

Sustained attention disturbance is another key element of the cognitive dysfunction in schizophrenia (Nuechterlein et al., 2004). Continuous Performance task results correlated significantly with gray matter concentration in left inferior frontal gyrus, left angular, supramarginal and postcentral gyri, as well as in left thalamus in first-episode schizophrenia patients (Salgado-Pineda et al., 2003).

Another key concept in schizophrenia is the impairment in *social cognition* – theory of mind, self-reference or working memory – i.e. abilities also linked with prefrontal cortex (Amodio and Frith, 2006), orbitofrontal and triangular parts in particular. Orbitofrontal cortex is involved in attribution of emotional valence to percieved stimuli: lateral parts were shown to mediate evaluation of punishment value while medial parts were linked with the evaluation of reward (Kringelbach and Rolls, 2004) – both functions seem to be impaired in schizophrenia and related to negative symptoms. Pars triangularis of the inferior frontal gyrus is linked with language skills and formal thought disorder or language disturbances are significant features of schizophrenia (Ceccherini-Nelli and Crow, 2004). It is also of importance that mirror neurons were located within pars triangularis. Activity of mirror neurons reflect observed action and disturbances of their function was also proposed to be a key abnormality in schizophrenia (Arbib and Mundehnk, 2005). Others view schizophrenia as a disorder of social cognition in general: the social brain hypothesis (Burns, 2006). In schizophrenia, gray matter reduction was observed in both medial and lateral orbitofrontal cortex, as well as in pars triangularis, even in first-episode patients (Venkatasubramanian et al., 2008). Yamada et al. (2007) studied the relationship between regional brain morphology and the ability to attribute emotional valence to different stimuli as assessed by Perception of Affect Task and found that the performance was positively correlated with gray matter concentration in medial frontal gyrus (BA 10), where a reduction of gray matter was present in schizophrenia subjects with consequent poor performance.

Symptomathology

As mentioned earlier, a considerable heterogeneity of structural findings persists. It is a question if they may reflect the phenomenological diversity of schizophrenia, i.e. if certain clinical subtypes correlate with distinct neurobiological features. Several studies investigated the effect of various clinical variables on the regional brain morphology.

First, there is a certain effect of the illness itself, i.e. subjects in which the illness lasts longer or who have more frequent psychotic exacerbation or more severe course of the illness have pronounced changes of brain morphology. Longer *duration of prodromal phase* of schizophrenia was associated with smaller gray matter density in anterior cingulate, medial and inferior frontal cortex, and insula (Lapin et al., 2007). Similarly, *duration of untreated psychosis* correlated with gray matter density decreases in temporal areas (BA 21, 37, 39) and occipital areas (BA 18, 19) (Lapin et al., 2006), and longer *duration of illness* was associated with lower gray matter volume in right medial temporal region including hippocampus, parahippocampal gyrus, in bilateral anterior cingulate cortex, and medial cerebellum and more gray matter volume in right globus pallidus (Velakoulis et al., 2002). Smaller lingual gyrus (BA 17) and larger precuneus (BA 7) were linked with greater number of previous psychotic episodes, but no association was found between gray matter in putamen and precuneus with antipsychotic exposure (Antonova et al., 2005). *Poor-outcome patients,* i.e. those who were continuously hospitalized or completely dependent on caregivers, unemployed and expressing severe negative and formal thought disorder, demonstrated significantly smaller gray matter volume in temporal and occipital, but not frontal cortical areas (Mitelman et al., 2003). In another group of chronic schizophrenia patients, whose functioning was classified by Global Assessment of Functioning (GAF), a significant negative correlation between the GAF score and regional gray matter was found in the left inferior frontal gyrus and left inferior parietal lobule (Wilke et al., 2001), i.e. the less gray matter in these regions the poorer outcome.

Second, certain clinical symptoms demonstrate association with specific neurobiologic substrate, reflecting either their specific pathophysiology or neurobiological heterogeneity of the condition. Such specific association is demonstrated for verbal hallucinations, insight and negative symptoms.

Comparison of patients with pronounced history of *verbal hallucinations* with non-hallucinating patients revealed gray matter reduction in left insula and adjacent temporal lobe (Shapleske et al., 2002). Intensity of auditory hallucinations correlated with left inferior frontal and right posterior gyri (García-Martí et al., 2008), in a different study using BPRS items to rate intensity of hallucination, negative correlation with hallucinations was found in the left superior (transverse) temporal gyrus, left thalamus, and left and right cerebellum (Neckelmann et al., 2006).

Insight is a concept with critical importance in schizophrenia. Poor insight is frequent finding in schizophrenia patients (Mintz et al., 2003) and the quality of the understanding of schizophrenia symptoms and the need of treatment seem to be crucial for the long-term outcome of the illness (Drake et al., 2007). Insight is linked with cognitive abilities – executive functions in particular (Laroy et al., 2000; Smith et al., 2000; Drake and Lewis, 2003) and thus it is not surprising that schizophrenia subjects with cognitive impairment may have difficulties to understand the consequences of their situation. The clinical observation of the association between executive dysfunction and the quality of insight suggest the involvement of prefrontal systems linked with perceptual and monitoring systems. Several studies investigated such connection between insight and prefrontal morphology: earlier studies found association with frontal lobe atrophy as defined from CT scans (Laroy et al., 2000), and a negative correlation between the score for the severity of 'lack of insight and judgment' and gray matter concentrations in the left posterior and right anterior cingulate and bilateral inferior temporal regions including the lateral fusiform gyri was found (Ha et al., 2004). However, Bassitt et al., (2007) who investigated the link between regional gray matter and quality of insight rated by a specific scale Unawareness of Mental Illness Scale in fifty schizophrenia subjects did not find any correlation.

Negative symptoms rated by BPRS were inversely correlated with gray matter volume in frontal areas BA 8, 9, 10, and temporal areas BA 20, 21, 22; the range of correlation magnitude was between -0.30 and -0.51 (Hazlett et al., 2008).

Recent large scale (175 schizophrenia patients and 177 healthy subjects) VBM study tried to resolve the neurobiological heterogeneity that is behind distinct clinical syndromes (negative, positive and disorganized) and simultaneously to detect areas of changes that are generally linked with schizophrenia, shared by all clinical subgroups (Koutsouleris et a., 2008).

Changes associated with *negative symptoms* were the most widespread and demonstrated the largest effect size. They were linked to gray matter density reduction in *frontal areas:* medial and lateral parts of superior frontal gyrus, middle frontal gyrus, inferior frontal gyrus (orbital, triangular, and opercular parts), gyrus rectus, and supplementary motor area, precentral gyrus, anterior and middle parts of cingulate gyrus; bilateral *insula; temporal areas:* bilateral superior, middle and inferior temporal gyri, fusiform gyrus, mediotemporal structures - left amygdala, bilateral hippocampus and parahippocampal gyrus; *parietal areas:* supramarginal gyrus, postcentral gyrus; and bilateral cerebellum (VI), left caudate and thalamus. No changes were present in occipital areas.

Positive symptoms were associated with reduction in *frontal areas*: middle, inferior frontal (orbital opercular and triangular parts) gyri, right gyrus rectus, precentral gyrus, rolandic operculum, anterior and middle cingulate gyrus; bilateral *insula; temporal areas*: superior temporal gyrus, left middle temporal gyrus; *parietal areas*: supramarginal gyrus; *occipital areas:* inferior occipital cortex; and bilateral *thalamus.* Although there were some changes in the frontal areas, the reduction in temporal areas and in the thalamus were more pronounced than in negative symptoms. Interestingly, no association was observed with mediotemporal limbic areas or cerebellum.

The disorganized symptoms were associated with reduction in *frontal areas:* inferior frontal gyrus, gyrus rectus, medial orbitofrontal cortex, anterior and middle cingulate gyrus, rolandic operculum; *insula; temporal areas*: temporal pole, superior and middle temporal gyri, fusiform gyrus, and left amygdala; *parietal areas*: supramarginal gyrus. No changes were observed in occipital, cerebellar or subcortical structures.

All three syndromes shared (as demonstrated by conjunction analysis) reduction in orbitofrontal areas, medial and lateral prefrontal cortices, inferior frontal gyrus, anterior cingulate gyrus, bilateral insula, temporal polar area, middle and inferior temporal cortex, rolandic operculum, and supramarginal gyrus. These areas seem to be common neurobiological substrate of schizophrenia, irrespective to the clinical manifestation.

Treatment

There are reports that antipsychotic agents may have some influence on the brain morphology. The evidence comes from animal, postmortem, and neuroimaging studies. Although there is a good evidence for the effect of antipsychotics (classical neuroleptics in most cases) in striatum (Harrison, 1999b), much fewer data are available for cortical areas, which are critical for the understanding how antipsychotics interfere with the pathophysiological processes in schizophrenia. Even in the striatum, the effect of antipsychotics on the pattern of synaptic pathology seems to be qualitatively different from the one associated with schizophrenia (Harrison, 1999b).

Present day evidence suggests that there might be a differential effect of first- and second-generation antispychotics on the *brain plasticity.* First-generation antipsychotics, haloperidol in particular, were demonstrated to be neurotoxic as they decrease levels of neurotrophic factors (Parikh et al., 2004; Pillai et al., 2006) and induce apoptosis (Ukai et al., 2004; Wei et al., 2006). Furthermore, no beneficial effect of first-generation antipsychotics on neurogenesis was observed (Mallberg et al., 2000; Wakade et al., 2002; Halim et al., 2004; Schmitt et al., 2004; Wang et al., 2004). Second-generation antipsychotics seem to be superior to classical neuroleptics in the case of neurogenesis potentiation and their anti-apoptotic properties (Quing et al., 2003; Wei et al., 2003). Olanzapine treatment for 28 days increased hippocampal neurogenesis (Kodama et al., 2004), olanzapine also led to proliferation in prefrontal cortex, which rather than neuronal proliferation represented increase in endothelial or glial cells (Wang et al., 2004). Positive effect was demonstrated also for risperidone (Wakade et al., 2002), paliperidone (Nasrallah and Pixley, 2006), and quetiapine (Luo et al., 2005). However, quite opposite to expectations, no effect on neurogenesis was demonstrated for clozapine (Halim et al., 2004; Schmitt et al., 2004). Olanzapine and risperidone reversed the BDNF and NGF reduction induced by haloperidol in rats (Parikh et al., 2004; Pillai et al., 2006). In humans, NGF levels were reduced in drug-naive patients, which were increased after the treatment with risperidone (Parikh et al., 2003).

The direct observation of the *effect of antipsychotics on the brain morphology* in antipsychotic-treated animals brought rather inconsistent and heterogeneous results. Earlier animal studies did not found changes of the neuronal morphology in the cortex of rats treated with perphenazine (Pakkenberg et al., 1973; Fog et al., 1976), or haloperidol when observed at the light microscopic level (Benes et al., 1985).

Following studies brought significant results: treatment-associated *gray matter volume* reduction was observed in left parietal cortex in macaque monkeys (Dorph-Petersen et al., 2005) after olanzapine or haloperidol treatment for 27 months. Widening of layer V in dorsolateral prerontal area 46 was observed after six-months of antipsychotic exposure (Selemon et al., 1999b). No changes of *neuronal number or density* were observed after half-year (Selemon et al., 1999) as well as one year-long treatment with typical or atypical antipsychotics in macaque monkeys (Konopaske et al., 2007). Studies using direct assessment of *neuropil* by electron microscopy showed loss of dendritic spines in layer VI of medial prefrontal cortex in rats treated with haloperidol (Benes et al., 1985; Klintzova et al., 1989). Chronic exposure to haloperidol or clozapine led to increase of axodendritic symmetric, i.e. inhibitory, synapses with the loss of asymmetric, i.e. excitatory, synapses in layer VI of medial prefrontal cortex in rats (Vincent et al., 1991). Haloperidol administration was also linked with increased immunoreactivity for GABA in medial prefrontal cortex of rats (Vincent 1994). These studies indicate that the drugs may induce reorganization of synapses in layer VI, perhaps preferentially the inhibitory ones. Haloperidol treatment-associated changes of cytoskeleton and dendritic spines proteins were observed also in rhesus monkeys: chronic exposure to haloperidol led to decrease of spinophilin, protein associated with dendritic spines, increase of microtubule-associated protein 2 (MAP2) phosphorylation (which reduces its ability to stabilize dendritic microtubules) in many cortical areas – prefrontal, orbital, cingulate, entorhinal – but not in primary visual cortex; no changes of vesicle-associated protein synaptophysin were observed (Lidow et al., 2001). However, human post-mortem studies did not reveal a substantial effect of antipsychotics on the morphology of cortical synapses (Harrison et al., 1999a, Harrison et al., 1999b).

Antipsychotic agents were also linked with *glial cells* changes – although again with inconsistent results. Treatment with haloperidol or olanzapine decreased glial cell numbers in parietal cortex (Konopaske et al., 2007), which was specific to astrocytes (Konopaske et al., 2008), and was accompanied by cortical volume reduction. Previous report of antipsychotic effect on glial cells that used the same methodology as in human studies showed just the opposite: in dorsolateral prefrontal cortex (BA 46) six-months exposure to atypical or typical antipsychotics led to increased glial cell density in layer IV and widening of cortical thickness in layer V (Selemon et al., 1999b). This study, however, used shorter duration of antipsychotic exposure and lower daily doses of antipsychotics than the Konopaske et al. studies. Nevertheless, the results are of importance because they demonstrate the possible correlate of neuroimaging findings of cortical increase in schizophrenia. In this context, predominant distribution of dopamine D2 receptors in layer V might be linked with the increase of layer V thickness (Vincent et al., 1993).

It is apparent that although some antipsychotic-associated changes seem to reflect certain features of brain morphology changes in schizophrenia leaving open the possibility, that at least some of the changes in schizophrenia are a consequence of the antipsychotic exposure, other, such as widening of cortical thickness, go against the pattern seen in schizophrenia. However, there is no evidence suggesting that any antipsychotic agent can reverse the pathological cortical changes in schizophrenia; at least no reports of layer III dendritic spine density increase were published. Such prove is, unfortunately, difficult to obtain, since it is hard to model the schizophrenia-associated neuropathology in animals, and antipsychotic drugs may not exert the same effect in the health, where only adverse effects are observed, as in the disease, where specific antipsychotic effect can prevail.

Neuroimaging studies seem to suggest that antipsychotic agents may have influence on brain morphology. ROI studies demonstrated the effect of classical neuroleptics on basal ganglia (Chakos et al., 1994), as well as some second generation antipsychotics (Massana et al., 2005).

As for *the effect on cortical areas*, little evidence is available. Garver et al. (2005) observed an increase of total gray matter by 20.6 (SD 11.4) cc in patients treated with second generation antipsychotics – risperidone or ziprasidone – for 28 days, with no changes in haloperidol-treated subjects. Lieberman et al. (2005) observed decreased rate of gray matter loss in olanzapin- in contrast to haloperidol-treated first-episode schizophrenia subjects. Molina et al. (2005) studied treatment-naive and chronic treatment-resistant schizophrenia patients for two years of treatment with risperidone (treatment naive subjects) or clozapine (treatment-resistant subjects). Treatment with both agents led to increase in frontal (by 9-12 %), parietal (by 8-11 %) and occipital (by 10-12 %) gray matter volume, only on clozapin total (by 4 %) and temporal (by 2 %) gray matter volume increased.

Regional specificity of the changes was investigated in a few studies using cross-sectional as well as longitudinal design. Dazzan et al. (2005) investigated the potential effect of different antipsychotic agents on brain morphology in a cross-sectional VBM study of first-episode psychosis subjects who were drug-free (n = 22), treated with classical neuroleptics (n = 32) or atypical antipsychotics (n = 30). Majority of the atypical antipsychotic treated subjects was given olanzapine (n = 21). The mean duration of treatment was 9 weeks for atypical antipsychotics and 8 weeks for classical neuroleptics. The first-episode psychosis project included patients with schizophrenia or schizophreniform psychosis, affective psychosis, or other psychotic disorders. The distribution of diagnostic categories was non-random in the three groups: atypical antipsychotic –exposed subjects were in 80% diagnosed with schizophrenia, in 7% with affective psychosis and in 13% with other psychosis. Classical neuroleptics-exposed subjects were in 47% schizophrenia subjects, in 47% diagnosed with affective psychosis, and in 6% with other psychosis. Drug-free subjects were diagnosed with schizophrenia only in 32%, in 41% with affective psychosis and in 27% with other psychosis. Subjects treated with classical neuroleptics had higher gray matter concentration in basal ganglia and clusters of gray matter reduction stretching across insula, inferior frontal gyrus (BA 47), and superior temporal gyrus (BA 22), across paracentral lobule (BA 4, 5), superior and medial frontal gyrus (BA 6, 31), and cingulate gyrus (BA 24), and across precuneus (BA 7) when compared with drug free subjects. Subject exposed to atypical antipsychotics had increased gray matter in thalamus when compared with drug free subjects. Direct comparison of the two treated groups showed gray matter reduction in middle temporal gyrus (BA 21) in classical neuroleptics-exposed patients. Due to the apparent diagnostic heterogeneity between the study groups the results may reflect differences in the neurobiology of different conditions rather than the effect of different kinds of treatment.

In a longitudinal study of 6-week treatment with risperidon in a small group of 15 neuroleptic-naive first-episode psychosis subjects a tiny increase of gray matter in BA 39 (superior and middle temporal gyrus) was observed (Girgis et al., 2006). However, the authors did not correct for multiple comparisons effect in a study with no a priori regional hypothesis, which brings the significant probability of the results being false positives. Another longitudinal assessment of 10 chronic patients treated for twelve weeks with second generation antipsychotic identified no changes in cortical or subcortical areas (McClure et al., 2008). Volumetric study of the effect of first as well second generation antipsychotics on the anterior cingulate during the treatment for 2-3 years yielded interesting results: increased anterior cingulate volume correlated with increased exposure to first generation antipsychotics, but negative correlation was found for exposure with second-generation agents. The increase of anterior cingulate volume was also correlated with greater improvement of positive symptoms (McCormick et al., 2005). These results are important for they demonstrate similar pattern of changes as seen in basal ganglia also for cortical structure. Anterior cingulate is interconnected with basal ganglia, and extrastriate dopamine D2 receptors are expressed here (Olsson et al., 2004); both findings may contribute to the anterior cingulate increase after first-generation antipsychotics. The interpretation of such increase is quite important in the light of the findings of gray matter increase in schizophrenia.

Thus, although there are data suggesting there is certain effect of antipsychotics on the brain morphology, the exact nature of this effect is not known and we cannot conclude that the effect of antipsychotics is beneficial in the sense of the reverse of basic neuropathological pattern of changes as present in schizophrenia. However, this pattern – reduced neuropil without the loss of neurons – leaves a chance open that there might be a treatment that may help remodel local neurocircuits and restore normal function in schizophrenia.

F: Specificity of the Morphological Changes

High-Risk Subjects

The patter of brain morphology changes described above is not entirely specific for schizophrenia subjects. Even subjects at high risk of development of schizophrenia show a discrete pattern of cortical reduction. Job et al. (2003) presented data from the Edinburgh High Risk Study, a project of compelling elaboration that recruited healthy siblings of schizophrenia patients at the time window for development of schizophrenia and followed them prospectively. The high risk subjects (n = 146) had reduced gray matter in the anterior cingulate bilaterally than healthy subjects. First episode patients (n = 34) had further reduced gray matter in the left and right cingulate gyrus, left medial, left and right inferior, and middle frontal gyrus (BA9, BA45), right precentral gyrus, in right hippocampus, amygdala, parahippocampal gyrus, middle temporal gyrus (BA 22, BA39), and in left postcentral gyrus (BA40). Another sample of high risk subjects (n = 40) form Early Detection and Intervention Centre for Mental Crises of Ludwig-Maximilians-University in Germany detected significant clusters of gray matter reduction in as good as the whole frontal cortex (medial, dorsolateral and ventrolateral, orbitofrontal parts, anterior cingulate, motor and supplementary motor cortex), temporal areas in superior, middle temporal gyrus, parietal supramarginal gyrus, postcentral gyrus and Rolandic operculum (Meisenzahl et al., 2008). High risk subjects who later developed psychoses had smaller gray matter volume in posterior cingulate, precuneus, superior parietal gyrus and increased gray matter in left supramarginal gyrus when compared with healthy controls. When compared with first-episode schizophrenia patients, relatively higher gray matter volume was observed in temporal lobe bilaterally and smaller gray matter volume in basal ganglia (Borgwardt et al., 2007).

Relatives

Gray matter changes are present even in healthy siblings of schizophrenia patients who did not develop schizophrenia. This finding is one of the features of intermediate phenotype, or *endophenotype,* reflecting neurobiological substrate of the illness that lies between genotype and clinical manifestation of the illness. In particular, Honea et al. (2008) studied 213 healthy siblings of schizophrenia subjects and found a trend (after stringent thresholding $p<0.05$ FWE corrected) for a gray matter reduction in medial frontal gyrus (BA 10). Without such stringent significance criteria the siblings shared gray matter reduction also in inferior frontal gyrus, paracingulate sulcus (BA 10), superior temporal gyrus (BA 22) and insula. Furthermore, hippocampal gray matter volume was significantly correlated within sibling pairs. In a smaller study, where the genetic liability to schizophrenia was quantified on a continuous scale, the liability was associated with gray matter volume in dorsolateral and ventrolateral cortex (McIntosh et al., 2006). More elegant approach to study the contribution of genome on the illness neurobiology is to study twins discordant for schizophrenia. In one such study Hulshof Pol et al. (2006) found that twins discordant for schizophrenia share reduction of gray matter density in the left medial orbitofrontal cortex, where differences between the schizophrenia-affected and healthy twins were less pronounced in monozygotic twin pairs than in dizygotic ones.

Schizotypal Disorder

Schizotypal disorder, a condition considered to be a member of schizophrenia-spectrum disorders, may represent the *genetic liability* for, or share some pathophysiological processes with schizophrenia – i.e. the patients with schizotypal disorder may share endophenotypes with schizophrenia subjects. Kawasaki et al. (2004) performed direct comparison of schizophrenia patients (n = 25), schizotypal subjects (n = 25) and healthy controls (n = 50) using VBM: schizotypal subjects demonstrated gray matter reduction in the left inferior frontal gyrus (BA47), insula, superior temporal gyrus (BA22), and medial temporal lobe (BA28). When compared with schizophrenia subjects, the schizotypal subjects had significantly more gray matter in orbitofrontal cortex (BA11). Reduction in inferior frontal gyrus and left medial temporal lobe were reduced in both schizophrenia and schizotypal disorder and therefore may represent the core substrate of vulnerability to schizophrenia. Comparison of only schizotypal women with healthy controls brought similar pattern of gray matter reduction: left inferior frontal gyrus, left superior, and middle temporal gyrus (BA 21, 22), right premotor cortex (BA6), and parietal areas (BA13, BA40) (Koo et al., 2006). Automatic ROI analysis of several Brodman's areas in schizophrenia (n = 57), schizotypal (n = 79) and healthy (n = 148) subjects found also quite similar pattern of changes: schizophrenia subjects showed gray matter reduction in many fronto-temporal areas (prefrontal area 10; cingulate areas 23, 24, 31; temporal areas 20, 21, 22), schizotypal subjects showed similar pattern of changes but of smaller magnitude (cingulate areas 23, 24, 31; temporal area 21). The difference between schizophrenia and schizotypal subjects was present in frontopolar region BA 10 where schizotypal subjects showed volume increase relative to healthy controls, and in superior temporal gyrus (BA 20, 22), where schizotypal subjects showed similar volume as healthy subjects whereas schizophrenia subjects showed reduction (Hazlett et al., 2008).

Bipolar Affective Disorder

There is a continuing debate on the similarities and differences between schizophrenia and bipolar disorder (Murray et al., 2004). It is then interesting to look at the similarities and differences in the brain morphology. Meta-analysis of volumetric studies with bipolar subjects showed no changes of brain morphology in bipolar patients as a whole, but substantial heterogeneity for left subgenual prefrontal cortex, bilateral amygdala and thalamus was noted, suggesting a possible existence of subgroups of patients with morphological abnormalities (Mc Donald et al., 2004). Bearden et al. (2007) found overall increase of the total gray matter by 6.6%, with regional increase of gray matter density in many cortical areas, notably in the heteromodal associative cortex: by 10 % or more in bilateral superior and middle frontal gyri, left ventrolateral prefrontal cortex, superior temporal cortex, retrosplenial and paracingulate cortex, subgenual coretx, and somatosensory cortex. This study found no area of gray matter density reduction. Moreover, the increase of gray matter density was explained by the effect of lithium treatment; patients not treated with lithium did not differ from healthy subjects. Similar increase of gray matter in the anterior cingulate, ventral prefrontal cortex, fusiform gyrus and primary and supplementary motor cortices in adult bipolar patients on various psychopharmacological treatment was reported (Adler et al., 2005). Direct comparison of first-episode schizophrenia and bipolar subjects showed significantly less gray matter in the left precentral/inferior frontal gyrus - BA 6/45, left anterior cingulate/medial frontal gyrus - BA 32/10, right superior frontal gyrus - BA 10, bilateral middle frontal gyrus – BA 9/46 in schizophrenia and significantly less gray matter in the left inferior/middle temporal gyrus - BA 20/21, right uncus - BA 20, and right anterior superior/middle temporal gyrus - BA 38/21 in the bipolar subjects. However, the bipolar subject showed significant reduction of gray matter in the right inferior frontal/precentral gyrus – BA 44/6, and in several temporal and parietal cortical areas when compared with healthy controls; in these areas the changes were present also in the schizophrenia subjects (Farrow et al., 2005). Gray matter reduction in the right inferior frontal gyrus and the left anterior cingulate was referred also in another sample of bipolar patients in which only minority of patients received lithium (Lyoo et al., 2004). This suggests that although the schizophrenia subjects show greater impairment, notably in the prefrontal cortex, the pattern of changes is not specific to schizophrenia and thus, the information is not useful in differential diagnosis between schizophrenia and bipolar disorder. On the histological level, there seem to be different abnormalities in bipolar disorder than those seen in schizophrenia (Harrison, 2002; Frey et al., 2004): the main positive findings include decreased glial density in subgenual prefrontal cortex – BA24 – and dorsolateral prefrontal cortex – BA 9, a reduction of non-pyramidal neurons in cingulate and hippocampus, and a higher occurrence of hyperintensities in white matter; however, clear cut between affective disorders and schizophrenia cannot be made.

Substance Abuse

As noted several times in the discussion of the findings of possible progression, abuse of psychoactive substances may contribute to the pattern of changes. Gray matter reduction was demonstrated in the alcohol- (Chandraud et al., 2007; Jang et al., 2007), opiate- (Lyoo et al., 2006), and cocaine-dependent patients (Franklin et al., 2002; Sim et al., 2007), or users of MDMA (Cowan et al., 2003). Alcohol-dependent patients had substantial reduction in prefrontal cortex (BA 9, 10), precentral gyrus (BA 6), cingulate gyrus (BA 32), temporal cortex (BA 19, 21, 22, 37), insula (BA 13), parietal cortex (BA 40), thalamus and cerebellum. Neuropsychological performance correlated significantly with the gray matter in the areas of gray matter reduction (Chandraud et al., 2007; Jang et al., 2007). Opiate-dependent patients showed gray matter concentration reduction in dorsolateral prefrontal cortex (BA 9, 10, 11, 47), insula (BA 13), superior temporal cortex (BA 21, 38), and mediotemporal structures (BA 28) (Lyoo et al., 2006). Cocaine-dependent patients had lower gray matter concentration in prefrontal cortex (BA 10), anterior cingulate, premotor cortex (BA 6, 8), insula, and superior temporal cortex (BA 20, 38), thalamus and cerebellum (Franklin et al., 2002; Sim et al., 2007). MDMA users had decreased gray matter in temporal (BA 21), frontal (BA 45) and cerebellum (Cowan et al., 2003). Of special interest are the findings of gray matter differences between smokers and non-smokers because high proportion of schizophrenia subjects smokes (Hughes et al., 1986). Smokers had significantly lower gray matter volume in the dorsolateral, ventrolateral prefrontal cortex, left cingulate and right cerebellum (Brody et al., 2004). Apparently, abuse of or dependence on psychoactive substances is linked with a very similar pattern of gray matter changes as manifest in schizophrenia, even in the first-episode subjects. They affect areas linked with higher order cognitive functions; however, the functional outcome of the affection depends on many factors: if they affect matured or developing brain, what is the exact nature of the pathology of local circuits caused by the particular pathological process etc.

Quite unique situation is in the case of a link between schizophrenia and *cannabis* use. Still unresolved issue is if cannabis use predisposes for or increase risk of the later schizophrenia development or if it reflects certain pathophysiological features of the illness (Newell et al., 2006) with consequent use of cannabis as a kind of automedication. Advocates may be found for both viewpoints. In this context studies that may shed light on the common pathways of schizophrenia neurobiology and cannabis use are of special interest. Bangalore et al. (2008) studied the link between the cannabis use and regional gray matter in first-episode schizophrenia who abused cannabis (n = 15), who did not (n = 24) and healthy controls (n = 42) without anamnesis of abuse. When compared with schizophrenia subjects without cannabis abuse, schizophrenia subjects abusing cannabis had smaller gray matter density in posterior cingulate, a region rich of CB1 receptors (Newell et al., 2006). Even heavy (more than 5 joints/day) and long term (more than 10 years) cannabis use alone, in subjects without schizophrenia or significant psychosis, was associated with bilateral hippocampal and amygdala volume in a ROI study (Yucel et al., 2008), i.e. in areas linked with pathopysiology of schizophrenia.

Neurotic and Stress Related Disorders

Obsessive-compulsive disorder is another condition considered to be of neurodevelopmental origin. Imaging studies refer a consistent pattern of gray matter in anterior cingulate gyrus (Valente et al., 2005; Carmona et al., 2007; Yoo et al., 2008), with reports of gray matter reduction in inferior and medial frontal gyrus, insula, and superior temporal gyrus (Yoo et al., 2008). However, even conditions considered to be consequences of sole psychological processes, such as *Panic disorder*, were shown to be linked with gray matter deficits. In panic disorder, reduction of gray matter density in the left parahippocampal gyrus (Massana et al., 2003) or bilateral putamen (Yoo et al., 2005) was reported. Similarly, life events, at least unfavorable ones exerting substantial stress, can also contribute to the brain morphology changes. This factor is marked in *Posttraumatic stress disorder* where gray matter reduction in anterior cingulate was reported (Yamasue et al., 2003). Moreover, even some *personality traits* may have neuroanatomical correlate: harm avoidance score correlated significantly with the gray matter in the left amygdala (Iidaka et al., 2006), a limbic structure where Rusch et al. (2003) reported significant reduction of gray matter in borderline personality disorder. Moreover, novelty seeking was associated with gray matter in the left medial frontal gyrus and reward dependence with caudate nucleus (Iidaka et al., 2006).

Histopathological Correlates of Similar Findings

The same pattern of neuroimaging findings does not speak about the same neuropathology. The final judge in the etiology and character of the neuroimaging findings is the histopathology. As demonstrated above, it seems that VBM studies in schizophrenia image the abundance of synaptic connections or neuropil. The histopathological meaning of neuroimaging findings in other psychiatric conditions is, unfortunately, unclear.

Apparently, not all changes in schizophrenia detected using imaging methods have support from neuropathological studies. This is because the neuropathological studies focused mainly on the limbic and prefrontal areas. On the other hand, the findings from neuroimaging studies inspire and guide the neuropathological investigation. Neuroimaging, however, brings information that cannot be achieved by neuropathological studies – such as dynamics of the changes. Both approaches are thus complementary and should be used together when trying to understand quite complex findings of brain morphology changes in schizophrenia and related conditions.

Conclusion

In schizophrenia, a somewhat widespread reduction of cortical gray matter exists. The changes are quite heterogeneous both in terms of intersubject and regional variability, with the most consistent and extensive findings being at hand for the dorsolateral prefrontal cortex. Its dysfunction leads to cognitive symptoms as well as to the dysregulation of the dopaminergic system, which predisposes those affected to psychotic episodes. However, the changes are not limited to the heteromodal associative cortex; changes were observed also in primary sensory or motor cortical areas. These findings substantiate the fact that schizophrenia is not only a disease of higher cognition; on the contrary, many signs and symptoms reflect motor (Kasparek et al., in press) or perceptual (Butler et al., 2008) dysfunction.

Neurobiologically, it corresponds to the loss of dendritic spines of layer III pyramidal neurons and interrelated changes in parvalbumin GABA-ergic cells, thalamocortical and dopaminergic projections. Such a pattern of cortical microcircuitry changes results in abnormal coordination of cortical pyramidal neuron activity. This dyscoordination is expressed on the level of neurophysiological abnormalities, such as reduced theta or gamma band oscillations during cognitive load.

It is apparent that the pattern of neuroimaging findings in schizophrenia is not disease-specific. Thus, the neuroimaging has limited value in the diagnostic or differential diagnostic process. However, in the context of established diagnoses, we are able to interpret the changes on the neuropathological level and we may use the information from neuroimaging methods in a specific and quite useful way, i.e., we may try to link the pattern of changes with clinical features of the illness or we may consider regionally-specific therapeutic approaches, such as rTMS for negative syndrome (Prikryl et al., 2007) or refractory hallucinations (Aleman et al., 2007).

Acknowledgment

Supported by a research project of the Ministry of Education, Youth and Sports of the Czech Republic no. MSM0021622404.

References

Adler, C; Levine, A; DelBello, M; Strakowski, S. Changes in gray matter volume in patients with bipolar disorder. *Biol. Psychiatry*, 2005, 58, 151-157.

Agartz, I; Sedvall, GC; Terenius, L; Kulle, B; Frigessi, A; Hall, H; Jonsson, EG. BDNF gene variant and brain morphology in schizophrenia. *American Journal of medical Genetics Part* B (Neuropsychiatric Genetics), 2006, 141B, 513-523.

Ahmed, B; Anderson, JC; Douglas, RJ; Martin, KAC; Nelson, JC; Polyneurronal innervation of spiny stellate neurons in cat visual cortex. *J. Comp. Neurol.*, 1994, 341, 39-49.

Akbarian, S; Kim, JJ; Potkin, SG; Hagman, JO; Tafazzoli, A; Bunney, WE Jr; Jones EG. Gene expression for glutamic acid decarboxylase is reduced without loss of neurons in prefrontal cortex of schizophrenics. *Arch. Gen. Psychiatry*, 1995, 52, 258-66.

Akil, M; Kolachana, BS; Rothmond, DA; Hyde, TM; Weinberger, DR; Kleinman, JE. Catechol-O-methyltransferase genotype and dopamine regulation in the human brain. *J. Neurosce,* 2003, 23, 2008-2013.

Aleman, A; Sommer, IE; Kahn, RS. Efficacy of slow repetitive transcranial magnetic stimulation in the treatment of resistant auditory hallucinations in schizophrenia: a meta-analysis. *J. Clin. Psychiatry*, 2007, 68, 416-21.

Alexander, GE; Goldman, PS. Functional development of the dorsolateral prefrontal cortex: An analysis utilizing reversible cryogenic depression. Brain Res, 1978, 143, 233-249.

Amodio, DM; Frith, CD. Meeting of minds: the medial frontal cortex and social cognition. *Nat. Rev. Neurosci.*, 2006, 7, 268-77.

Antonova, E; Sharma, T; Morris, R; Kumari, V. The relationship between brain structure and neurocognition in schizophrenia: a selective review. *Schizophr. Res.*, 2004, 70, 117-45.

Antonova, E; Kumari, V; Morris, R; Halari, R; Anilkumar, A; Mehrotra, R; Sharma, T. The relationship of structural alterations to cognitive deficits in schizophrenia: a voxel-based morphometry study. *Biol. Psychiatry*, 2005, 58, 457–467.

Arbib, MA; Mundhenk, TN. Schizophrenia and the mirror system: an essay. *Neuropsychologia*, 2005, 43, 268-80.

Arnsten, AFT; Cai, JX; Murphy, BL; Goldman-Rakic, PS. Dopamine D1 receptor mechanisms in the cognitive performance of young adult and aged monkeys. *Psychopharmacology*, 1994, 116, 143-151.

Baaré, WF; Hulshoff Pol, HE; Hijman, R; Mali, WP; Viergever, MA; Kahn, RS. Volumetric analysis of frontal lobe regions in schizophrenia: relation to cognitive function and symptomatology. *Biol. Psychiatry,* 1999, 45, 1597-605.

Bangalore, SS; Prasad, KMR; Montrose, DM; Goradia, DD; Diwadkar, VA; Keshavan, MS. Cannabis use and brain structural alterations in first episode schizophrenia — a region of interest, voxel based morphometric study. *Schizophrenia Res.*, 2008, 99, 1–6.

Bayer, TA; Falkai, P; Maier, W. Genetic and non-genetic vulnerability factors in schizophrenia: The basis of the "two-hit hypothesis". *J. Psychiatry Res.*, 1999, 33, 543-548.

Beal, MF; Brouillet, E; Jenkins, B. Neurochemical and histological characterization of striatal excitotoxic lesions produced by the mitochondrial toxin 3-nitropropionic acid. *J. Neurosci.*, 1993, 13, 4181-4191.

Bearden, CE; Thompson, PM; Dalwani, M; Hayashi, KM; Lee, AD; Nicoletti, M; Trankhtenbroit, M; Glahn, DC; Brambilla, P; Sassi, RB; Mallinger, AG; Frank, E; Kupfer, D; Soares, JC. Greater cortical gray matter density in lithium-treated patients with bipolar disorder. *Biol. Psychiatry*, 2007, 62, 7-16.

Beasly, CL; Reynolds, GP. Parvalbumin-immunoreactive neurons are reduced in the prefrontal cortex of schizophrenia. *Schizophr. Res.*, 1997, 24, 349-355.

Ben-Schachar, D; Zuk, R; Gazawi, H; Ljuboncic, P. Dopamine toxicity involves mitochondrial complex I inhibition: implications to dopamine-related neuropsychiatric disorders. *Biochem. Pharmacol.*, 2004, 67, 1965-1974.

Benes, FM; Paskevich, PA; Davidson, J; Domesick, VB. Synaptic rearangements in medial prefrontal cortex of haloperidol-treated rats. *Brain Res.*, 1985, 348, 15-20.

Benes; FM; McSparren, J; Bird, ED; SanGiovanni, JP; Vincent, SL. Deficits in small interneurons in prefrontal and cingulate cortices of schizophrenic and schizoaffective patients. *Arch. Gen. Psychiatry*, 1991, 48, 996-1001.

Benes; FM; Todtenkopf, MS; Taylor, JB. A shift in tyrosine hydroxylase-immunoreactive varicosities (TH-IRv) form pyramidal (PN) to nonpyramidal (NP) neurons occurs in layer II of the anterior cingulate cortex of schizophrenics. *Soc. Neurosci. Abst.*, 1995, 21, 259.

Benes, FM; Vincent, SL; Marie, A; Khan, Y. Up-regulation of GABAA receptor binding on neurons of the prefrontal cortex in schizophrenic subjects. *Neuroscience*, 1996, 75, 1021-31.

Benes, FM. The role of stress and dopamine-GABA interactions in the vulnerability for schizophrenia. *J. Psychiatr. Res.*, 1997, 31, 257-275.

Berger, GE; Wood, S; McGorry, PD. Incipient neurovulnerability and neuroprotection in early psychosis. *Psychopharmacol. Bul.l*, 2003, 37, 79-101.

Bertolino, A; Saunders, RC; Mattay, VS; Bachevalier, J; Frank, JA; Weinberger, DR. Altered development of prefrontal neurons in rhesus monkeys with neonatal mesial temporo-limbic lesions: a proton magnetic resonance spectroscopic imaging study. *Cereb. Cortex*, 1997, 7, 740-8.

Bertolino, A; Knable, MB; Saunders, RC; Callicott, JH; Kolachana, B; Mattay, VS; Bachevalier, J; Frank, JA; Egan, M; Weinberger, DR. The relationship between dorsolateral prefrontal N-acetylaspartate measures and striatal dopamine activity in schizophrenia. *Biol. Psychiatry*, 1999, 45, 660-7.

Bertolino, A; Breier, A; Callicott, JH; Adler, C; Mattay, VS; Shapiro, M; Frank, JA; Pickar, D; Weinberger, DR. The relationship between dorsolateral prefrontal neuronal N-acetylaspartate and evoked release of striatal dopamine in schizophrenia. *Neuropsychopharmacology*, 2000; 22, 125-32.

Bilder, RM; Bogerts, B; Ashtari, M; Wu, H; Alvir, JM; Jody, D; Reiter, G; Bell, L; Lieberman, JA. Anterior hippocampal volume reductions predict frontal lobe dysfunction in first episode schizophrenia. *Schizophr. Res.*, 1995, 17, 47-58.

Blatow, M; Rozov, A; Katona, I; Hormuzdi, SG; Meyer, AH; Whittington, MA; Caputi, A; Monyer, H. A novel network of multipolar bursting interneurons generates theta frequency oscillations in neocortex. *Neuron*, 2003, 38, 805-17.

Bogerts, B. The neuropathology of schizophrenic diseases: historical aspects and present knowledge. *Eur. Arch. Psychiatry Clin. Neurosci.*, 1999, 249(suppl. 4), IV/2-IV/13.

Bourgeois, JP; Goldman-Rakic, PS; Rakic, P. Synaptogenesis in the prefrontal cortex of rhesus monkeys. *Cereb. Cortex*, 1994, 4, 78-96.

Braff, DL; Freedman, R; Schork, NJ; Gottesman, II. Deconstructing schizophrenia: an overview of the use of endophenotypes in order to understand a complex disorder. *Schizophr. Bull.*, 2007; 33; 21-32.

Broadbelt; K; Byne, W; Jones, LB. Evidence for a decrease in basilar dendrites of pyramidal cells in schizophrenic medial prefrontal cortex. *Schizophr. Res.*, 2002, 58, 75-81.

Brody, AL; Mandelkern, MA; Jarvik, ME; Lee, GS; Smith, EC; Huang, JC; Bota, RG; Bartzokis, G; London, ED. Differences between smokers and nonsmokers in regional gray matter volumes and densities. *Biol. Psychiatry*, 2004, 55, 77–84.

Bonilha, L; Molnar, C; Horner, MD; Anderson, B; Forster, L; George, MS; Nahas, Z. Neurocognitive deficits and prefrontal cortical atrophy in patients with schizophrenia. *Schizophrenia Res.*, 2008; 101; 142-151.

Borgwardt, SJ; McGuire, PK; Aston, J; Berger, G; Dazzan, P; Gschwandtner, U; Pfluger, M; D'Souza, M; Radue, EW; Riecher-Rossler, A. Structural brain abnormalities in individuals with an at-riskmental state who later develop psychosis. *Br. J. Psychiatry*, 2007, 191 (suppl . 51); 69-75.

Brock, JW; Prasad, C. Alterations in dendritic spine density in the rat brain associated with protein malnutrition. *Dev. Brain Res.*, 1992, 66, 266-269.

Bromet, EJ; Naz, B; Fochtmann, LB; Carlson, GA; Tanenberg-Karant, M. Long-term diagnostic stability and outcome in recent first-episode cohort studies of schizophrenia. *Schizophrenia Bulletin,* 2005, 31, 639–649.

Bryan, GK; Riesen, AH. Deprived somatosensory-motor experience in stump-tailed monkey neocortex: dendritic spine density and dendritic branching of layer IIIb pyramidal cells. *J. Comp. Neurol.,* 1989, 286, 208-217.

Burns J. The social brain hypothesis of schizophrenia. *World Psychiatry*, 2006, 5, 77-81.

Butler, PD; Silverstein, SM; Dakin, SC. Visual perception and its impairment in schizophrenia. *Biol. Psychiatry*, 2008, 64, 40-7.

Cahn, W; Hulshoff Pol, HE; Lems, EB; van Haren, NE; Schnack, HG; van der Linden, JA; Schothorst, PF; van Engeland, H; Kahn, RS. Brain volume changes in first-episode schizophrenia: a 1-year follow-up study. *Arch. Gen. Psychiatry*, 2002, 59, 1002-10.

Cannon, TD; Hennah, W; van Erp, TG; Thompson, PM; Lonnqvist, J; Huttunen, M; Gasperoni, T; Tuulio-Henriksson, A; Pirkola, T; Toga, AW; Kaprio, J; Mazziotta, J; Peltonen, L. Association of DISC1/TRAX haplotypes with schizophrenia, reduced prefrontal gray matter, and impaired short- and long-term memory. *Arch. Gen. Psychiatry*, 2005, 62, 1205-13.

Carmona, S; Bassas, N; Rovira, M; Gispert, JD; Soliva, JC; Prado, M; Tomas, J; Bulbena, A; Vilarroya, O. Pediatric OCD structural brain deficits in conflict monitoring circuits: A voxel-based morphometry study. *Neuroscience Letters*, 2007, 421, 218–223.

Ceccherini-Nelli A; Crow TJ. Disintegration of the components of language as the path to a revision of Bleuler's and Schneider's concepts of schizophrenia. Linguistic disturbances compared with first-rank symptoms in acute psychosis. *Br. J. Psychiatry*, 2003, 182, 233-40.

Chakos, MH; Lieberman, JA; Bilder, RM; et al. Increase in caudate nuclei volumes of first-episode schizophrenic patients taking antipsychotic drugs. *Am. J. Psychiatry*, 1994, 151, 1430-1436.

Chanraud, S; Martelli, C; Delain, F; Kostogianni, N; Douaud, G; Aubin, HJ; Reynaud, M; Martinot, JL. Brain morphometry and cognitive performance in detoxified alcohol-dependents with preserved psychosocial functioning. *Neuropsychopharmacology*, 2007, 32, 429–438.

Cho, RY; Konecky, RO; Carter, CS. Impairments in frontal cortical gamma synchrony and cognitive control in schizophrenia. *Proc. Natl. Acad. Sci. USA*, 2006, 103, 19878-83.

Cobb, SR; Buhl, EH; Halasy, K; Paulsen, O; Somogyi, P. Synchronization of neuronal activity in hippocampus by individual GABAergic interneurons. *Nature*, 1995, 378, 75-8.

Connor, JR; Diamond, MC. A comparison of dendritic spine number and type on pyramidal neurons of the visual cortex of old adult rats from social or isolated environments. *J. Comp. Neurol.*, 1982, 210, 99-106.

Cowan, RL; Lyoo, IK; Sunga, SM; Ahna, KH; Kima, MJ; Hwang, J; Hagaa, E; Vimal, RLP; Lukas, SE; Renshaw, PF. Reduced cortical gray matter density in human MDMA (Ecstasy) users: a voxel-based morphometry study. *Drug and Alcohol Dependence*, 2003, 72, 225–235.

Crow, TJ; Ball, J; Bloom, SR, Brown, R; Bruton, CJ; Colter, N; Frith, CD; Johnstone, EC; Owens, DG; Roberts, GW. Schizophrenia as an anomaly of development of cerebral asymmetry. A postmortem study and a proposal concerning the genetic basis of the disease. *Arch. Gen. Psychiatry*, 1989, 46,1145-50.

Datta, S; Brunet, A; Greenberg, M. Cell survival: A play in three AKTs. *Gene Dev.*, 1999, 13, 2905-2927.

Davidson, L; McGlashan, TH. The varied outcomes of schizophrenia. *Can. J. Psychiatry*, 1997, 42, 34-43.

Dazzan, P; Morgan, KD; Orr, K; Hutchinson, G; Chitnis, X; Suckling, J; Fearon, P; McGuire ,PK; Mallett, RM; Jones, PB; Leff, J; Murray, RM. Different effects of typical and atypical antipsychotics on grey matter in first episode psychosis: the ÆSOP study. *Neuropsychopharmacology*, 2005, 30, 765–774.

de Haan, L. Bakker, JM. Overview of neuropathological theories of schizophrenia: from degeneration to progressive developmental disorder. *Psychopathology*, 2004, 37, 1-7.

DeFelipe, J; Farinas, I. The pyramidal neuron of the cerebral cortex: morphological and chemical characteristics of the synaptic inputs. *Prog. Neurobiol.,* 1992, 39, 563-607.

Deutch, AY. The effects of dopamine denervation on prefrontal cortical structure and reversal by atypical antipsychotic drugs. *Biol. Psychiatry*, 2005, 57, 82S.

Deutch, AY; Jing, D. Prefrontal cortical dopamine denervation decreases dendritic spine density in pyramidal neurons. *Schizophr. Res.*, 2003, 60, 56.

Deutsch, S; Rosse, R; Schwartz, B; Mastropaolo, J. A revised excitotoxic hypothesis of schizophrenia: therapeutic implications. *Clin. Neuropharmacol.*, 2001, 24, 43-49.

Dorph-Petersen, K-A; Pierri, JN; Sun, Z; Sampson, AR; Lewis, DA. Stereological analysis of the mediodorsal thalamic nucleus in schizophrenia: volume; neuron number; and cell types. *J. Comp. Neurol.*, 2004, 472, 449-462.

Dorph-Petersen, KA; Pierri, JN; Perel, JM; Sun, Z; Sampson, AR; Lewis, DA. The influence of chronic exposure to antipsychotic medications on brain size before and after tissue fixation: a comparison of haloperidol and olanzapine in macaque monkeys. *Neuropsychopharmacology*, 2005, 30, 1649-1661.

Drake, RJ; Lewis, W. Insight and neurocognitive deficits in schizophrenia. *Schizophr. Res.*, 2003, 62, 165–173.

Drake, RJ; Dunn, G; Tarrier, N; Bentall, RP; Haddock, G; Lewis, SW. Insight as a predictor of the outcome of first-episode nonaffective psychosis in a prospective cohort study in England. *J. Clin. Psychiatry,* 2007, 68, 81-6.

Eastwood, SL; Cairns, NJ; Harrison, PJ. Synaptophysin gene expression in schizophrenia. Investigation of synaptic pathology in the cerebral cortex. *Br. J. Psychiatry*, 2000,176, 236-42.

Ellison-Wright, I; Glahn, DC; Laird, AR; Thelen, SM; Bullmore, E. The anatomy of first-episode and chronic schizophrenia: an anatomical likelihood estimation meta-analysis. *Am. J. Psychiatry*, 2008, AiA, 1-9.

Erickson, SE; Lewis, DA. Cortical connections of the lateral mediodorsal thalamus in cynomolgus monkeys. *J. Comp. Neurol.,* 2004, 473, 107-127.

Farber, N; Jiang, X; Dikranian, K; et al. Muscimol prevents NMDA antagonist neurotoxicity by activating GABA-A receptors in several brain regions. *Brain Res.*, 2003, 993, 90-100.

Farrow, TFD; Whitford, TJ; Williams, LM; Gomes, L; Harris, AWF. Diagnosis-related regional gray matter loss over two years in first episode schizophrenia and bipolar disorder. *Biol. Psychiatry*, 2005, 58(9), 713-23.

Feinberg, I. Schizophrenia: caused by a fault in programmed synaptic elimination during adolescence? *J. Psychiatr. Res.*, 1982, 17, 319-334.

Ferrer, I; Fabregues, I; Rairiz, J; et al. Decreased number of dendritic spines on cortical pyramidal spines on cortical pyramidal neurons in human chronic alcoholism. *Neurosci. Lett.,* 1986, 69, 115-9.

Fiscus, RR. Involvement of cyclic GMP and protein kinase G in the regulation of apoptosis and survival in neurol cells. *Neurosignals*, 2002, 11, 175-190.

Fleischhaker, C; Schulz, E; Tepper, K; Martin, M; Hennighausen, K; Remschmidt, H. Long-term course of adolescent schizophrenia. *Schizophrenia Bulletin*, 2005, 31, 769–780.

Flores, G; Alquicer, G; Silva-Goméz, AB; Zaldivar, G; Stewart, J; Quirion, R; Srivastava, LK. Alterations in dendritic morphology of prefrontal cortical and nucleus accumbens neurons in post-pubertal rats after neonatal excitotoxic lesions of the ventral hippocampus. *Neuroscience,* 2005, 133, 463-70.

Fog, R; Pakkenberg, H; Juul, P; Bock, E; Jorgensen, OS; Andersen, J. High-dose treatment of rats with perphenazine enanthate. *Psychopharmacology* (Berl), 1976, 50, 305-7.

Ford, JM; Mathalon, DH; Whitfield, S; Faustman, WO; Roth, WT. Reduced communication between frontal and temporal lobes during talking in schizophrenia. *Biol. Psychiatry*, 2002, 51, 485-92.

Franklin, TR; Acton, PD; Maldjian, JA; Gray, JD; Croft, JR; Dackis, CA; O'Brien, CP; Childress, AR. Decreased gray matter concentration in the insular; orbitofrontal; cingulate; and temporal cortices of cocaine patients. *Biol. Psychiatry*, 2002, 51, 134–142.

Frey, BN; da Fonseca, MMR; Machado-Vieira, R; Soarese, JC; Kapczinski, F. Neuropathological and neurochemical abnormalities in bipolar disorder. *Rev. Bras. Pisquistr*; 2004, 26, 180-8.

Friston, KJ; Frith, CD. Schizophrenia: A disconnection syndrome? *Clin. Neurosci.*, 1995, 3, 89-97.

García-Martí, G; Aguilar, EJ; Lull, JJ; Martí-Bonmatí, L; Escartí, MJ; Manjón, JV; Moratal, D; Robles, M; Sanjuán, J. Schizophrenia with auditory hallucinations: a voxel-based morphometry study. *Prog. Neuropsychopharmacol. Biol. Psychiatry*, 2008, 32, 72-80.

Garden, GA; Budd, SL; Tsai, E; Hanson, L; Kaul, M; D'Emilia, DM; Friedlander, RM; Yuan, J; Masliah, E; Lipton, SA. Caspase cascades in human immunodeficiency virus-associated neurodegeneration. *J. Neurosci.,* 2002, 22, 4015-4024.

Garey, LJ; Ong, WY, Patel, PS; Kanani, M; Davis, A; Mortimer, AM; Barnes, TRE; Hirsch, SR. Reduced dendritic spine density on cerebral cortical pyramidal neurons in schizophrenia. *J. Neurol. Neurosurg. Psychiatry*, 1998, 65, 446-453.

Garver, DL; Holcomb, JA; Christensen, JD. Cerebral cortical gray expansion associated with two second-generation antipsychotics. *Biol. Psychiatry*, 2005, 58, 62-6.

Gilman, CP; Mattson, MG. Do apoptotic mechanisms regulate synaptic plasticity and growth-cone motility? *Neuromolecular. Med.*, 2002, 2, 197-214.

Girgis, RR; Diwadkar, VA; Nutche, JJ; Sweeney, JA; Keshavan, MS; Hardan, AY. Risperidone in first-episode psychosis: a longitudinal; exploratory voxel-based morphometric study. *Schizophr. Res.,* 2006, 82, 89-94.

Giuliani, NR; Calhoun, VD; Pearlson, GD; Francis, A; Buchanan, RW. Voxel-based morphometry versus region of interest: a comparison of two methods for analyzing gray matter differences in schizophrenia. *Schizophr. Res*., 2005, 74, 135-47.

Glantz, LA; Lewis, DA. Reduction of synaptophysin immunoreactivity in the prefrontal cortex of subjects with schizophrenia. Regional and diagnostic specificity. *Arch. Gen. Psychiatry,* 1997, 54, 943-52.

Glantz, LA; Lewis, DA. Decreased dendritic spine density on prefrontal cortical pyramidal neurons in schizophrenia. *Arch. Gen. Psychiatry*, 2000, 57, 65-73.

Glantz, LA; Gilmore, JH; Lieberman, JA; Jarskog, LF. Apoptotic mechanisms and the synaptic pathology of schizophrenia. *Schizophrenia Res.,* 2006, 81: 4-63.

Goldman-Rakic, PS; Leranth, C; Williams, SM; Mons, N; Geffard, M. Dopamine synaptic complex with pyramidal neurons in primate cerebral cortex. *Proc. Natl. Acad. Sci. USA*, 1989, 86, 9015:9019.

Guidotti, A; Auta, J; Davis, JM; Di-Giorgi-Gerevini, V; Dwivedi, Y; Grayson, DR; Impagnatiello, F; Pandey, G; Pesold, C; Sharma, R; Uzunov, D; Costa, E. Decrease in reelin and glutamic acid decarboxylase67 (GAD67) expression in schizophrenia and bipolar disorder: a postmortem brain study. *Arch. Gen. Psychiatry*, 2000, 57, 1061-9.

Guo, ZH; Mattson, MP. Neurotrophic factors protect cortical synaptic terminals against amyloid and oxidative stress-induced impairment of glucose transport; glutamate transport and mitochondrial function. *Cereb Cortex,* 2000, 10, 50-57.

Gurling, HM; Critchley, H; Datta, SR; McQuillin, A; Blaveri, E; Thirumalai, S; Pimm, J; Krasucki, R; Kalsi, G; Quested, D; Lawrence, J; Bass, N; Choudhury, K; Puri, V; O'Daly, O; Curtis, D; Blackwood, D; Muir, W; Malhotra, AK; Buchanan, RW; Good, CD; Frackowiak, RS; Dolan, RJ. Genetic association and brain morphology studies and the chromosome 8p22 pericentriolar material 1 (PCM1) gene in susceptibility to schizophrenia. *Arch. Gen. Psychiatry*, 2006, 63, 844-54.

Ha, TH; Youn, T; Ha, KS; Rho, KS; Lee, JM; Kim, IY; Kim, SI; Kwon, JS. Gray matter abnormalities in paranoid schizophrenia and their clinical correlations. *Psychiatry Res*, 2004, 132, 251-60.

Halim, ND; Weickert, CS; McClintock, BW; et al. Effects of chronic haloperidol and clozapine treatment on neurogenesis in the adult rat hippocampus. *Neuropsychopharmacology*, 2004, 29, 1063-1069.

Harrison, PJ. Neuropathology of schizophrenia. A critical review of the data and their interpretation. *Brain,* 1999a, 122, 593-624.

Harrison, PJ. The neuropathological effects of antipsychotic drugs. *Schizophr. Res.*; 1999b, 40, 87-99.

Harrison, PJ. The neuropathology of primary mood disorder. *Brain*, 2002, 125, 1428-1449.

Harrison, PJ. The hippocampus in schizophrenia: a review of the neuropathological evidence and its pathophysiological implications. *Psychopharmacology,* 2004, 174, 151-162.

Hashimoto, T; Volk, DW; Eggan, SM; Mirnics, K; Pierri, JN; Sun, Z; Sampson, AR; Lewis, DA. Gene expression deficits in a subclass of GABA neurons in the prefrontal cortex of subjects with schizophrenia. *J. Neurosci.,* 2003, 23, 6315-26.

Hashimoto, T; Bergen, SE; Nguyen, QL; Xu, B; Monteggia, LM; Pierri, JN; Sun, Z; Sampson, AR; Lewis, DA. Relationship of brain-derived neurotrophic factor and its receptor TrkB to altered inhibitory prefrontal circuitry in schizophrenia. J. *Neurosci.*, 2005, 25, 372-83.

Hazlett, EA; Buchsbaum, MS; Haznedar, MM; Newmark, R; Goldstein, KE; Zelmanova, Y; Glanton, CF; Torosjan, Y; New, AS; Lo, JN; Mitropoulou, V; Siever, LJ. Cortical gray and white matter volume in unmedicated schizotypal and schizophrenia patients. Schizophr Res, 2008, 101, 111-23.

Ho, B; Milev, P; O'Leary, DS; Librant, A; Andreasen, NC; Wassink, TH. Cognitive and magnetic resonance imaging brain morphometric correlates of brain-derived neurotrophic factor Val66Met gene polymorphism in patients with schizophrenia and healthy volunteers. *Arch. Gen. Psychiatry*, 2006, 63, 731-740.

Hof, PR; Haroutunian, V; Friedrich Jr, VL; Byne, W; Buitron, C; Perl, DP. Loss and altered spatial distribution of oligodendrocytes in the superior frontal gyrus in schizophrenia. *Biol. Psychiatry*, 2003, 53, 1075-1085.

Hoffman, RE; Dobscha, SK. Cortical pruning and the development of schizophrenia: A computer model. *Schizophr. Bull.*, 1989, 15, 477-490.

Honea, R; Crow, TJ; Passingham, D; Mackay, CE. Regional deficits in brain volume in schizophrenia: a meta-analysis of voxel-based morphometry studies. *Am. J. Psychiatry,* 2005, 162, 2233-2245.

Honea, RA; Meyer-Lindenberg, A; Hobbs, KB; Pezawas, L; Mattay, VS; Egan, MF; Verchinski, B; Passingham, RE; Weinberger, DR; Callicott, JH. Is gray matter volume an intermediate phenotype for schizophrenia? A voxel-based morphometry study of patients with schizophrenia and their healthy siblings. *Biol. Psychiatry*, 2008, 63, 465-74.

Honer, WG; Falkai, P; Young, C; Wang, T; Xie, J; Bonner, J; Hu, L; Boulianne, GL; Luo, Z; Trimble, WS. Cingulate cortex synaptic terminal proteins and neural cell adhesion molecule in schizophrenia. *Neuroscience*, 1997, 78, 99-110.

Hughes, JR; Hatsukami, DK; Mitchell, JE; Dahlgren, IA. Prevalence of smoking among psychiatric outpatients. *Am. J. of Psychiatry*, 1986, 143, 993-997.

Hulshoff Pol, HE; Schnack, HG; Mandl, RC; Brans, RG; van Haren, NE; Baaré, WF; van Oel, CJ; Collins, DL; Evans, AC; Kahn, RS. Gray and white matter density changes in monozygotic and same-sex dizygotic twins discordant for schizophrenia using voxel-based morphometry. *Neuroimage*, 2006, 31, 482-8.

Iidakaa, T; Matsumotob, A; Ozakia, N; Suzukic, T; Iwatac, N; Yamamotod, Y; Okadad, T; Sadato, T. Volume of left amygdala subregion predicted temperamental trait of harm avoidance in female young subjects. A voxel-based morphometry study. *Brain Res*, 2006, 1125, 85–93.

Iritani, S. Neuropathology of schizophrenia: A mini review. *Neuropathology*, 2007, 27, 604-608.

Jang, DP; Namkoong, K; Kimb, JJ; Park, S; Kime, IY; Kime, SI; Kima, YB; Choa, ZH; Lee, E. The relationship between brain morphometry and neuropsychological performance in alcohol dependence. *Neuroscience Letters*, 2007, 428, 21–26.

Jarskog, LF; Glantz, LA; Gilmore, JH; Lieberman, JA. Apoptotic mechanisms in the pathophysiology of schizophrenia. Prog Neuro-psychopharmacol *Biol. Psychiatry*, 2005, 29, 846-858.

Job, DE; Whalley, HC; McConnel, S; Glabus, M; Johnstone, EC; Lawrie, SM. Voxel-based morphometry of grey matter densities in subjects at high risk of schizophrenia. *Schizophrenia Res.*, 2003, 64, 1– 13.

Jobe, TH; Harrow, M: Long-term outcome of patients with schizophrenia: a review. *Can. J. Psychiatry*, 2005, 50, 892-900.

Johnstone, EC; Crow, TJ; Frith, CD; Husband, J; Kree,l L. Cerebral ventricular size and cognitive impairment in chronic schizophrenia. *Lancet*, 1976, 2, 924-6.

Jones, LB; Johnson, N; Byne, W. Alteration in MAP2 immunocytochemistry in area 9 and 32 of schizophrenic prefrontal cortex. *Psychiatry Res.*, 2002, 114, 137-48.

Kalus, P; Senitz, D; Beckmann, H. Altered distribution of parvalbumin-immunoreactive local circuit neurons in the anterior cingulate cortex of schizophrenic patients. *Psychiatry Res.*, 1997, 75, 49-59.

Kasai, K; Shenton, ME; Salisbury, DF; Hirayasu, Y; Onitsuka, T; Spencer, MH; Yurgelun-Todd, DA; Kikinis, R; Jolesz, FA; McCarley, RW. Progressive decrease of left Heschl gyrus and planum temporale gray matter volume in first-episode schizophrenia: a longitudinal magnetic resonance imaging study. *Arch. Gen. Psychiatry*, 2003, 60, 766-75.

Kasparek, T; Prikryl, R; Mikl, M; Schwarz, D; Ceskova, E; Krupa, P. Prefrontal but not temporal grey matter changes in males with first-episode schizophrenia. *Prog. Neuropsychopharmacol. Biol. Psychiatry*, 2007, 31,151–157.

Kasparek, T; Prikryl, R; Schwarz, D; Tronerová, S; Ceskova, E; Mikl, M; Vanicek, J. Movement sequencing abilities and basal ganglia morphology in first-episode schizophrenia. *World Journal of Biological Psychiatry*, 2008 January 30. [Epub ahead of print]

Kawasaki, Y; Suzuki, M; Nohara, S; Hagino, H; Takahashi, T; Matsui, M; Yamashita, I; Chitnis, XA; McGuire, PK; Seto, H; Kurachi, M. Structural brain differences in patients with schizophrenia and schizotypal disorder demonstrated by voxel-based morphometry. *Eur. Arch. Psychiatry Clin. Neurosci.*, 2004, 254, 406–414.

Keshavan, MS; Anderson, S; Pettegrew, JW. Is schizophrenia due to excessive synaptic pruning in the prefrontal cortex? The Feinberg hypothesis revisited. *J. Psychiatr. Res.*, 1994, 28, 239-65.

Keller, SS; Wilke, M; Wieshmann, UC; Sluming, VA; Roberts, N. Comparison of standard and optimized voxel-based morphometry for analysis of brain changes associated with temporal lobe epilepsy. *Neuroimage*, 2004, 23, 860–868.

Klintzova, AJ; Haselhorst, U; Uranova, NA; Schenk, H; Istomin, VV. The effects of haloperidol on synaptic plasticity in rat's medial prefrontal cortex. *J. Hirnforsch*, 1989, 30, 51-7.

Kodama, M; Jujioka, T; Duman, RS. Chronic olanzapine or fluoxetine administration increases all proliferation in hippocampus and prefrontal cortex of adult rat. *Biol. Psychiatry*, 2004, 56, 570-580.

Konopaske, GT; Dorph-Petersen, KA; Pierri, JN; Wu, Q; Sampson, AR; Lewis, DA. Effect of chronic exposure to antipsychotic medication on cell numbers in the parietal cortex of macaque monkeys. *Neuropsychopharmacology*, 2007, 32, 1216-1223.

Kolluri, N; Sun, Z; Sampson, A; Lewis, DA. Lamina-specific reductions in dendritic spine density in the prefrontal cortex of subjects with schizophrenia. *Am. J. Psychiatry*, 2005, 162, 1200-1202.

Konopaske, GT; Dorph-Petersen, KA; Pierri, JN; Wu, Q; Sampson, AR; Lewis, DA. Effect of chronic exposure to antipsychotic medication on cell numbers in the parietal cortex of macaque monkeys. *Neuropsychopharmacology*, 2007, 32, 1216-1223.

Konopaske, GT; Dorph-Petersen, KA; Sweet, RA; Pierri, JN; Wei, Z; Sampson, AR; Lewis, DA. Effect of chronic exposure on astrocyte and oligodendrocyte numbers in macaque monkeys. *Biol. Psychiatry,* 2008, 63, 759-762.

Koo, MS; Dickey, CC; Park, HJ; Kubicki, M; Ji, NY; Bouix, S; Pohl, KM; Levitt, JJ; Nakamura, M; Shenton, ME; McCarley, RW. Smaller neocortical gray matter and larger sulcal cerebrospinal fluid volumes in neuroleptic-naive women with schizotypal personality disorder. *Arch. Gen. Psychiatry*, 2006, 63, 1090-1100.

Koutsouleris, N; Gaser, C; Jäger, M; Bottlender, R; Frodl, T; Holzinger, S; Schmitt, GJ; Zetzsche, T; Burgermeister, B; Scheuerecker, J; Born, C; Reiser, M; Möller, HJ;

Meisenzahl, EM. Structural correlates of psychopathological symptom dimensions in schizophrenia: a voxel-based morphometric study. *Neuroimage*, 2008, 39, 1600-12.

Kringelbach, ML; Rolls, ET. The functional neuroanatomy of the human orbitofrontal cortex: evidence from neuroimaging and neuropsychology. *Prog. Neurobiol.,* 2004, 72, 341-72.

Laird, AR; Fox, PM; Price, CJ; Glahn, DC; Uecker, AM; Lancaster, JL; Turkeltaub, PE; Kochunov, P; Fox, PT: ALE meta-analysis: controling the false discovery rate and performing statistical contrasts. *Hum. Brain Mapp*, 2005, 25, 155-164.

Lappin, JM; Morgan, K; Morgan, C; Hutchison, G; Chitnis, X; Suckling, J; Fearon, P; McGuire, PK; Jones, PB; Leff, J; Murray, RM; Dazzan, P. Gray matter abnormalities associated with duration of untreated psychosis. *Schizophr. Res.,* 2006, 83, 145-53.

Lappin, JM; Dazzan, P; Morgan, K; Morgan, C; Chitnis, X; Suckling, J; Fearon, P; Jones, PB; Leff, J; Murray, RM; McGuire, PK. Duration of prodromal phase and severity of volumetric abnormalities in first-episode psychosis. *Br. J. Psychiatry Suppl.*, 2007, 51, s123-7.

Laroi, F; Fannemel, M; Rønneberg, U; Flekkoy, K; Opjordsmoen, S; Dullerud, R; Haakosen, M. Unawareness of illness in chronic schizophrenia and its relationship to structural brain measures and neuropsychological tests. *Psychiat. Res.*, 2000, 100, 49–58.

Lee, DE. Reduced inhibitory capacity in prefrontal cortex of schizophrenics. *Arch. Gen. Psychiatry,* 1995, 52, 267-268.

Levitt, JB; Lewis, DA; Yoshioka, T; Lund, JS. Topography of pyramidal neuron intrinsic connections in macaque monkey prefrontal cortex (areas 9 and 46). *J. Comp. Neurol.*, 1993, 338, 360-367.

Lewis, DA. Development of the prefrontal cortex during adolescence: Insights into vulnerable neural circuits in schizophrenia. *Neuropsychopharmacology*, 1997, 16, 385-398.

Lewis, DA; Cruz, DA; Melchitzky, DS; Pierri, JN. Lamina-specific deficits in parvalbumin-immunoreactive varicosities in the prefrontal cortex of subjects with schizophrenia: evidence for fewer projections from the thalamus. *Am. J. Psychiatry,* 2001, 158, 1411-22.

Lewis, DA; Hashimoto, T; Volk, DW. Cortical inhibitory neurons and schizophrenia. *Nature Reviews Neuroscience,* 2005, 6, 312-324.

Lidow, MS; Song, ZM; Castner, SA; Allen, PB; Greengard, P; Goldman-Rakic, PS. Antipsychotic treatment induces alterations in dendrite- and spine-associated proteins in dopamine-rich areas of the primate cerebral cortex. *Biol. Psychiatry*, 2001, 49, 1-12.

Lieberman, JA; Sheitman, BB; Kinon, BJ. Neurochemical sensitization in the pathophysiology of schizophrenia: Deficits and dysfuntion in neuronal regulation and plasticity. *Neuropsychopharmacol.*, 1997, 17, 205-229.

Lieberman, J; Chakos, M; Wu, H; Alvir, J; Hoffman, E; Robinson, D; Bilder, R. Longitudinal study of brain morphology in first episode schizophrenia. *Biol. Psychiatry*, 2001, 49, 487-99.

Lieberman, JA; Tollefson, GD; Charles, C; Zipursky, R; Sharma, T; Kahn, RS; Keefe, RS; Green, AI; Gure, RE; McEvoy, J; Perkins, D; Hamer, RM; Gu, H; Tohen, M. Antipsychotic drug effects on brain morphology in first-episode psychosis. *Arch. Gen. Psychiatry*, 2005, 62, 361-370.

Lipska, BK; Jaskiw, GE; Weinberger, DR. Postpubertal emergence of hyperresponsiveness to stress and to amphetamine after neonatal excitotoxic hippocampal damage: a potential animal model of schizophrenia. *Neuropsychopharmacology,* 1993, 9, 67-75.

Lipska, BK; Swerdlow, NR; Geyer, MA; Jaskiw, GE; Braff, DL; Weinberger, DR. Neonatal excitotoxic hippocampal demage in rats causes post-pubertal changes of prepulse-inhibition of startle and its disruption by apomorphine. *Psychopharmacology* (Berl.), 1995, 122, 35-43.

Lipska, BK; Weinberger, DR. Genetic variation in vulnerability to the behavioral effects of neonatal hippocampal demage in rats. *Proc. Natl. Acad. Sci. USA*, 1995, 92, 8906-8910.

Lipska, BK; Lerman, DN; Khaing, ZZ; Weickert, CS; Weinberger, DR. Gene expression in dopamine and GABA systems in an animal model of schizophrenia: effects of antipsychotic drugs. *Eur. J. Neurosci.,* 2003, 18, 391-402.

Lund, JS; Holbach, S. Postnatal development of thalamic recipient neurons in monkey striate cortex: I. A comparison of spine acquisition and dendritic growth of layer 4C alpha and beta spiny stellate neurons. *J. Comp. Neurol.,* 1991, 309, 115-128.

Lund, JS; Yoshioka, T; Lewitt, JB. Comparison of intrinsic connectivity in different areas of macaque monkey cerebral cortex. *Cereb Cortex*, 1993, 3, 148-162.

Luo, Y; Umegaki, H; Wang, X; et al. Dopammine induces apoptosis through an oxidation-involved SAPK-JNK activation pathway. *J. Biol. Chem.,* 1998, 273, 3756-3764.

Lyoo, IK; Kim, MJ; Stoll, AL; Demopulos, CM; Parow, AM; Dager ,SR; et al. Frontal lobe gray matter density decreases in bipolar I disorder. *Biol. Psychiatry,* 2004, 55, 648-651.

Lyoo, IK; Pollack, MH; Silveri, MM; Ahn, KH; Diaz, CI; Hwang, J; Kim, SJ; Yurgelun-Todd, DA; Kaufman, MJ; Renshaw, PF. Prefrontal and temporal gray matter density decreases in opiate dependence. *Psychopharmacology*, 2006, 184, 139–144.

Mahadik, S; Evans, D; Lal, H. Oxidative stress and role of antioxidant and omega-3 essential fatty acid supplementation in schizophrenia. *Prog. Neuropharmacol. Biol. Psychiatry,* 2001, 25, 463-493.

Malberg, JE; Eisch, AJ; Nestler, EJ; et al. Chronic antidepressant treatment increases neurogenesis in the adult rat hippocampus. *J. Neurosci.*, 2000, 20, 9104-9110.

Massana, G; Serra-Grabulosa, JM; Salgado-Pineda, P; Gastó, C; Junqué, C; Massana, J; Mercader, JM. Parahippocampal gray matter density in panic disorder: a voxel-based morphometric study. *Am. J. Psychiatry,* 2003, 160, 566–568.

Massana, G; Salgado-Pineda, P; Junqué, C; Pérez, M; Baeza, I; Pons, A; Massana, J; Navarro, V; Blanch, J; Morer, A; Mercader, JM; Bernardo, M. Volume changes in gray matter in first-episode neuroleptic-naive schizophrenic patients treated with risperidone. *J. Clin. Psychopharmacol.*, 2005, 25, 111-7.

Maynard, TM; Sikich, L; Lieberman, JA; LaMantia, AS. Neural development; cell-cell signaling; and the „Two-hit" hypothesis of schizophrenia. *Schizophrenia Bull.*, 2001, 27, 457-476.

McClure, RK; Carew, K; Greeter, S; Maushauer, E; Steen, G; Weinberger, DR. Absence of regional brain volume change in schizophrenia associated with short-term atypical antipsychotic treatment. *Schizophrenia Res.,* 2008, 98, 29–39.

McCormick, L; Decker, L; Nopoulos, P; Ho, BC; Andreasen, N. Effects of atypical and typical neuroleptics on anterior cingulate volume in schizophrenia. *Schizophr. Res.,* 2005, 80, 73-84.

McDonald, C; Zanelli, J; Rabe-Heketh, S; Ellison-Wright, I; Kalidindi, S; Murray, RM; Kennedy, N. Meta-analysis of magnetic resonance imaging brain morphometry studies in bipolar disorder. Biol Psychiatry, 2004, 56, 411-7.

McIntosh, AM; Job, DE; Moorhead, WJ; Harrison, LK; Whalley, HC; Johnstone, EC; Lawrie, SM. Genetic liability to schizophrenia or bipolar disorder and its relationship to brain structure. *Am. J. Med. Genet. B Neuropsychiatr. Genet.,* 2006, 141B, 76-83.

Meda, SA; Giuliani, NR; Calhoun, VD; Jagannathan, K; Schretlen, DJ; Pulver, A; Cascella, N; Keshavan, M; Kates, W; Buchanan, R; Sharma, T; Pearlson, GD. A large scale (N=400) investigation of gray matter differences in schizophrenia using optimized voxel-based morphometry. *Schizophr Res*., 2008, 101, 95-105.

Meisenzahl, EM; Koutsouleris, N; Gaser, C; Bottlender, R; Schmitt, GJE; McGuire, P; Decker, P; Burgermeister, B; Born, C; Reiser, M; Möller, HJ. Structural brain alterations in subjects at high-risk of psychosis: A voxel-based morphometric study. *Schizophr. Res.,* 2008, doi:10.1016/j.schres.2008.02.023.

Melchitzky, DS; Sasack, SR; Pucak, ML; Lewis, DA. Synaptic targets of pyramidal neuron axon collaterals providing horizontal connections in monkey prefrontal cortex. Soc. *Neurosci. Abstr*., 1995, 21: 409.

Melchitzky, DS; Sesack, SR; Lewis, DA. Parvalbumin-immunoreactive axon terminals in macaque monkey and human prefrontal cortex: laminar; regional; and target specificity of type I and type II synapses. *J. Comp. Neurol*., 1999, 408, 11-22.

Melchitzky, DS; González-Burgos, G; Barrionuevo, G; Lewis, DA. Synaptic targets of the intrinsic axon collaterals of supragranular pyramidal neurons in monkey prefrontal cortex. *J. Comp. Neurol.,* 2001, 430, 209-21.

Melchitzky, DS; Lewis, DA. Pyramidal neuron local axon terminals in monkey prefrontal cortex: differential targeting of subclasses of GABA neurons. *Cereb. Cortex*; 2003, 13, 452-60.

Mintz, AR; Dobson, KS; Romney, DM. Insight in schizophrenia: a meta-analysis. *Schizophr Res.;* 2003, 61, 75–88.

Mirnics, K; Middleton, FA; Marquez, A; Lewis, DA; Levitt, P. Molecular characterization of schizophrenia viewed by microarray analysis of gene expression in prefrontal cortex. *Neuron*., 2000, 28, 53-67.

Mitelman, SA; Shihabuddin, L; Brickman, AM; Hazlett, EA; Buchsbaum, MS. MRI assessment of gray and white matter distribution in Brodmann's areas of the cortex in patients with schizophrenia with good and poor outcomes. *Am. J. Psychiatry*, 2003, 160, 2154-68.

Morris, HM; Hashimoto, T; Lewis, DA. Alterations in somatostatin mRNA expression in the dorsolateral prefrontal cortex of subjects with schizophrenia or schizoaffective disorder. *Cereb Cortex*, 2008 Jan 17. [Epub ahead of print]

Moser, M-B; Trommald, M; Andersen, P. An increase in dendritic spine density on hippocampal CA1 pyramidal cells following spatial learning in adult rats suggests the formation of new synapses. *Proc. Natl. Acad. Sci. USA*, 1994, 91, 12673-12675.

Murray, RM; Lewis, SW. Is schizophrenia a neurodevelopmental disorder? *BMJ*, 1987, 295, 681-682.

Murray, RM. Neurodevelopmental schizophrenia: the rediscovery of dementia praecox. *Br. J. Psychiatry*, 1994, 25, 6-12.

Murray, RM; Sham, P; Van Os, J; Zanelli, J; Cannon, M; McDonald, C. A developmental model for similarities and dissimilarities between schizophrenia and bipolar disorder. *Schizophr. Res.*, 2004, 71, 405-16.

Narr, KL; Bilder, RM; Toga, AW; Woods, RP; Rex, DE; Szeszko, PR; Robinson, D; Sevy, S; Gunduz-Bruce, H; Wang, YP; DeLuca, H; Thompson, PM. Mapping cortical thickness and gray matter concentration in first episode schizophrenia. *Cerebral. Cortex*, 2005, 15, 708-719.

Nasrallah, HA; Pixley, S. The atypical antipsychotic paliperidone induces neurogenesis in the rat brain: a controlled study. *Neuropsychopharmacology,* 2006, 31, S126-S127.

Newell, KA; Deng, C; Huang, XF. Increased cannabinoid receptor density in the posterior cingulate cortex in schizophrenia. *Exp. Brain Res*, 2006, 172, 556–560.

Nuechterlein, KH; Barch, DM; Gold, JM; Goldberg, TE; Green, MF; Heaton, RK. Identification of separable cognitive factors in schizophrenia. *Schizophr. Res.*, 2004, 72, 29-39.

Ohnishi, T; Hashimoto, R; Mori, T; Nemoto, K; Moriguchi, Y; Lida, H; Noguchi, H; Nakabayashi, T; Hori, H; Ohmor, M; Tsukue, R; Anami, K; Hirabayashi, N; Harada, S; Arima, K; Satoh, O; Kunugi, H. The association between the Val158Met polymorphism of the catechol-O-methyl transferase gene and morphological abnormalities of the brain in chronic schizophrenia. *Brain,* 2006, 129, 399-410.

Neckelmann, G; Specht, K; Lund, A; Ersland, L; Smievoll, AI; Neckelmann, D; Hugdahl, K. MR morphometry analysis of grey matter volume reduction in schizophrenia: association with hallucinations. Int J Neurosci, 2006, 116, 9-23.

Olsson, H; Halldin, C; Farde, L. Differentiation of extrastriatal dopamine D2 receptor density and affinity in the human brain using PET. *Neuroimage*, 2004, 22, 794-803.

Pakkenberg, H; Fog, R; Nilakantan, B. The long-term effect of perphenazine enanthate on the rat brain. Some metabolic and anatomical observations. *Psychopharmacologia*, 1973, 29, 329-36.

Pakkenberg, B. Post-mortem study of chronic schizophrenic brains. *Br. J. Psychiatry*, 1987, 151, 744-52.

Pakkenberg P. Pronounced reduction of total neuron number in mediodorsal thalamic nucleus and nucleus accumbens in schizophrenics. *Arch. Gen. Psychiatry*, 1990, 47, 1023-1028.

Pakkenberg, B. Total nerve cell number in neocortex in chronic schizophrenics and controls estimated using optical dissectors. *Biol. Psychiatry,* 1993, 34, 768-72.

Pantelis, C; Velakoulis, D; McGorry, PD; Wood, SJ; Suckling, J; Phillips, LJ; Yung, AR; Bullmore, ET; Brewer, W; Soulsby, B; Desmond, P; McGuire, PK. Neuroanatomical abnormalities before and after onset of psychosis: a corss-sectional and longitudinal MRI comparison. *Lancet,* 2003, 361, 281-288.

Parikh, V; Ekams, DR; Khan, MM; et al. NGF in never-medicated first-episode psychotic and medicated chronic schizophrenic patients: possible implications for treatment outcome. *Schizophr Res.* 2003, 60, 117-123.

Parikh, V; Khan, MN; Mahadik, SP. Olanzapine counteracts the reduction of BDNF and TrkB receptors in rat hippocampus produced by haloperidol. *Neurosci. Lett.*, 2004, 356, 135-139.

Perlman, WR; Weickert, CS; Akil, M; Kleinman, JE. Postmortem investigations of the pathophysiology of schizophrenia: the role of susceptibility genes. *J. Psychiatry Neurosci.,* 2004, 29(4), 287-93.

Pierri, JN; Volk, CLE; Auh, S; Sampson, A; Lewis, DA. Decreased somal size of deep layer 3 pyramidal neurons in the prefrontal cortex in subjects with schizophrenia. *Arch. Gen. Psychiatry*, 2001, 58, 466-473.

Pillai, A; Terry, A; Mahadik, SP. Differential effects of long-term treatment with typical and atypical antipsychotics on NGF and BDNF levels in rat striatum and hippocampus. *Schizophr. Res*., 2006, 82, 95-106.

Popken, GJ; Bunney, WE Jr, Potkin, SG; Jones, EG. Subnucleus-specific loss of neurons in medial thalamus of schizophrenics. *Proc. Natl. Acad. Sci. USA*, 2000, 97, 9276-80.

Powers, RE. The neuropathology of schizophrenia. *Journal of Neuropathology and experimental neurology,* 1999, 58(7), 679-690.

Prikryl, R; Kasparek, T; Skotakova, S; Ustohal, L; Kucerova, H; Ceskova E. Treatment of negative symptoms of schizophrenia using repetitive transcranial magnetic stimulation in a double-blind; randomized controlled study. *Schizophr Res.,* 2007, 95, 151-7.

Quing, H; Xu, H; Wei, Z; Gibson, K; Li, XM. The ability of atypical antipsychotic drugs vs. haloperidol to protect PC12 cells against MPP-induced apoptosis. *Eur. J. Neurosci*., 2003, 17, 1563-1570.

Radewicz, K; Garey, LJ; Gentleman, SM; Reynolds, R. Increase in HLA-DR immunoreactive microglia in frontal and temporal cortex of chronic schizophrenics. *J. Neuropathol. Exp. Neurol.,* 2000, 59, 137-50.

Radley, JJ; Rocher, AB; Miller, M; Janssen, WG; Liston, C; Hof, PR; McEwen, BS; Morrison, JH. Repeated stress induces dendritic spine loss in the rat medial prefrontal cortex. *Cereb Cortex*, 2006, 16, 313-20.

Rajkowska, G; Selemon, LD; Rakic, PS. Neuronal and glial somal size in prefrontal cortex: a postmortem morphometric study of schizophrenia and Huntington disease. *Arch. Gen. Psychiatry*, 1998, 55, 215-24.

Reig, S; Moreno, C; Moreno, D; Burdalo, M; Janssen, J; Parellada, M; Zabala, A; Desco, M; Arango, C. Progression of brain volume changes in adolescent-onset psychosis. *Schizophr Bull.,* 2008 Jan 24. [Epub ahead of print]

Roberts, GW. Schizophrenia: a neuropathological perspective. *Br. J. Psychiatry*, 1991, 158, 8-17.

Rusch, N; van Elst, LT; Ludaescher, P; Wilke, M; Huppertz, JH; Thiel, T; Schmahl, C; Bohus, M; Lieb, K; Heßlinger, B; Hennig, J; Eberta, D. A voxel-based morphometric MRI study in female patients with borderline personality disorder. *NeuroImage,* 2003, 20, 385–392.

Rusch, N; Spoletini, I; Wilke, M; Bria, P; Di Paola, M; Di Iulio, F; Martinotti, G; Caltagirone, C; Spalletta, G. Prefrontal-thalamic-cerebellar gray matter networks and executive functioning in schizophrenia. *Schizophr. Res*., 2007, 93, 79-89.

Salgado-Pineda, P; Baeza, I; Perez-Gomez, M; Vendrell, P; Junque, C; Bargallo, N; Bernardo, M. Sustained attention impairment correlates to gray matter decreases in first episode neuroleptic-naive schizophrenic patients. *Neuroimage*, 2003, 19, 365-375.

Salisbury, DF; Kuroki, N; Kasai, K; Shenton, ME; McCarley, RW. Progressive and interrelated functional and structural evidence of post-onset brain reduction in schizophrenia. *Arch. Gen.Psychiatry*, 2007, 64, 521-9.

Sams-Dodd, F; Lipska, BK; Weinberger, DR. Neonatal lesions of the rats ventral hippocampus result in hyperlocomotion and deficits of social behavior in adulthood. *Psychopharmacology* (Berl.), 1997, 132, 303-310.

Sastry, PS; Rao, KS. Apoptosis and the nervous system. *J. Neurochem*., 2000, 74, 1-20.

Saunders, RC; Kolachana, BS; Bachevalier, J; Weinberger, DR. Neonatal lesions of the medial temporal lobe disrupt prefrontal cortical regulation of striatal dopamine. *Nature,* 1998, 393, 169-71.

Saze, T; Hirao, K; Namiki, C; Fukuyama, H; Hayashi, T; Murai, T. Insular volume reduction in schizophrenia. *Eur. Arch. Psychiatry Clin. Neurosci*., 2007, 257, 473-9.

Schmitt, A; Weber, S; Jatzko, A; et al. Hippocampal volume and cell proliferation after acute and chronic clozapine or haloperidol treatment. *J. Neural. Transm*, 2004, 111, 91-100.

Selemon, LD; Rajakowska, G; Goldman-Rakic, PS. Abnormally high neuronal density in the schizophrenic cortex. A morphometric analysis of prefrontal area 9 and occipital area 17. *Arch. Gen. Psychiatry,* 1995, 52, 805-18.

Selemon, LD; Rajkowska, G; Goldman-Rakic, PS. Elevated neuronal density in prefrontal area 46 in brains from schizophrenic patients: application of a three dimensional; stereologic counting method. *J. Comp. Neurol.,* 1998, 392, 402-12.

Selemon, LD; Goldman-Rakic, PS. The reduced neuropil hypothesis: a circuit based model of schizophrenia. *Biol. Psychiatry*, 1999a, 45, 17-25.

Selemon, LD; Lidow, MS; Goldman-Rakic, PS. Increased volume and glial density in primate prefrontal cortex associated with chronic antipsychotic drug exposure. *Biol. Psychiatry*, 1999b, 46, 161-172.

Selemon, LD; Lidow MS; Goldman-Rakic, PS. Increased volume and glial density in primate prefrontal cortex associated with chronic antipsychotic drug exposure. *Biol. Psychiatry,* 1999b, 46, 161-172.

Selemon, LD; Kleinman, JE; Herman, MM; Goldman-Rakic, PS. Smaller frontal gray matter volume in postmortem schizophrenic brains. *Am. J. Psychiatry*, 2002, 159, 1983-1991.

Selemon, LD; Mrzljak, J; Kleinman, JE; Herman, MM; Goldman-Rakic, PS. Regional specificity in the neuropathologic substrates of schizophrenia: a morphometric analysis of Broca's area 44 and area 9. *Arch. Gen. Psychiatry*, 2003, 60, 69-77.

Selemon, LD; Begovic, A; Goldman-Rakic, PS; Castner, SA. Amphetamine sensitization alters dendritic morphology in prefrontal cortical pyramidal neurons in the non-human primate. *Neuropsychopharmacology*, 2007, 32, 919-31.

Sesack, SR; Bressler, CN; Lewis, DA: Ultrastructural associations between dopamine terminals and local circuit neurons in the monkey prefrontal cortex: A study of calretinin-immunoreactive cells. *Neurosci. Lett*, 1995a, 200, 9-12.

Sesack, SR; Snyder, CL; Lewis, DA: Axon terminals immunolabeled for dopamine or tyrosine hydroxylase synapse on GABA-immunoreactive dendrites in rat and monkey cortex. *J. Comp. Neurol.*; 1995b, 363, 264-280.

Shapleske, J; Rossell, SL; Chitnis, XA; Suckling, J; Simmons, A; Bullmore, ET; Woodruff, PW; David, AS. A computational morphometric MRI study of schizophrenia: effects of hallucinations. *Cereb Cortex*, 2002, 12, 1331-41.

Sim, ME; Lyoo, IK; Streeter, CC; Covell, J; Sarid-Segal, O; Ciraulo, DA; Kim, MJ; Kaufman, MJ; Yurgelun-Todd, DA; Renshaw, PF. Cerebellar gray matter volume correlates with duration of cocaine use in cocaine-dependent subjects. *Neuropsychopharmacology*, 2007, 32, 2229–2237.

Smiley, JF; Williams, SM; Szigeti, K; Goldman-Rakic, PS. Light and electron microscopic characterization of dopamine-immunoreactive axons in human cerebral cortex. *J. Comp. Neurol.*, 1992, 321, 325-335.

Smith, TE; Hull, JW; Israel, LM; Willson, DF. Insight; symptoms; and neurocognition in schizophrenia and schizoaffective disorder. *Schizophr. Bull.*, 2000, 26,193–200.

Spencer, KM; Nestor, PG; Niznikiewicz, MA; Salisbury, DF; Shenton, ME; McCarley, RW. Abnormal neural synchrony in schizophrenia. *J. Neurosci.*, 2003, 23, 7407-11.

Stark, AK; Uylings, HB; Sanz-Arigita, E; Pakkengerg, B. Glial cell loss in the anterior cingulate cortex; a subregion of the prefrontal cortex; in subjects with schizophrenia. *Am. J. Psychiatry*, 2004, 161, 882-887.

Sweet, RA; Pierri, JN; Auh, S; Sampson, AR; Lewis ,DA. Reduced pyramidal cell somal volume in auditory association cortex of subjects with schizophrenia. *Neuropsychopharmacology*, 2003, 28, 599-609.

Sweet, RA; Henteleff, RA; Zhang, W; Sampson, AR; Lewis, DA. Reduced dendritic spine density in auditory cortex of subjects with schizophrenia. *Neuropsychopharmacology,* 2008 May 7. [Epub ahead of print]

Szabadics, J; Lorincz, A; Tamás, G. Beta and gamma frequency synchronization by dendritic gabaergic synapses and gap junctions in a network of cortical interneurons. *J. Neurosci*, 2001, 21, 5824-31.

Szeszko, PR; Strous, RD; Goldman, RS; Ashtari, M; Knuth, KH; Lieberman, JA; Bilder, RM. Neuropsychological correlates of hippocampal volumes in patients experiencing a first episode of schizophrenia. *Am. J. Psychiatry*, 2002, 159, 217-26.

Tamás, G; Buhl, EH; Lörincz, A; Somogyi, P. Proximally targeted GABAergic synapses and gap junctions synchronize cortical interneurons. *Nat. Neurosci.*, 2000, 3, 366-71.

Thompson, PM; Vidal, C; Giedd, JN; Gochman, P; Blumenthal, J; Nicolson, R; Toga, AW; Rapoport, JL. Mapping adolescent brain change reveals dynamic wave of accelerated gray matter loss in very early-onset schizophrenia. *Proc. Natl. Acad. Sci. USA,* 2001, 98, 11650-5.

Thune, JJ; Uylings, HB; Pakkenberg, B. No deficit in total number of neurons in the prefrontal cortex in schizophrenics. *J. Psychiatry Res.*, 2001, 35, 15-21.

Ukai, W; Ozawa, H; Tateno, M; et al. Neurotoxic potentiation of haloperidol in comparison with risperidon: implications of AKT-mediated signal changes by haloperidol. *J. Neural. Transm*, 2004, 111, 667-681.

Velakoulis, D; Wood, SJ; Smith, DJ; Soulsby, B; Brewer, W; Leeton, L; Desmond, P; Suckling, J; Bullmore, ET; McGuire, PK; Pantelis, C. Increased duration of illness is associated with reduced volume in right medial temporal/anterior cingulate grey matter in patients with chronic schizophrenia. *Schizophr. Res*., 2002, 57, 43-9.

Valente, AA; Miguel, EC; Castro, CC; Amaro, E; Duran, FLS; Buchpiguel, CA; Chitnis, X; McGuire, PK; Busatto, GF. Regional gray matter abnormalities in obsessive-compulsive disorder: a voxel-based morphometry study. *Biol. Psychiatry*, 2005, 58, 479–487.

Valverde, F. Apical dendritic spines of the visual cortex and light deprivation in the mouse. *Exp. Brain Res.*, 1967, 3, 337-352.

van Haren, NE; Hulshoff Pol, HE; Schnack, HG; Cahn, W; Mandl, RC; Collins, DL; Evans, AC; Kahn, RS. Focal gray matter changes in schizophrenia across the course of the illness: a 5-year follow-up study. *Neuropsychopharmacology*, 2007, 32, 2057-66.

Venkatasubramanian, G; Jayakumar, PN; Gangadhar, BN; Keshavan, MS. Automated MRI parcellation study of regional volume and thickness of prefrontal cortex (PFC) in antipsychotic-naïve schizophrenia. *Acta Psychiatr. Scand,* 2008, 117, 420-31.

Vincent, SL; McSparren, J; Wang, RY; Benes, FM. Evidence for ultrastructural changes in cortical axodendritic synapses following long-term treatment with haloperidol or clozapine. *Neuropsychopharmacology,* 1991, 5, 147-155.

Vincent, SL; Khan, Y; Benes, FM. Cellular distribution of dopamine D1 and D2 receptors in rat medial prefrontal cortex. *J. Neurosci.,* 1993, 13, 2552-2564.

Vincent, SL; Adamec, E; Sorensen, I; Benes,FM. The effects of chronic haloperidol administration on GABA-immunoreactive axon terminals in rat medial prefrontal cortex. *Synapse,* 1994, 17, 26-35.

Volk, DW; Austin, MC; Pierri, JN; Sampson, AR; Lewis, DA. Decreased glutamic acid decarboxylase67 messenger RNA expression in a subset of prefrontal cortical gamma-aminobutyric acid neurons in subjects with schizophrenia. *Arch. Gen. Psychiatry*, 2000, 57, 237-45.

Volk, D; Austin, M; Pierri, J; Sampson, A; Lewis, D. GABA transporter-1 mRNA in the prefrontal cortex in schizophrenia: decreased expression in a subset of neurons. *Am. J. Psychiatry*, 2001, 158, 256-65.

Volk, DW; Pierri, JN; Fritschy, JM; Auh, S; Sampson, AR; Lewis, DA. Reciprocal alterations in pre- and postsynaptic inhibitory markers at chandelier cell inputs to pyramidal neurons in schizophrenia. *Cereb Cortex,* 2002, 12, 1063-70.

Volk, DW; Lewis, DA. Effects of a mediodorsal thalamus lesion on prefrontal inhibitory circuitry: implications for schizophrenia. *Biol. Psychiatry*; 2003; 53: 385-9.

Wakade, CG; Mahadik, S; Waller, JL; Chiu, FC. Atypical neuroleptics stimulate neurogenesis in adult rat brain. *J. Neurosci. Res*., 2002, 69, 72-79.

Wang, HD; Dunnavant, FD; Jarman, R; et al. Effects of antipsychotic drugs on neurogenesis in the forebrain of adult rat. *Neuropsychopharmacology*, 2004, 29, 1230-1238.

Wei, Z; Mousseau, DD; Richardson, JS; Dyck, LE; Li, XM. Atypical antipsychotics attenuate neurotoxicity of beta-amyloid 925-35) by modulating Bax and Bcl-X(l/s) expression and localization. *J. Neurosci. Res*., 2003, 74, 942-947.

Wei, Z; Moussem, DD; Dai, Y; et al. Haloperidol induces apoptosis via the delta-2 receptor system and BCI-XS. *Psychogenomics J*., 2006, 6, 279-288.

Weinberger, DR. Implications of normal brain development for the pathogenesis of schizophrenia. *Arch. Gen. Psychiatry*, 1987, 44, 660-669.

Weinberger, DR; Berman, KF; Suddath, R; Torrey, EF. Evidence of dysfunction of a prefrontal-limbic network in schizophrenia: a magnetic resonance imaging and regional cerebral blood flow study of discordant monozygotic twins. *Am. J. Psychiatry*, 1992, 149, 890-7.

Weinberger, DR. Schizophrenia. From neuropathology to neurodevelopment. *Lancet,* 1995, 346, 552-557.

Weinberger, DR; McClure, RK. Neurotoxicity; neuroplasticity; and magnetic resonance imaging morphometry: what is happening in the schizophrenic brain? *Arch. Gen. Psychiatry*, 2002, 59, 553-558.

Whitford, TJ; Farrow, TF; Gomes, L; Brennan, J; Harris, AW; Williams, LM. Grey matter deficits and symptom profile in firsts episode schizophrenia. *Psychiatry Res.,* 2005, 139, 229-238.

Whitford, TJ; Grieve, SM; Farrow, TF; Gomes, L; Brennan, J; Harris, AW; Gordon, E; Williams, LM. Progressive grey matter atrophy over the first 2-3 years of illness in first-episode schizophrenia: a tensor-based morphometry study. *Neuroimage*, 2006, 32, 511-519.

Williams, GV; Goldman-Rakic, PS. Modulation of memory fields by dopamine D1 receptors in prefrontal cortex. *Nature,* 1995, 376, 572-575.

Wilke, M; Kaufmann, C; Grabner, A; Pütz, B; Wetter, TC; Auer, DP. Gray matter-changes and correlates of disease severity in schizophrenia: a statistical parametric mapping study. *Neuroimage*, 2001, 13, 814-24.

Woo, TU; Pucak, ML; Kye, CH; Matus, CV; Lewis, DA. Peripubertal refinement of the intrinsic and associational circuitry in monkey prefrontal cortex. *Neuroscience*, 1997, 80,1149-58.

Woo, TU; Whitehead, RE; Melchitzky, DS; Lewis, DA. A subclass of prefrontal gamma-aminobutyric acid axon terminals are selectively altered in schizophrenia. *Proc. Natl. Acad. Sci USA*, 1998, 95, 5341-6.

Wood, SJ; Pantelis, C; Velakoulis, D; Yücel, M; Fornito, A; McGorry, PD. Progressive changes in the development toward schizophrenia: studies in subjects at increased symptomatic risk. *Schizophr Bull*, 2008, 34, 322-9.

Woods, TB. Is schizophrenia a progressive neurodevelopmental disorder? Towards a unitary pathogenetic mechanism. *Am. J. Psychiatry,* 1998, 155, 1661-1670.

Wooley, CS; Gould, E; Frankfurt, M; McEwen, BS. Naturally occuring fluctuation in dendritic spine density on adult hippocampal pyramidal neurons. *J. Neurosci.*, 1990, 10, 4035-4039.

Wright, IC; Rabe-Hesketh, S; Woodruff, PWR; David, AS; Murray, RM; Bullmore, ET. Meta-analysis of regional brain volumes in schizophrenia. *Am. J. Psychiatry*, 2000, 157, 16-25.

Yamada, M; Hirao, K; Namiki, C; Hanakawa, T; Fukuyama, H; Hayashi, T; Murai, T. Social cognition and frontal lobe pathology in schizophrenia: a voxel-based morphometric study. *Neuroimage*, 2007, 35, 292-8.

Yamasue, H; Kasai, K; Iwanami, A; Ohtani, T; Yamada, H; Abe, O; Kuroki, N; Fukuda, R; Tochigi, M; Furukawa, S; Sadamatsu, M; Sasaki, T; Aoki, S; Ohtomo, K; Asukai, N; Kato, N. Voxel-based analysis of MRI reveals anterior cingulate gray-matter volume reduction in posttraumatic stress disorder due to terrorism. *PNAS*, 2003, 100, 9039–9043.

Yoo, HK; Kim, MJ; Kim, SJ; Sung, YH; Sim, ME; Lee, YS; Song, SY; Kee, BS; Lyoo, IK. Putaminal gray matter volume decrease in panic disorder: an optimized voxel-based morphometry study. *European Journal of Neuroscience*, 2005, 22, 2089–2094;

Yoo, SY; Roh, MS; Choi, JS; Kang, DH; Ha, TH; Lee, JM; Kim, IY; Kim, SI; Kwon, JS. Voxel-based morphometry study of gray matter abnormalities in obsessive-compulsive disorder. *J. Korean Med. Sci.,* 2008, 23, 24-30.

Yücel, M; Solowij, N; Respondek, C; Whittle, S; Fornito, A; Pantelis, C; Lubman, DI. Regional Brain Abnormalities Associated With Long-term Heavy Cannabis Use. *Arch. Gen. Psychiatry*, 2008, 65, 694-701.

In: Prefrontal Cortex: Roles, Interventions and Traumas
Editors: Lorenzo LoGrasso and Giovanni Morretti
ISBN 978-1-60692-415-0

Chapter 2

Prefrontal Cholinergic Receptors: Their Role in the Pathology of Schizophrenia

M. Udawela, E. Scarr and B. Dean
Rebecca L Cooper Research Laboratories,
Mental Health Research Institute of Victoria,
Parkville, VIC, Australia

Abstract

There is a growing body of evidence to suggest that alterations in the cholinergic systems of the central nervous system are important in the pathology of schizophrenia. This data has arisen from studies into preclinical and clinical pharmacology, patient treatment, post-mortem neurochemistry and neuroimaging of patients with the disorder. The neuropharmacology of antipsychotics used to treat the disorder first led scientists to investigate changes in both the neurotransmitters and their receptors that are targeted by these therapeutic agents. These investigations have revealed that some atypical antipsychotics increase acetylcholine release in the prefrontal cortex, possibly contributing to improvements seen in some of the cognitive dysfunction for these drugs. Whilst there are data that show that some current atypical antipsychotic drugs have some impact on negative symptoms and cognitive deficits, none of these drugs are truly effective in treating these symptoms. Thus, in schizophrenia, various components within the cholinergic system are being investigated as potential targets for drugs that might effectively reverse these symptoms that are currently treatment-resistant. In this regard, post-mortem studies have revealed that patients with schizophrenia have low levels of cholinergic muscarinic receptors (CHRMs) in the CNS, and it is now well established that CHRM1 is decreased in the dorsolateral prefrontal cortex from subjects with the disorder; this receptor deficit is believed to play an important role in the cognitive dysfunctions associated with the disease. Recent information from basic research, in particular from studies using *CHRM*$^{-/-}$ mice, has enabled us to develop hypotheses as to what the functional consequences of deficits in CHRMs might be. Several lines of evidence also suggest a pathophysiological function for nicotinic acetylcholine receptors in schizophrenia. Nicotine administration has been shown to improve cognition in patients with schizophrenia. In the prefrontal cortex this receptor is thought to affect cognition through its activation-dependent effects on dopamine D_1 receptor mediated neurotransmission. Thus, both muscarinic and nicotinic receptors are viable drug targets with respect to cognitive deficits in schizophrenia. Using previous findings, in combination with our own data, we are now beginning to understand the specific changes in the various neurotransmitter receptors in the brains of schizophrenic patients, the functional effects of these changes and the roles the receptors may play in the pathology of the disorder.

Introduction

Schizophrenia is a debilitating mental illness, affecting approximately 1% of the population [1]. Importantly, CHRM antagonists have been extensively used to control the extrapyramidal side effects associated with the first generation of antipsychotic drugs [2] but it is now becoming clear that the cholinergic receptors may be a target for drugs to alleviate the symptoms of schizophrenia. The symptoms of schizophrenia can be broadly divided into positive symptoms, such as hallucinations and delusions, negative symptoms, such as social withdrawal and lack of motivation, and cognitive deficits, which can include impairments in attention/information processing, problem-solving, speed of processing, working memory and verbal and visual learning and memory [3, 4]. Whilst the positive symptoms have proven malleable to treatment with antipsychotic drugs, the negative symptoms and cognitive deficits are still essentially resistant to available treatments [5, 6]. This in part could be due to schizophrenia being a syndrome, rather than a distinct disease with a single pathology, with the different diseases within the syndrome showing differential responsiveness to available drugs. Thus, a major challenge is to be able to dissect the syndrome of schizophrenia into its components, to understand the pathologies of these biologically distinct entities and to design effective treatments for each disorder. Perhaps the most pressing need is for treatments for the cognitive deficits associated with schizophrenia as these are now recognised as the most debilitating symptoms associated with the disorder [7-9].

Cognitive Impairment

Despite the relationship between cognitive deficits and schizophrenia being identified almost a century ago [10], overall treatment of these symptoms remains inadequate [11]. Whilst some atypical antipsychotics offer slight cognitive benefit in patients with schizophrenia, even the patients who benefit from antipsychotic drug treatment continue to exhibit pronounced cognitive impairments [12-16]. There is evidence that dysfunction of the pre-frontal cortex (PFC) is responsible for cognitive impairments in schizophrenia [17, 18]. As stated earlier, cognitive deficits are a better predictor of the functional outcome in patients with schizophrenia compared to other symptoms of the disease [19-21], with these deficits now believed to be the most debilitating symptom for patients with schizophrenia to assimilate back into society. Thus there is a great need for new generation therapeutics, directed towards improving cognition.

Neuroimaging Studies, Cognition and Schizophrenia

Functional neuroimaging studies were first performed on patients with schizophrenia in 1974, using the ^{133}Xenon clearance method [22], and showed that, while whole brain cerebral blood flow was not different compared to healthy volunteers, there was a reduced gradient of frontal to posterior blood flow in patients with schizophrenia, termed 'hypofrontality'. This was replicated in other studies using both ^{133}Xenon [23, 24] and positron emission tomography (PET) [25, 26]. However, hypofrontality was not observed in all investigations [27-30], which may have been due to the lack of behavioural control over the subjects' mental activity. Subsequent studies overcame this by performing cognitive activation tasks during imaging, the most common being the Wisconsin Card Sorting Test, which measures concept formation, cognitive flexibility, feedback processing and working memory [23, 31-33]. These studies revealed a lack of the normal increase in blood flow in the dorsolateral pre-frontal cortex (DLPFC) during cognitive challenge in patients with schizophrenia compared to control subjects. This occurred in patients both on and off medication and did not appear to be due to global cortical dysfunction [34]. These findings are indicative of a potential role for the DLPFC in the cognitive deficits of schizophrenia.

To further characterise the changes in cerebral blood flow seen in schizophrenia to sub regions within the frontal cortex, and to link these to the distinct components of cognitive impairment, investigators later utilised various tasks that could allow differentiation of cognitive components, together with functional magnetic resonance imaging (fMRI). These tasks included working memory tasks such as N-back and Sternberg paradigm, as many of the cognitive deficits observed in schizophrenia have been attributed to working memory abnormalities [18, 34-36], as well as response inhibition tasks such as the Stroop and AX-type continuous performance task. In agreement with the ^{133}Xenon studies, the majority of the fMRI studies demonstrated hypoactivity of the DLPFC in subjects with schizophrenia during working memory tasks compared to matched controls [37-39]. Once more, the results from all the studies were not in agreement; some revealed no difference between control and schizophrenia groups [40], whilst others showed hyperactivity in this region in schizophrenia [41, 42]. More recent studies indicated that the degree of DLPFC activation is linked to performance during various executive and working memory tasks, with good performance associated with relatively greater DLPFC activity and marked behavioural deficits associated with relatively reduced DLPFC signal [39, 41, 43, 44], which could account for inconsistencies seen in other studies.

A recent quantitative meta-analysis by Glahn *et al.* [45] on 12 neuroimaging studies that used the N-back working memory paradigm, where subjects are required to monitor a series of quickly changing stimuli and indicate when the current stimulus is the same as the one presented *n* trials previously [46], confirmed hypoactivity of the DLPFC (Brodmann's Area, BA 9), rostral PFC (BA 11) and right ventrolateral/insular cortex (BA 13), but also revealed abnormally increased activation in the right dorsomedial PFC (BA 9), anterior cingulate (BA 32) and left frontal pole (BA 10) regions in patients with schizophrenia [45]. It was proposed that in these patients adjacent brain regions are being recruited in an effort to compensate for the impaired DLPFC activity during working memory tasks [45, 47].

The notion that changes in functionality of the DLPFC and other areas of the cortex are important in schizophrenia is supported by structural neuroimaging studies. Thus, abnormalities in the rostral medial PFC/orbito-fontal cortex have been observed in some studies [48]. These include a reduction in grey matter [49-51] and increased mean diffusivity [52], as well as reduced neuropil fraction and reduced grey-level index in the rostral PFC (BA 10) [53]. Several cognitive abilities associated with BA 10 are impaired in schizophrenia such as impairments in mentalising, episodic memory, prospective memory, source memory and multitasking, and these are suggested to be associated with particular symptoms [48]. Studies using fMRI have also shown reduced activity in the anterior cingulate gyrus in schizophrenia compared to healthy subjects during a wide range of tasks [54-60]. Although not all imaging studies have reported this finding, reduced activation in the anterior cingulate gyrus appears to be consistent during tasks which reliably activate this region in healthy subjects, such as Stroop; which measures reaction time to determine interference in attention, Go-No-Go; which measures a participants capacity for sustained attention and response control and Verbal Fluency, and during incorrect responding [45, 61].

The attenuated frontal lobe activation observed in patients with schizophrenia can be normalised with antipsychotic treatment. For example, it was shown using PET that haloperidol, a first generation antipsychotic, increased regional cerebral blood flow (rCBF) in part of the right DLPFC (BA 8/9) while reducing rCBF in several other cortical regions: in the ventrolateral frontal cortex (BA 47) on the left, the dorsolateral frontal cortex (BA 44 and 45) on the right, and the occipital cortex (BA 17/18), bilaterally. The second generation antipsychotic, clozapine, increased rCBF in several neocortical regions: the dorsolateral frontal cortex, bilaterally in BA 46 and on the left in BA 6 and 9. Clozapine decreased rCBF in ventrolateral frontal cortex (BA 47), bilaterally, and in parts of the superior frontal cortex (BA 10) and the sensory motor cortex (BA 4) [62]. Substitution of risperidone for typical antipsychotic drugs increased functional activation in the right PFC during working memory task performance [63]. However minimal performance improvement was observed in these cases, which could be due to the small sample sizes, low level of cognitive impairment at study entry or the simplicity of the task [62-64].

The Cholinergic System in Schizophrenia

The dopamine hypothesis of schizophrenia has been held for the last three decades [65, 66] and is based on the observation that stimulation of the dopaminergic system with drugs such as amphetamine often leads to transient psychotic symptoms, while blocking the dopamine D_2 receptor with antagonists leads to reduced positive symptoms in subjects with schizophrenia [66-69]. Dopamine receptor dysfunction has also been linked to cognitive dysfunction in patients with schizophrenia, with a decrease in D_1 receptor-like binding, as measured with PET, in the PFC of patients with schizophrenia, which correlated with cognitive dysfunction [70]. Significantly, chronic blockade of D_2 receptors leads to a decrease in D_1 receptors in the PFC region, along with impairments in working memory, in non-human primates [71]. This raised the possibility that effective treatment for psychoses may contribute to the impaired cognitive functioning seen in subjects with schizophrenia.

Despite a large body of pharmacological evidence supporting the dopamine hypothesis, it cannot account for the whole range of symptoms seen in schizophrenia. It is therefore significant that some of the earliest forms of treatment for schizophrenia involved modulation of the cholinergic system using agents such as atropine and hyoscine to treat positive symptoms [2, 10, 72]. However, with the advent of antipsychotic drugs, interest in these therapeutic agents waned and these treatments were never widely used except in the case of CHRM antagonists, which were used to control the side effects produced by antipsychotic drug treatment [2, 73]. Interest in targeting the CHRMs in the treatment of schizophrenia has seen a resurgence since it became clear that one of the actions of clozapine, the archetypal second generation atypical antipsychotic drug [74], is to antagonise that family of receptors [75-80]. The pharmacology of clozapine was of keen interest because it i) does not cause extrapyramidal side effects or tardive dyskinesia [81, 82], ii) was effective in otherwise treatment-refractory patients [74], iii) can cause some alleviation of negative symptoms [83, 84] and iv) has cognitive enhancing effects [85, 86]. More recently it has been shown that the major metabolite of clozapine, *N*-desmethylclozapine (NDMC), is a potent partial agonist at the muscarinic cholinergic M1 receptor (CHRM1) [87]. Moreover, it has been shown in subjects with schizophrenia that improvement in cognitive deficits after treatment with clozapine correlates with a higher plasma NDMC / clozapine ratio [87]. This suggests that the cognitive improvement associated with clozapine could have been due to NDMC stimulating CHRM1. Other atypical antipsychotic drugs, which have been shown to impact on cognitive deficits compared to typical drugs, significantly increased ACh release in the medial PFC, an effect not observed with typical antipsychotics [88]. These data suggest that all atypical antipsychotic drugs can indirectly target the cholinergic system even though they do not bind to any CHRMs. This could be why some of these drugs may prove partially effective in the treatment of cognitive impairments associated with the disease. However, data from NDMC, and previous studies showing that muscarinic antagonists can worsen neurocognitive impairment [89, 90], would suggest that direct stimulation of CHRMs will be the best approach to treating the cognitive deficits associated with schizophrenia.

Underpinning the notion that targeting cholinergic receptors will be a useful therapeutic approach to treating schizophrenia is a body of evidence indicating that the cholinergic system may be disrupted in schizophrenia [91]. This evidence mainly comes from post-mortem studies, which have revealed decreased nicotinic and muscarinic acetylcholine receptor availability or expression in the cortex and hippocampus of individuals with schizophrenia [92-101]. These are supported by a study showing decreased activity of choline acetyltransferase, which catalyses the synthesis of ACh, measured post-mortem, in correlation with a patient history of poorer cognitive functioning [102]. These findings suggest that the processing of acetylcholine may also be abnormal in subjects with schizophrenia. This concept fits with the first of more recent attempts to treat schizophrenia, which has been to use inhibitors of acetylcholine esterase, an enzyme that rapidly breaks down acetylcholine in the synapse, to indirectly increase levels of acetylcholine. This approach is supported by experiments in rodents where it has been shown that combining atypical antipsychotic drug treatment with cholinesterase inhibitors increased the concentration of ACh in the medial PFC by 2- to 3- fold [88]. This outcome could explain why treatment with galantamine, an acetylcholinesterase inhibitor, produces cognitive enhancement in subjects with schizophrenia [103, 104]. Unfortunately outcomes from subsequent studies using various acetylcholine esterase inhibitors have been inconsistent. Whilst targeting cholinesterase gives a non-focussed approach to improving cognitive deficits in schizophrenia, efforts are also being made to directly target specific muscarinic receptors to improve cognitive impairments [11, 105].

Muscarinic Receptors in Schizophrenia

CHRMs are G-protein coupled receptors found on cholinergic and non-cholinergic cells, where they function as both auto- and hetero- receptors [106-108]. There have been five subtypes identified (CHRM1-5) which are encoded by distinct genes, show different pharmacological properties and are expressed in regionally varying concentrations throughout the CNS [109-113]. As these receptors display a broad range of functions, it has been difficult to determine which CHRM subtypes are involved in the pathology of schizophrenia and / or may be useful therapeutic targets.

Initial studies of CHRM expression in post-mortem CNS looked at [^{3}H]-quinuclidinyl benzilate ([^{3}H]QNB) binding in the frontal cortex from subjects with schizophrenia and showed no significant differences [114]. However [^{3}H]QNB binds to all 5 CHRM subtypes [115], thus there was no change in global CHRM expression in this cortical region. A more comprehensive study measuring [^{3}H]QNB binding in the orbito-frontal and medial frontal cortices from 6 schizophrenia subjects receiving antipsychotic drugs up until death (on-drug), 6 schizophrenia subjects who had not received antipsychotic drugs for at least 40 days prior to death (off-drug) and 10 control subjects showed an increase in receptor number in the orbito-frontal cortex in all schizophrenia subjects compared to controls [116]. The study also revealed that the on-drug group showed a significant increase in receptor number and a significant decrease in affinity in both areas, while the off-drug group showed no significant differences in any binding parameters compared to controls [116]. These results were confirmed in a follow up study, performed on the same subjects, showing increased [^{3}H]QNB binding in the PFC from on drug schizophrenia subjects compared to off drug and control subjects [117]. Therefore it was suggested that differences in CHRM density were a result of long-term antipsychotic use.

Later studies gave a more specific picture of changes in CHRM density in the CNS of people with schizophrenia by utilising pirenzepine, which binds to CHRM1 and to a lesser extent to CHRM4 [118]. Using [^{3}H]pirenzepine, we and others showed decreased binding in the caudate-putamen [119, 120], hippocampus [92] and PFC in schizophrenia [93]. Importantly, we showed that levels of CHRM1 protein and mRNA, but not CHRM4, are decreased in BA 9, indicating the CHRM1 was responsible for the decreased [^{3}H]pirenzepine observed in this region [94]. This picture is made a little complex by our findings that, whilst there was no decrease in CHRM1 or CHRM4 protein or [^{3}H]pirenzepine binding in BA 40, mRNA was decreased for both receptor subtypes, indicating that the pattern of receptor expression observed in BA 9 does not extend to all regions of the PFC. Furthermore, there were no changes in levels of CHRM2 or 3 protein with diagnosis in either BA 9 or BA 40 in the same cohort [121], further indicating that CHRM1 is the receptor predominantly changed in BA 9 in schizophrenia. A change in CHRM1 mRNA was also shown by Mancama *et al.* [98] in BA 6 from subjects with the disorder. Taken together these studies indicate that CHRM1 has important implications in schizophrenia pathology, and thus specifically targeting CHRM1 may prove beneficial in treating cognition with the additional benefit of limited side effects. This hypothesis gains support from data showing that a polymorphism in the *CHRM1* gene in subjects with schizophrenia is associated with higher levels of cognitive impairment [122]. Furthermore, studies in *CHRM1* knockout mice have shown that deletion of this receptor leads to disturbances in learning, memory [123] and circadian rhythms [124], functions that are affected in subjects with schizophrenia [125, 126]. Perhaps the most convincing data supporting this hypothesis comes from the study showing that xanomeline (3-[3-hexyloxy-1,2,5-thiadiazo-4-yl]-1,2,5,6-tetrahydro-1-methylpyridine), a CHRM1/4 selective agonist, has antipsychotic effects and improves cognitive deficits in subjects with schizophrenia [127, 128]. On the other hand, recent data have shown that CHRM4 is more likely the cause of decreased [^{3}H]pirenzepine binding in the hippocampus in schizophrenia, as CHRM4 but not CHRM1 mRNA was decreased in this region [100], where it may be involved in schizophrenia pathology linked to the hippocampus, such as psychosis. Together, these data suggest that decreases in CHRMs in schizophrenia are region and subtype specific, and that different CHRMs may play different roles in the pathology of schizophrenia.

One concern regarding these studies is that changes in CHRM expression may be a result of treatment with antipsychotics, as many of the patients used in these studies had a record of receiving antipsychotic drugs. However, we found no significant correlation between experimental variables and final recorded antipsychotic drug dose [94, 129]. Moreover, the effect of antipsychotics on receptor expression has been examined in rats treated with haloperidol and chlorpromazine; these studies indicated these drugs do not significantly influence either CHRM expression or density [93, 119, 130, 131]. Thus, alterations in CHRMs are likely an entity of the disease rather than an effect of drug use. To date there has been one study performed on medication free subjects that strongly supports the hypothesis that changes in the CHRMs are involved in the pathology of schizophrenia. This study used [^{123}I]iodoquinuclidynyl benzilate, which binds with high affinity to all five CHRM subtypes, and showed decreased binding *in vivo* in cortical and sub-cortical regions in medication free schizophrenia subjects compared to matched controls. The results also showed a significant inverse correlation between level of binding and severity of positive symptoms, suggesting the levels of CHRMs may be associated with symptom levels [99].

Given the numerous roles CHRMs play in a variety of functions, it is imperative to find agents directed at the specific subtypes relevant to the symptoms of interest. Both natural and exogenous ligands of the CHRMs bind to a site that is highly conserved among the receptor subtypes and thus show very low selectivity to the subtypes [132]. Some antagonists, on the other hand, display good selectivity due to their bulky structure, allowing them to interact with amino acids adjacent to the classic (orthosteric) binding site that are less well conserved.

However, the smaller orthosteric agonists display poor selectivity as they only interact with a few key amino acids in this site [133]. One approach to increasing ligand selectivity is to use allosteric modulators; an allosteric site can be found on all 5 subtypes of CHRMs [115]. A huge selection of structurally divergent modulators has been described for the different receptor subtypes, including gallamine and alcuronium [134-143]. These can increase or decrease the affinity of agonists and antagonists, including ACh, in a selective manner. Recently, a novel structural class of agonists was identified that are potent and selective for CHRM1, the first to be described being xanomeline [144-147]. These exhibit 'functional selectivity' in that they bind with comparable affinity to all 5 muscarinic subtypes but mainly activate CHRM1 [145]. They are believed to bind to an additional, less conserved 'ectopic' site that is important for receptor activation. However, the precise molecular mechanisms of these agents are still not fully understood [133]. The actions of this class of agonists are promising for treating cognitive deficits, offering a new approach to selectively targeting CHRMs.

In order to determine whether decreases in cortical CHRMs might be related to CHRM1 genotype, or possibly define a subgroup of schizophrenia patients, we performed [H^3]pirenzepine binding in the DLPFC from 80 subjects with schizophrenia and 74 age sex matched control subjects. Interestingly, Kernel density estimation on the binding data revealed two distinct populations among schizophrenia subjects, but not controls, where one group represented 26% of the schizophrenic subjects showing a 74% reduction in mean cortical [H^3]pirenzepine binding compared to control subjects, and were termed the 'muscarinic receptor-deficit schizophrenia' [148]. This segregation showed no correlation with CHRM1 sequence, gender, age, suicide, duration of illness or drug treatment [148]. This is interesting in terms of identifying one of the specific disease entities that make up schizophrenia, and perhaps identifying patients that may respond to some forms of treatments better than others. It would be interesting to see if such patients show altered cognitive behaviours compared to other schizophrenic patients, as indeed findings from previous studies have suggested a link between the level of CHRM expression and severity of symptoms [99].

There is a great deal of evidence demonstrating that the dopaminergic and muscarinic systems interact with each other [149]. For example, *in vivo*, xanomeline increased striatal levels of dopamine metabolites [144]. Studies in rats showed that the cognitive deficits produced by the muscarinic antagonist scopolamine could be reversed by the mixed dopamine D_1-D_2 blocker haloperidol [150]. This was later shown to be due to D_1 and not D_2 blockade [151]. Thus, it is possible that disruption of the interaction between the muscarinic and dopaminergic systems may cause symptoms of schizophrenia. It has been suggested that the balance of dopamine/ACh is of central importance to the pathophysiology of schizophrenia and that increased muscarinic ACh activity may be an attempt to maintain this balance [91]. This model also proposes that this compensatory increase in the muscarinic cholinergic system exerts a damping effect on the positive symptoms while adversely increasing the negative symptoms [91].

Nicotinic Receptors in Schizophrenia

Acetylcholine also acts through another family of receptors, the nicotinic acetylcholine receptors (nAChRs) [152]. The nAChRs are non-selective ligand-gated ion channels, opened by the binding of ACh, but can also be opened by nicotine. nAChRs are present in the CNS and periphery and are made up of pentamers of α, β, γ, δ and ε subunits, each sub-unit being a single gene product [153, 154]. Importantly, only the α_2-α_9 and β_2-β_4 sub-units are expressed in the CNS [154]. The two most predominant CNS nAChRs are $\alpha_4\beta_2$, which is the high affinity receptor, and the receptor made up entirely of α_7 subunits, which is the low affinity receptor [155-158], both of which have been shown to be reduced in schizophrenia [96, 97, 101]. Interestingly, there is an increased rate of smoking in subjects with schizophrenia compared to the general population, up to 90%, and compared to any other psychiatric illness [159]. This has been suggested to reflect self-medication [160-162]; signifying that nAChRs could constitute a drug target for the disorder.

Nicotine affects many aspects of behavior including locomotion, conception, anxiety, learning and memory [163]. Nicotine administration can enhance cognition in patients with schizophrenia, particularly attention [164-172]. Effects of nicotine in schizophrenia, however, do not extend to all areas of cognition. Thus, targeting this system alone would not be an effective form of treatment but it is one that may prove useful in combination with other therapeutics. Another concern with nicotinic agents is the rapid desensitisation observed with repeated administrations of nicotine, which renders nicotine ineffective over time [165, 167, 168, 172-174]. This has prompted research into exploring less toxic partial agonists and allosteric modulators of nAChRs as potential agents for cognitive enhancement, which would be less likely to cause rapid receptor desensitisation. The desensitisation of nicotinic receptors may also explain the ineffectiveness seen in attempts to treat schizophrenia symptoms with anticholinergic agents.

Neurobiological and genetic studies identified the α_7 nicotinic receptor as a potential contributor to the pathology of schizophrenia. Functional polymorphisms in the promoter region of α_7 have shown genetic linkage to the disease [175, 176], while the α_7 receptor was shown to be reduced in the PFC from patients with schizophrenia [97]. Furthermore, rodent studies have shown that α_7 antagonists induce sensory gating deficits (inability to respond appropriately to multiple sensory stimuli) [177] similar to those seen in schizophrenia [178-180]. Sensory gating deficits have been suggested to strongly impact cognitive performance [181-184], and have also been shown to be normalized by cigarette smoking [185]. Hence, drugs directed to the α_7 receptor may alleviate some of the cognitive deficits in schizophrenia. In further support of this, clinical response to clozapine was shown to be higher in schizophrenic subjects who smoke compared to non smokers, and furthermore, treatment with clozapine caused a decrease in smoking behaviours in patients [186, 187], suggesting that nicotinic receptors may also mediate the effects of clozapine. Animal studies have indicated that increased P50 auditory response inhibition by clozapine is mediated by stimulation of α_7 nicotinic receptors [188, 189]. This receptor is, therefore, a highly studied target for the development of drugs to treat cognitive deficits.

A series of α_7 agonists have been developed, one of which is the partial agonist 3-2,4-dimethoxybenzylidene anabaseine (DMZB-A) [190-192]. This compound improved auditory gating deficits in rodents and improved memory in several animal models [193, 194]. In humans, DMZB-A enhanced cognitive functions, particularly attention, in healthy volunteers [195], and in a small proof of concept trial, showed improvement in neurocognition as well as P50 inhibition in subjects with schizophrenia [196]. More recently, the selective α_7 agonist 2-methyl-5-(6-phenyl-pyridazin-3-yl)-octahydro-pyrrolo[3,4-c]pyrrole (A-582941) was shown in rats to activate brain regions involved in working memory and attention; the medial PFC and the ventral/lateral orbitofrontal cortex [197]. The effect was greater in juvenile rats than adult rats, which may be relevant in the treatment of juvenile onset schizophrenia [197]. Although results with α_7 agonists have been promising, the concern of desensitisation of the receptor with long term use remains, thus further development of partial agonists or allosteric modulators is warranted [11, 198]. Galantamine, a cholinesterase inhibitor, which is also an allosteric potentiator of α_7 nicotinic receptors, did not cause α_7 receptor desensitisation, and was effective in enhancing cognition in patients who smoked [199]. This suggests that combining allosteric modulators of the nicotinic receptor with anticholinesterase inhibitors may overcome issues with receptor desensitisation when targeting this receptor.

The $\alpha_4\beta_2$ nicotinic receptor is also likely to be involved in cognition [200], and is also reduced in the hippocampus, cortex and caudate of patients with schizophrenia [101]. These receptors are more sensitive to nicotine than the α_7 receptor, and are thought to account for 90% of the high affinity nicotine binding sites in the rat brain [155]. Agonists of $\alpha_4\beta_2$ have been shown to stimulate the release of dopamine and acetylcholine in the hippocampus and frontal cortex in rats [201]. Furthermore, agonists of this receptor can improve memory in rats and monkeys [201-203]. Thus the $\alpha_4\beta_2$ receptor may also be a potential therapeutic target for treating cognitive symptoms of schizophrenia by several mechanisms. Other nicotinic receptors may also be involved in cognition, however this is difficult to determine given the lack of selective agents to these other receptors.

There is evidence that the role of both the α_7 and $\alpha_4\beta_2$ receptors in cognitive impairments in schizophrenia is mediated through the dopamine receptor system. Unlike haloperidol's reversal effect on CHRM antagonist induced cognitive deficit, this drug potentiated the deficits induced by the nicotinic antagonist mecamylamine [204]. This action was due to dopamine D_2 blockade, since the mecamylamine induced deficit was potentiated by the selective D_2 blocker raclopride, but not the D_1 blocker SCH 23390 [205], and reversed by D_2 but not D_1 agonism [206]. Combined treatment of gallantamine and the neuroleptic drug risperidone showed synergistic improvement of cognitive impairment and increased extracellular concentration of dopamine in the medial PFC in mice. These effects were blocked by a dopamine D_1 receptor antagonist and a nAChR antagonist but not a CHRM antagonist [207], indicating these drugs act independently of the CHRM system, and that when taken in combination may enhance cognition in schizophrenia patients.

It has been suggested that interactions of nicotine with the NMDA glutamate system may play an important role in cognitive functions. This comes from studies showing pre-treatment with the NMDA antagonist MK801 reduced high-affinity nicotinic receptor upregulation induced by repeated nicotine injections in rats, preventing behavioural sensitization [208], and nicotine could reverse MK-801 induced attention deficits [209, 210], while *in vitro* studies have shown that nicotine reduces MK-801 binding to NMDA receptors [211, 212]. These effects were shown to be regionally selective throughout the brain [213].

There is also some evidence of synergistic interactions between the nicotinic and CHRM systems, both at the level of receptor regulation and the functional level [149, 214-216]. In rat brain, administration of scopolamine increased both muscarinic and nicotinic receptors in the frontoperietal cortex [214]. Furthermore, combined scopolamine and mecamylamine treatment acted in a greater than additive fashion in disrupting cognitive function in rats [149]. This action was attenuated by the D_2 agonist LY 171555 but not the D_1 antagonist SCH 23390 [149]. In humans, combined blockade of both receptor types with scopolamine and mecamylamine produced a large impairment in early visual information processing, while selective blockade of the CHRM alone produced only a small impairment and blockade of the nAChR alone showed no impairment [217]. A similar effect was also observed on other cognitive functions, including working memory, visual attention and psychomotor speed [218]. Thus treatments that can reverse the effects of combined blockade of the muscarinic and nicotinic receptors may be useful in treating cognitive deficits.

Conclusion

Schizophrenia is a complex disease with a broad spectrum of symptoms. It is now believed that several neurotransmitter systems in addition to dopamine are involved, and the disease may be a result of interactions between dopamine and these other neurotransmitter systems. This concept suggests that efficacious treatment of schizophrenia may require a combination of therapies, directed at the various neurotransmitter systems involved, to address the wide range of symptoms associated with the disorder. Studies on the PFC of schizophrenia subjects indicate that the cholinergic system may play an important role in the pathology of schizophrenia, particularly in relation to cognitive functioning, identifying possible new targets for improved therapeutics. Our identification of MRDS suggests that different patients may respond differently to various drugs depending on their biochemical profile, and that identifying which patients would benefit from different types of drugs may be the key to effectively treating this debilitating disorder.

References

[1] Black, Andraeson. *Textbook of Psychiatry*. 2nd ed. Washington, DC: The American Psychiatric Press; 1994.

[2] Tandon, R. Cholinergic aspects of schizophrenia. *Br. J. Psychiatry Suppl.* 1999(37):7-11.

[3] Goldberg, T. E., Gold, J. M., Greenberg, R., Griffin, S., Schulz, S. C., Pickar, D., et al. Contrasts between patients with affective disorders and patients with schizophrenia on a neuropsychological test battery. *Am. J. Psychiatry* 1993;150(9):1355-62.

[4] Nuechterlein, K. H., Barch, D. M., Gold, J. M., Goldberg, T. E., Green, M. F., Heaton, R. K. Identification of separable cognitive factors in schizophrenia. *Schizophr. Res.* 2004;72(1):29-39.

[5] Tandon, R., Belmaker, R. H., Gattaz, W. F., Lopez-Ibor, J. J., Jr., Okasha, A., Singh, B., et al. World Psychiatric Association Pharmacopsychiatry Section statement on comparative effectiveness of antipsychotics in the treatment of schizophrenia. *Schizophr Res.* 2008;100(1-3):20-38.

[6] Heinrichs, R. W. The primacy of cognition in schizophrenia. *Am. Psychol.* 2005;60(3):229-42.

[7] Peuskens, J., Demily, C., Thibaut, F. Treatment of cognitive dysfunction in schizophrenia. *Clin. Ther.* 2005;27 Suppl A:S25-37.

[8] Prouteau, A., Verdoux, H., Briand, C., Lesage, A., Lalonde, P., Nicole, L., et al. Cognitive predictors of psychosocial functioning outcome in schizophrenia: a follow-up study of subjects participating in a rehabilitation program. *Schizophr. Res.* 2005;77(2-3):343-53.

[9] Chen, E. Y., Hui, C. L., Dunn, E. L., Miao, M. Y., Yeung, W. S., Wong, C. K., et al. A prospective 3-year longitudinal study of cognitive predictors of relapse in first-episode schizophrenic patients. *Schizophr. Res.* 2005;77(1):99-104.

[10] Kraepelin, E. Dementia Praecox and Paraphrenia (1919). 1st ed. New York: Thoemmes Continuum; 1971.

[11] Gray, J. A., Roth, B. L. Molecular targets for treating cognitive dysfunction in schizophrenia. *Schizophr. Bull.* 2007;33(5):1100-19.

[12] Bilder, R. M., Goldman, R. S., Volavka, J., Czobor, P., Hoptman, M., Sheitman, B., et al. Neurocognitive effects of clozapine, olanzapine, risperidone, and haloperidol in patients with chronic schizophrenia or schizoaffective disorder. *Am. J. Psychiatry* 2002;159(6):1018-28.

[13] Harvey, P. D., Keefe, R. S. Studies of cognitive change in patients with schizophrenia following novel antipsychotic treatment. *Am. J. Psychiatry* 2001;158(2):176-84.

[14] Purdon, S. E., Jones, B. D., Stip, E., Labelle, A., Addington, D., David, S. R., et al. Neuropsychological change in early phase schizophrenia during 12 months of treatment with olanzapine, risperidone, or haloperidol. The Canadian Collaborative Group for research in schizophrenia. *Arch. Gen. Psychiatry* 2000;57(3):249-58.

[15] Keefe, R. S., Silva, S. G., Perkins, D. O., Lieberman, J. A. The effects of atypical antipsychotic drugs on neurocognitive impairment in schizophrenia: a review and meta-analysis. *Schizophr. Bull.* 1999;25(2):201-22.

[16] Woodward, N. D., Purdon, S. E., Meltzer, H. Y., Zald, D. H. A meta-analysis of neuropsychological change to clozapine, olanzapine, quetiapine, and risperidone in schizophrenia. *Int. J. Neuropsychopharmacol* 2005;8(3):457-72.

[17] Weinberger, D. R. A connectionist approach to the prefrontal cortex. *J. Neuropsychiatry Clin. Neurosci.* 1993;5(3):241-53.

[18] Goldman-Rakic, P. S. Working memory dysfunction in schizophrenia. *J. Neuropsychiatry Clin. Neurosci.* 1994;6(4):348-57.

[19] Meltzer, H. Y. Dimensions of outcome with clozapine. *Br. J. Psychiatry Suppl.* 1992(17):46-53.

[20] Green, M. F. What are the functional consequences of neurocognitive deficits in schizophrenia? *Am. J. Psychiatry* 1996;153(3):321-30.

[21] Green, M. F., Braff, D. L. Translating the basic and clinical cognitive neuroscience of schizophrenia to drug development and clinical trials of antipsychotic medications. *Biol Psychiatry* 2001;49(4):374-84.

[22] Ingvar, D. H., Franzen, G. Distribution of cerebral activity in chronic schizophrenia. *Lancet* 1974;2(7895):1484-6.

[23] Berman, K. F., Zec, R. F., Weinberger, D. R. Physiologic dysfunction of dorsolateral prefrontal cortex in schizophrenia. II. Role of neuroleptic treatment, attention, and mental effort. *Arch. Gen. Psychiatry* 1986;43(2):126-35.

[24] Mathew, R. J., Wilson, W. H., Tant, S. R., Robinson, L., Prakash, R. Abnormal resting regional cerebral blood flow patterns and their correlates in schizophrenia. *Arch. Gen. Psychiatry* 1988;45(6):542-9.

[25] Buchsbaum, M. S., Ingvar, D. H., Kessler, R., Waters, R. N., Cappelletti, J., van Kammen, D. P., et al. Cerebral glucography with positron tomography. Use in normal subjects and in patients with schizophrenia. *Arch. Gen. Psychiatry* 1982;39(3):251-9.

[26] Volkow, N. D., Wolf, A. P., Van Gelder, P., Brodie, J. D., Overall, J. E., Cancro, R., et al. Phenomenological correlates of metabolic activity in 18 patients with chronic schizophrenia. *Am. J. Psychiatry* 1987;144(2):151-8.

[27] Catafau, A. M., Parellada, E., Lomena, F. J., Bernardo, M., Pavia, J., Ros, D., et al. Prefrontal and temporal blood flow in schizophrenia: resting and activation technetium-99m-HMPAO SPECT patterns in young neuroleptic-naive patients with acute disease. *J. Nucl. Med.* 1994;35(6):935-41.

[28] Ebmeier, K. P., Lawrie, S. M., Blackwood, D. H., Johnstone, E. C., Goodwin, G. M. Hypofrontality revisited: a high resolution single photon emission computed tomography study in schizophrenia. *J. Neurol. Neurosurg. Psychiatry* 1995;58(4):452-6.

[29] Gur, R. E., Resnick, S. M., Gur, R. C., Alavi, A., Caroff, S., Kushner, M., et al. Regional brain function in schizophrenia. II. Repeated evaluation with positron emission tomography. *Arch. Gen. Psychiatry* 1987;44(2):126-9.

[30] Gur, R. E., Resnick, S. M., Alavi, A., Gur, R. C., Caroff, S., Dann, R., et al. Regional brain function in schizophrenia. I. A positron emission tomography study. *Arch Gen Psychiatry* 1987;44(2):119-25.

[31] Berman, K. F., Illowsky, B. P., Weinberger, D. R. Physiological dysfunction of dorsolateral prefrontal cortex in schizophrenia. IV. Further evidence for regional and behavioral specificity. *Arch. Gen. Psychiatry* 1988;45(7):616-22.

[32] Weinberger, D. R., Berman, K. F., Illowsky, B. P. Physiological dysfunction of dorsolateral prefrontal cortex in schizophrenia. III. A new cohort and evidence for a monoaminergic mechanism. *Arch. Gen. Psychiatry* 1988;45(7):609-15.

[33] Weinberger, D. R., Berman, K. F., Zec, R. F. Physiologic dysfunction of dorsolateral prefrontal cortex in schizophrenia. I. Regional cerebral blood flow evidence. *Arch. Gen. Psychiatry* 1986;43(2):114-24.

[34] Ragland, J. D., Yoon, J., Minzenberg, M. J., Carter, C. S. Neuroimaging of cognitive disability in schizophrenia: search for a pathophysiological mechanism. *Int. Rev. Psychiatry* 2007;19(4):417-27.

[35] Cohen, J. D., Braver, T. S., O'Reilly, R. C. A computational approach to prefrontal cortex, cognitive control and schizophrenia: recent developments and current challenges. *Philos Trans R Soc. Lond B Biol. Sci.* 1996;351(1346):1515-27.

[36] Silver, H., Feldman, P., Bilker, W., Gur, R. C. Working memory deficit as a core neuropsychological dysfunction in schizophrenia. *Am. J. Psychiatry* 2003;160(10):1809-16.

[37] Barch, D. M., Carter, C. S., Braver, T. S., Sabb, F. W., MacDonald, A., 3rd, Noll, D. C., et al. Selective deficits in prefrontal cortex function in medication-naive patients with schizophrenia. *Arch. Gen. Psychiatry* 2001;58(3):280-8.

[38] Callicott, J. H., Ramsey, N. F., Tallent, K., Bertolino, A., Knable, M. B., Coppola, R., et al. Functional magnetic resonance imaging brain mapping in psychiatry: methodological issues illustrated in a study of working memory in schizophrenia. *Neuropsychopharmacology* 1998;18(3):186-96.

[39] Perlstein, W. M., Carter, C. S., Noll, D. C., Cohen, J. D. Relation of prefrontal cortex dysfunction to working memory and symptoms in schizophrenia. *Am. J. Psychiatry* 2001;158(7):1105-13.

[40] Honey, G. D., Bullmore, E. T., Sharma, T. De-coupling of cognitive performance and cerebral functional response during working memory in schizophrenia. *Schizophr. Res.* 2002;53(1-2):45-56.

[41] Callicott, J. H., Bertolino, A., Mattay, V. S., Langheim, F. J., Duyn, J., Coppola, R., et al. Physiological dysfunction of the dorsolateral prefrontal cortex in schizophrenia revisited. *Cereb Cortex* 2000;10(11):1078-92.

[42] Manoach, D. S., Gollub, R. L., Benson, E. S., Searl, M. M., Goff, D. C., Halpern, E., et al. Schizophrenic subjects show aberrant fMRI activation of dorsolateral prefrontal cortex and basal ganglia during working memory performance. *Biol. Psychiatry* 2000;48(2):99-109.

[43] Ragland, J. D., Gur, R. C., Glahn, D. C., Censits, D. M., Smith, R. J., Lazarev, M. G., et al. Frontotemporal cerebral blood flow change during executive and declarative memory tasks in schizophrenia: a positron emission tomography study. *Neuropsychology* 1998;12(3):399-413.

[44] Ramsey, N. F., Koning, H. A., Welles, P., Cahn, W., van der Linden, J. A., Kahn, R. S. Excessive recruitment of neural systems subserving logical reasoning in schizophrenia. *Brain* 2002;125(Pt 8):1793-807.

[45] Glahn, D. C., Ragland, J. D., Abramoff, A., Barrett, J., Laird, A. R., Bearden, C. E., et al. Beyond hypofrontality: a quantitative meta-analysis of functional neuroimaging studies of working memory in schizophrenia. *Hum. Brain Mapp.* 2005;25(1):60-9.

[46] Gevins, A., Cutillo, B. Spatiotemporal dynamics of component processes in human working memory. *Electroencephalogr. Clin. Neurophysiol.* 1993;87(3):128-43.

[47] Tan, H. Y., Sust, S., Buckholtz, J. W., Mattay, V. S., Meyer-Lindenberg, A., Egan, M. F., et al. Dysfunctional prefrontal regional specialization and compensation in schizophrenia. *Am. J. Psychiatry* 2006;163(11):1969-77.

[48] Dumontheil, I., Burgess, P. W., Blakemore, S. J. Development of rostral prefrontal cortex and cognitive and behavioural disorders. *Dev. Med Child Neurol* 2008;50(3):168-81.

[49] Narr, K. L., Toga, A. W., Szeszko, P., Thompson, P. M., Woods, R. P., Robinson, D., et al. Cortical thinning in cingulate and occipital cortices in first episode schizophrenia. *Biol. Psychiatry* 2005;58(1):32-40.

[50] Yamada, M., Hirao, K., Namiki, C., Hanakawa, T., Fukuyama, H., Hayashi, T., et al. Social cognition and frontal lobe pathology in schizophrenia: a voxel-based morphometric study. *Neuroimage* 2007;35(1):292-8.

[51] Riffkin, J., Yucel, M., Maruff, P., Wood, S. J., Soulsby, B., Olver, J., et al. A manual and automated MRI study of anterior cingulate and orbito-frontal cortices, and caudate nucleus in obsessive-compulsive disorder: comparison with healthy controls and patients with schizophrenia. *Psychiatry Res.* 2005;138(2):99-113.

[52] Rose, S. E., Chalk, J. B., Janke, A. L., Strudwick, M. W., Windus, L. C., Hannah, D. E., et al. Evidence of altered prefrontal-thalamic circuitry in schizophrenia: an optimized diffusion MRI study. *Neuroimage* 2006;32(1):16-22.

[53] Black, J. E., Kodish, I. M., Grossman, A. W., Klintsova, A. Y., Orlovskaya, D., Vostrikov, V., et al. Pathology of layer V pyramidal neurons in the prefrontal cortex of patients with schizophrenia. *Am. J. Psychiatry* 2004;161(4):742-4.

[54] Boksman, K., Theberge, J., Williamson, P., Drost, D. J., Malla, A., Densmore, M., et al. A 4.0-T fMRI study of brain connectivity during word fluency in first-episode schizophrenia. *Schizophr. Res.* 2005;75(2-3):247-63.

[55] Laurens, K. R., Kiehl, K. A., Ngan, E. T., Liddle, P. F. Attention orienting dysfunction during salient novel stimulus processing in schizophrenia. *Schizophr. Res.* 2005;75(2-3):159-71.

[56] Holcomb, H. H., Lahti, A. C., Medoff, D. R., Weiler, M., Dannals, R. F., Tamminga, C. A. Brain activation patterns in schizophrenic and comparison volunteers during a matched-performance auditory recognition task. *Am. J. Psychiatry* 2000;157(10):1634-45.

[57] Rubia, K., Russell, T., Bullmore, E. T., Soni, W., Brammer, M. J., Simmons, A., et al. An fMRI study of reduced left prefrontal activation in schizophrenia during normal inhibitory function. *Schizophr Res.* 2001;52(1-2):47-55.

[58] Dehaene, S., Artiges, E., Naccache, L., Martelli, C., Viard, A., Schurhoff, F., et al. Conscious and subliminal conflicts in normal subjects and patients with schizophrenia: the role of the anterior cingulate. *Proc. Natl. Acad. Sci. USA* 2003;100(23):13722-7.

[59] Heckers, S., Weiss, A. P., Deckersbach, T., Goff, D. C., Morecraft, R. J., Bush, G. Anterior cingulate cortex activation during cognitive interference in schizophrenia. *Am. J. Psychiatry* 2004;161(4):707-15.

[60] Kerns, J. G., Cohen, J. D., MacDonald, A. W., 3rd, Johnson, M. K., Stenger, V. A., Aizenstein, H., et al. Decreased conflict- and error-related activity in the anterior cingulate cortex in subjects with schizophrenia. *Am. J. Psychiatry* 2005;162(10):1833-9.

[61] Raedler, T. J., Bymaster, F. P., Tandon, R., Copolov, D., Dean, B. Towards a muscarinic hypothesis of schizophrenia. *Mol Psychiatry* 2007;12(3):232-46.

[62] Lahti, A. C., Holcomb, H. H., Weiler, M. A., Medoff, D. R., Tamminga, C. A. Functional effects of antipsychotic drugs: comparing clozapine with haloperidol. *Biol. Psychiatry* 2003;53(7):601-8.

[63] Honey, G. D., Bullmore, E. T., Soni, W., Varatheesan, M., Williams, S. C., Sharma, T. Differences in frontal·cortical activation by a working memory task after substitution of risperidone for typical antipsychotic drugs in patients with schizophrenia. *Proc. Natl. Acad. Sci. USA* 1999;96(23):13432-7.
[64] Nahas, Z., George, M. S., Horner, M. D., Markowitz, J. S., Li, X., Lorberbaum, J. P., et al. Augmenting atypical antipsychotics with a cognitive enhancer (donepezil) improves regional brain activity in schizophrenia patients: a pilot double-blind placebo controlled BOLD fMRI study. *Neurocase* 2003;9(3):274-82.
[65] Meltzer, H. Y., Stahl, S. M. The dopamine hypothesis of schizophrenia: a review. *Schizophr. Bull.* 1976;2(1):19-76.
[66] Carlsson, A. Antipsychotic drugs and catecholamine synapses. *J. Psychiatr Res.* 1974;11:57-64.
[67] Seeman, P., Lee, T., Chau-Wong, M., Wong, K. Antipsychotic drug doses and neuroleptic/dopamine receptors. *Nature* 1976;261(5562):717-9.
[68] Kapur, S., Remington, G. Dopamine D(2) receptors and their role in atypical antipsychotic action: still necessary and may even be sufficient. *Biol. Psychiatry* 2001;50(11):873-83.
[69] Creese, I., Burt, D. R., Snyder, S. H. Dopamine receptor binding predicts clinical and pharmacological potencies of antischizophrenic drugs. *Science* 1976;192(4238):481-3.
[70] Okubo, Y., Suhara, T., Suzuki, K., Kobayashi, K., Inoue, O., Terasaki, O., et al. Decreased prefrontal dopamine D1 receptors in schizophrenia revealed by PET. *Nature* 1997;385(6617):634-6.
[71] Castner, S. A., Williams, G. V., Goldman-Rakic, P. S. Reversal of antipsychotic-induced working memory deficits by short-term dopamine D1 receptor stimulation. *Science* 2000;287(5460):2020-2.
[72] Pfeiffer, C. C., Jenney, E. H. The inhibition of the conditioned response and the counteraction of schizophrenia by muscarinic stimulation of the brain. *Ann. N Y Acad Sci.* 1957;66(3):753-64.
[73] Bilder, R. M. Neurocognitive impairment in schizophrenia and how it affects treatment options. *Can J Psychiatry* 1997;42(3):255-64.
[74] Kane, J., Honigfeld, G., Singer, J., Meltzer, H. Clozapine for the treatment-resistant schizophrenic. A double-blind comparison with chlorpromazine. *Arch. Gen. Psychiatry* 1988;45(9):789-96.
[75] Zorn, S. H., Jones, S. B., Ward, K. M., Liston, D. R. Clozapine is a potent and selective muscarinic M4 receptor agonist. *Eur. J. Pharmacol.* 1994;269(3):R1-2.
[76] Zeng, X. P., Le, F., Richelson, E. Muscarinic m4 receptor activation by some atypical antipsychotic drugs. *Eur. J. Pharmacol.* 1997;321(3):349-54.
[77] Bymaster, F. P., Shannon, H. E., Rasmussen, K., DeLapp, N. W., Ward, J. S., Calligaro, D. O., et al. Potential role of muscarinic receptors in schizophrenia. *Life Sci.* 1999;64(6-7):527-34.
[78] Michal, P., Lysikova, M., El-Fakahany, E. E., Tucek, S. Clozapine interaction with the M2 and M4 subtypes of muscarinic receptors. *Eur. J. Pharmacol.* 1999;376(1-2):119-25.

[79] Meltzer, H. Y., Chai, B. L., Thompson, P. A., Yamamoto, B. K. Effect of scopolamine on the efflux of dopamine and its metabolites after clozapine, haloperidol or thioridazine. *J. Pharmacol. Exp. Ther.* 1994;268(3):1452-61.

[80] Olianas, M. C., Maullu, C., Onali, P. Mixed agonist-antagonist properties of clozapine at different human cloned muscarinic receptor subtypes expressed in Chinese hamster ovary cells. *Neuropsychopharmacology* 1999;20(3):263-70.

[81] Gross, H., Hackl, H., Kaltenbaeck. Results of double-blind study of clozapine and thioridazine. In: VII CINP Congress; 1970; Prague; 1970.

[82] Casey, D. E. Clozapine: neuroleptic-induced EPS and tardive dyskinesia. *Psychopharmacology (Berl)* 1989;99 Suppl:S47-53.

[83] Brar, J. S., Chengappa, K. N., Parepally, H., Sandman, A. R., Kreinbrook, S. B., Sheth, S. A., et al. The effects of clozapine on negative symptoms in patients with schizophrenia with minimal positive symptoms. *Ann. Clin. Psychiatry* 1997;9(4):227-34.

[84] Llorca, P. M., Lancon, C., Farisse, J., Scotto, J. C. Clozapine and negative symptoms. An open study. *Prog. Neuropsychopharmacol Biol. Psychiatry* 2000;24(3):373-84.

[85] Hagger, C., Buckley, P., Kenny, J. T., Friedman, L., Ubogy, D., Meltzer, H. Y. Improvement in cognitive functions and psychiatric symptoms in treatment-refractory schizophrenic patients receiving clozapine. *Biol. Psychiatry* 1993;34(10):702-12.

[86] Goldberg, T. E., Weinberger, D. R. The effects of clozapine on neurocognition: an overview. *J. Clin. Psychiatry* 1994;55 Suppl B:88-90.

[87] Weiner, D. M., Meltzer, H. Y., Veinbergs, I., Donohue, E. M., Spalding, T. A., Smith, T. T., et al. The role of M1 muscarinic receptor agonism of N-desmethylclozapine in the unique clinical effects of clozapine. *Psychopharmacology (Berl)* 2004;177(1-2):207-16.

[88] Ichikawa, J., Dai, J., O'Laughlin, I. A., Fowler, W. L., Meltzer, H. Y. Atypical, but not typical, antipsychotic drugs increase cortical acetylcholine release without an effect in the nucleus accumbens or striatum. *Neuropsychopharmacology* 2002;26(3):325-39.

[89] Hagan, J. J., Jansen, J. H., Broekkamp, C. L. Blockade of spatial learning by the M1 muscarinic antagonist pirenzepine. *Psychopharmacology (Berl)* 1987;93(4):470-6.

[90] Bartus, R. T., Johnson, H. R. Short-term memory in the rhesus monkey: disruption from the anti-cholinergic scopolamine. *Pharmacol. Biochem. Behav.* 1976;5(1):39-46.

[91] Tandon, R., Greden, J. F. Cholinergic hyperactivity and negative schizophrenic symptoms. A model of cholinergic/dopaminergic interactions in schizophrenia. *Arch. Gen. Psychiatry* 1989;46(8):745-53.

[92] Crook, J. M., Tomaskovic-Crook, E., Copolov, D. L., Dean, B. Decreased muscarinic receptor binding in subjects with schizophrenia: a study of the human hippocampal formation. *Biol. Psychiatry* 2000;48(5):381-8.

[93] Crook, J. M., Tomaskovic-Crook, E., Copolov, D. L., Dean, B. Low muscarinic receptor binding in prefrontal cortex from subjects with schizophrenia: a study of Brodmann's areas 8, 9, 10, and 46 and the effects of neuroleptic drug treatment. *Am. J. Psychiatry* 2001;158(6):918-25.

[94] Dean, B., McLeod, M., Keriakous, D., McKenzie, J., Scarr, E. Decreased muscarinic1 receptors in the dorsolateral prefrontal cortex of subjects with schizophrenia. *Mol. Psychiatry* 2002;7(10):1083-91.

[95] Deng, C., Huang, X. F. Decreased density of muscarinic receptors in the superior temporal gyrusin schizophrenia. *J. Neurosci. Res.* 2005;81(6):883-90.

[96] Freedman, R., Hall, M., Adler, L. E., Leonard, S. Evidence in postmortem brain tissue for decreased numbers of hippocampal nicotinic receptors in schizophrenia. *Biol. Psychiatry* 1995;38(1):22-33.

[97] Guan, Z. Z., Zhang, X., Blennow, K., Nordberg, A. Decreased protein level of nicotinic receptor alpha7 subunit in the frontal cortex from schizophrenic brain. *Neuroreport* 1999;10(8):1779-82.

[98] Mancama, D., Arranz, M. J., Landau, S., Kerwin, R. Reduced expression of the muscarinic 1 receptor cortical subtype in schizophrenia. *Am. J. Med. Genet B Neuropsychiatr Genet.* 2003;119B(1):2-6.

[99] Raedler, T. J., Knable, M. B., Jones, D. W., Urbina, R. A., Gorey, J. G., Lee, K. S., et al. In vivo determination of muscarinic acetylcholine receptor availability in schizophrenia. *Am. J. Psychiatry* 2003;160(1):118-27.

[100] Scarr, E., Sundram, S., Keriakous, D., Dean, B. Altered hippocampal muscarinic M4, but not M1, receptor expression from subjects with schizophrenia. *Biol. Psychiatry* 2007;61(10):1161-70.

[101] Breese, C. R., Lee, M. J., Adams, C. E., Sullivan, B., Logel, J., Gillen, K. M., et al. Abnormal regulation of high affinity nicotinic receptors in subjects with schizophrenia. *Neuropsychopharmacology* 2000;23(4):351-64.

[102] Powchik, P., Davidson, M., Haroutunian, V., Gabriel, S. M., Purohit, D. P., Perl, D. P., et al. Postmortem studies in schizophrenia. *Schizophr Bull.* 1998;24(3):325-41.

[103] Lee, S. W., Lee, J. G., Lee, B. J., Kim, Y. H. A 12-week, double-blind, placebo-controlled trial of galantamine adjunctive treatment to conventional antipsychotics for the cognitive impairments in chronic schizophrenia. *Int. Clin. Psychopharmacol* 2007;22(2):63-8.

[104] Schubert, M. H., Young, K. A., Hicks, P. B. Galantamine improves cognition in schizophrenic patients stabilized on risperidone. *Biol. Psychiatry* 2006;60(6):530-3.

[105] Buchanan, R. W., Freedman, R., Javitt, D. C., Abi-Dargham, A., Lieberman, J. A. Recent advances in the development of novel pharmacological agents for the treatment of cognitive impairments in schizophrenia. *Schizophr Bull* 2007;33(5):1120-30.

[106] Raiteri, M., Leardi, R., Marchi, M. Heterogeneity of presynaptic muscarinic receptors regulating neurotransmitter release in the rat brain. *J. Pharmacol. Exp. Ther.* 1984;228(1):209-14.

[107] Wamsley, J. K., Zarbin, M. A., Kuhar, M. J. Distribution of muscarinic cholinergic high and low affinity agonist binding sites: a light microscopic autoradiographic study. *Brain Res. Bull.* 1984;12(3):233-43.

[108] Vizi, E. S., Kobayashi, O., Torocsik, A., Kinjo, M., Nagashima, H., Manabe, N., et al. Heterogeneity of presynaptic muscarinic receptors involved in modulation of transmitter release. *Neuroscience* 1989;31(1):259-67.

[109] Bonner, T. I., Buckley, N. J., Young, A. C., Brann, M. R. Identification of a family of muscarinic acetylcholine receptor genes. *Science* 1987;237(4814):527-32.

[110] Bonner, T. I., Young, A. C., Brann, M. R., Buckley, N. J. Cloning and expression of the human and rat m5 muscarinic acetylcholine receptor genes. *Neuron* 1988;1(5):403-10.

[111] Bonner, T. I. New subtypes of muscarinic acetylcholine receptors. *Trends Pharmacol. Sci.* 1989;Suppl:11-5.

[112] Bonner, T. I. The molecular basis of muscarinic receptor diversity. *Trends Neurosci* 1989;12(4):148-51.

[113] Peralta, E. G., Ashkenazi, A., Winslow, J. W., Smith, D. H., Ramachandran, J., Capon, D. J. Distinct primary structures, ligand-binding properties and tissue-specific expression of four human muscarinic acetylcholine receptors. *Embo. J.* 1987;6(13):3923-9.

[114] Bennett, J. P., Jr., Enna, S. J., Bylund, D. B., Gillin, J. C., Wyatt, R. J., Snyder, S. H. Neurotransmitter receptors in frontal cortex of schizophrenics. *Arch Gen Psychiatry* 1979;36(9):927-34.

[115] Ellis, J., Huyler, J., Brann, M. R. Allosteric regulation of cloned m1-m5 muscarinic receptor subtypes. *Biochem. Pharmacol.* 1991;42(10):1927-32.

[116] Watanabe, S., Nishikawa, T., Takashima, M., Toru, M. Increased muscarinic cholinergic receptors in prefrontal cortices of medicated schizophrenics. *Life Sci.* 1983;33(22):2187-96.

[117] Toru, M., Watanabe, S., Shibuya, H., Nishikawa, T., Noda, K., Mitsushio, H., et al. Neurotransmitters, receptors and neuropeptides in post-mortem brains of chronic schizophrenic patients. *Acta Psychiatr. Scand.* 1988;78(2):121-37.

[118] Levey, A. I., Kitt, C. A., Simonds, W. F., Price, D. L., Brann, M. R. Identification and localization of muscarinic acetylcholine receptor proteins in brain with subtype-specific antibodies. *J. Neurosci.* 1991;11(10):3218-26.

[119] Dean, B., Crook, J. M., Opeskin, K., Hill, C., Keks, N., Copolov, D. L. The density of muscarinic M1 receptors is decreased in the caudate-putamen of subjects with schizophrenia. *Mol. Psychiatry* 1996;1(1):54-8.

[120] Crook, J. M., Dean, B., Pavey, G., Copolov, D. The binding of [3H]AF-DX 384 is reduced in the caudate-putamen of subjects with schizophrenia. *Life Sci.* 1999;64(19):1761-71.

[121] Scarr, E., Keriakous, D., Crossland, N., Dean, B. No change in cortical muscarinic M2, M3 receptors or [35S]GTPgammaS binding in schizophrenia. *Life Sci.* 2006;78(11):1231-7.

[122] Liao, D. L., Hong, C. J., Chen, H. M., Chen, Y. E., Lee, S. M., Chang, C. Y., et al. Association of muscarinic m1 receptor genetic polymorphisms with psychiatric symptoms and cognitive function in schizophrenic patients. *Neuropsychobiology* 2003;48(2):72-6.

[123] Hamilton, S. E., Loose, M. D., Qi, M., Levey, A. I., Hille, B., McKnight, G. S., et al. Disruption of m1 receptor gene ablates muscarinic receptor-dependent current regulation and seizure activity in mice. *Proc. Natl. Acad. Sci. USA* 1997;94 (24):133116.

[124] Gillette, M. U., Buchanan, G. F., Artinian, L., Hamilton, S. E., Nathanson, N. M., Liu, C. Role of the M1 receptor in regulating circadian rhythms. *Life Sci.* 2001;68(22-23):2467-72.

[125] Heinrichs, R. W., Zakzanis, K. K. Neurocognitive deficit in schizophrenia: a quantitative review of the evidence. *Neuropsychology* 1998;12(3):426-45.

[126] Keshavan, M. S., Reynolds, C. F., 3rd, Miewald, M. J., Montrose, D. M., Sweeney, J. A., Vasko, R. C., Jr., et al. Delta sleep deficits in schizophrenia: evidence from automated analyses of sleep data. *Arch. Gen. Psychiatry* 1998;55(5):443-8.

[127] Mirza, N. R., Peters, D., Sparks, R. G. Xanomeline and the antipsychotic potential of muscarinic receptor subtype selective agonists. *CNS Drug Rev.* 2003;9(2):159-86.

[128] Shekhar, A., Potter, W. Z., Lienemann, J., Sundblad, K., Lightfoot, J., Herrera, J. Efficacy of zanomeline, a slelctive muscarinic agonist, in treating schizphrenia: a double-blind, placebo controlled study. In: 40th Annual Meeting ACNP; 2001 December 9-13, 2001; Hawaii; 2001.

[129] Dean, B. Role of muscarinic receptors in the pathology of schizophrenia. *Am J Med Genet B Neuropsychiatr Genet* 2004;126B(1):8-9.

[130] Zavitsanou, K., Nguyen, V. H., Han, M., Huang, X. F. Effects of typical and atypical antipsychotic drugs on rat brain muscarinic receptors. *Neurochem Res.* 2007;32(3):525-32.

[131] Han, M., Newell, K., Zavitsanou, K., Deng, C., Huang, X. F. Effects of antipsychotic medication on muscarinic M1 receptor mRNA expression in the rat brain. *J. Neurosci. Res* 2008;86(2):457-64.

[132] Hulme, E. C., Lu, Z. L., Saldanha, J. W., Bee, M. S. Structure and activation of muscarinic acetylcholine receptors. *Biochem. Soc. Trans* 2003;31(Pt 1):29-34.

[133] Jakubik, J., Michal, P., Machova, E., Dolezal, V. Importance and prospects for design of selective muscarinic agonists. *Physiol. Res.* 2008.

[134] Jager, D., Schmalenbach, C., Prilla, S., Schrobang, J., Kebig, A., Sennwitz, M., et al. Allosteric small molecules unveil a role of an extracellular E2/transmembrane helix 7 junction for G protein-coupled receptor activation. *J. Biol. Chem.* 2007;282(48):34968-76.

[135] Jakubik, J., Bacakova, L., el-Fakahany, E. E., Tucek, S. Subtype selectivity of the positive allosteric action of alcuronium at cloned M1-M5 muscarinic acetylcholine receptors. *J. Pharmacol. Exp. Ther.* 1995;274(3):1077-83.

[136] Jakubik, J., Bacakova, L., El-Fakahany, E. E., Tucek, S. Positive cooperativity of acetylcholine and other agonists with allosteric ligands on muscarinic acetylcholine receptors. *Mol. Pharmacol.* 1997;52(1):172-9.

[137] Lazareno, S., Birdsall, N. J. Detection, quantitation, and verification of allosteric interactions of agents with labeled and unlabeled ligands at G protein-coupled receptors: interactions of strychnine and acetylcholine at muscarinic receptors. *Mol. Pharmacol.* 1995;48(2):362-78.

[138] Lazareno, S., Dolezal, V., Popham, A., Birdsall, N. J. Thiochrome enhances acetylcholine affinity at muscarinic M4 receptors: receptor subtype selectivity via cooperativity rather than affinity. *Mol Pharmacol* 2004;65(1):257-66.

[139] Mohr, K., Trankle, C., Holzgrabe, U. Structure/activity relationships of M2 muscarinic allosteric modulators. *Receptors Channels* 2003;9(4):229-40.

[140] Proska, J., Tucek, S. Mechanisms of steric and cooperative actions of alcuronium on cardiac muscarinic acetylcholine receptors. *Mol. Pharmacol.* 1994;45(4):709-17.

[141] Tucek, S., Jakubik, J., Dolezal, V., el-Fakahany, E. E. Positive effects of allosteric modulators on the binding properties and the function of muscarinic acetylcholine receptors. *J. Physiol Paris* 1998;92(3-4):241-3.

[142] Tucek, S., Musilkova, J., Nedoma, J., Proska, J., Shelkovnikov, S., Vorlicek, J. Positive cooperativity in the binding of alcuronium and N-methylscopolamine to muscarinic acetylcholine receptors. *Mol. Pharmacol.* 1990;38(5):674-80.

[143] Dolezal, V., Tucek, S. The effects of brucine and alcuronium on the inhibition of [3H]acetylcholine release from rat striatum by muscarinic receptor agonists. *Br. J. Pharmacol.* 1998;124(6):1213-8.

[144] Bymaster, F. P., Wong, D. T., Mitch, C. H., Ward, J. S., Calligaro, D. O., Schoepp, D. D., et al. Neurochemical effects of the M1 muscarinic agonist xanomeline (LY246708/NNC11-0232). *J. Pharmacol. Exp. Ther.*1994;269(1):282-9.

[145] Shannon, H. E., Bymaster, F. P., Calligaro, D. O., Greenwood, B., Mitch, C. H., Sawyer, B. D., et al. Xanomeline: a novel muscarinic receptor agonist with functional selectivity for M1 receptors. *J. Pharmacol. Exp. Ther.* 1994;269(1):271-81.

[146] Spalding, T. A., Trotter, C., Skjaerbaek, N., Messier, T. L., Currier, E. A., Burstein, E. S., et al. Discovery of an ectopic activation site on the M(1) muscarinic receptor. *Mol. Pharmacol.* 2002;61(6):1297-302.

[147] Langmead, C. J., Fry, V. A., Forbes, I. T., Branch, C. L., Christopoulos, A., Wood, M. D., et al. Probing the molecular mechanism of interaction between 4-n-butyl-1-[4-(2-methylphenyl)-4-oxo-1-butyl]-piperidine (AC-42) and the muscarinic M(1) receptor: direct pharmacological evidence that AC-42 is an allosteric agonist. *Mol. Pharmacol.* 2006;69(1):236-46.

[148] Scarr, E., Cowie, T. F., Kanellakis, S., Sundram, S., Pantelis, C., Dean, B. Decreased cortical muscarinic receptors define a subgroup of subjects with schizophrenia. *Mol Psychiatry* 2008.

[149] Levin, E. D., Rose, J. E., McGurk, S. R., Butcher, L. L. Characterization of the cognitive effects of combined muscarinic and nicotinic blockade. *Behav. Neural. Biol.* 1990;53(1):103-12.

[150] McGurk, S. R., Levin, E. D., Butcher, L. L. Cholinergic-dopaminergic interactions in radial-arm maze performance. *Behav. Neural. Biol.* 1988;49(2):234-9.

[151] Levin, E. D. Scopolamine interactions with D1 and D2 antagonists on radial-arm maze performance in rats. *Behav. Neural. Biol.* 1988;50(2):240-5.

[152] Itier, V., Bertrand, D. Neuronal nicotinic receptors: from protein structure to function. *FEBS Lett* 2001;504(3):118-25.

[153] Paterson, D., Nordberg, A. Neuronal nicotinic receptors in the human brain. *Prog Neurobiol.* 2000;61(1):75-111.

[154] Le Novere, N., Changeux, J. P. Molecular evolution of the nicotinic acetylcholine receptor: an example of multigene family in excitable cells. *J. Mol. Evol.* 1995;40(2):155-72.

[155] Flores, C. M., Rogers, S. W., Pabreza, L. A., Wolfe, B. B., Kellar, K. J. A subtype of nicotinic cholinergic receptor in rat brain is composed of alpha 4 and beta 2 subunits and is up-regulated by chronic nicotine treatment. *Mol. Pharmacol.* 1992;41(1):31-7.

[156] Hill, J. A., Jr., Zoli, M., Bourgeois, J. P., Changeux, J. P. Immunocytochemical localization of a neuronal nicotinic receptor: the beta 2-subunit. *J. Neurosci.* 1993;13(4):1551-68.

[157] Zoli, M., Le Novere, N., Hill, J. A., Jr., Changeux, J. P. Developmental regulation of nicotinic ACh receptor subunit mRNAs in the rat central and peripheral nervous systems. *J. Neurosci.* 1995;15(3 Pt 1):1912-39.

[158] Wada, E., Wada, K., Boulter, J., Deneris, E., Heinemann, S., Patrick, J., et al. Distribution of alpha 2, alpha 3, alpha 4, and beta 2 neuronal nicotinic receptor subunit mRNAs in the central nervous system: a hybridization histochemical study in the rat. *J. Comp. Neurol.* 1989;284(2):314-35.

[159] Nisell, M., Nomikos, G. G., Svensson, T. H. Nicotine dependence, midbrain dopamine systems and psychiatric disorders. *Pharmacol. Toxicol.* 1995;76(3):157-62.

[160] Glassman, A. H. Cigarette smoking: implications for psychiatric illness. *Am. J. Psychiatry* 1993;150(4):546-53.

[161] Dalack, G. W., Healy, D. J., Meador-Woodruff, J. H. Nicotine dependence in schizophrenia: clinical phenomena and laboratory findings. *Am. J. Psychiatry* 1998;155(11):1490-501.

[162] Kumari, V., Postma, P. Nicotine use in schizophrenia: the self medication hypotheses. *Neurosci. Biobehav. Rev.* 2005;29(6):1021-34.

[163] Decker, M. W., Brioni, J. D., Bannon, A. W., Arneric, S. P. Diversity of neuronal nicotinic acetylcholine receptors: lessons from behavior and implications for CNS therapeutics. *Life Sci.* 1995;56(8):545-70.

[164] Adler, L. E., Olincy, A., Waldo, M., Harris, J. G., Griffith, J., Stevens, K., et al. Schizophrenia, sensory gating, and nicotinic receptors. *Schizophr. Bull.* 1998;24(2):189-202.

[165] Depatie, L., O'Driscoll, G. A., Holahan, A. L., Atkinson, V., Thavundayil, J. X., Kin, N. N., et al. Nicotine and behavioral markers of risk for schizophrenia: a double-blind, placebo-controlled, cross-over study. *Neuropsychopharmacology* 2002;27(6):1056-70.

[166] Avila, M. T., Sherr, J. D., Hong, E., Myers, C. S., Thaker, G. K. Effects of nicotine on leading saccades during smooth pursuit eye movements in smokers and nonsmokers with schizophrenia. *Neuropsychopharmacology* 2003;28(12):2184-91.

[167] Harris, J. G., Kongs, S., Allensworth, D., Martin, L., Tregellas, J., Sullivan, B., et al. Effects of nicotine on cognitive deficits in schizophrenia. *Neuropsychopharmacology* 2004;29(7):1378-85.

[168] Myers, C. S., Robles, O., Kakoyannis, A. N., Sherr, J. D., Avila, M. T., Blaxton, T. A., et al. Nicotine improves delayed recognition in schizophrenic patients. *Psychopharmacology (Berl)* 2004;174(3):334-40.

[169] Sacco, K. A., Termine, A., Seyal, A., Dudas, M. M., Vessicchio, J. C., Krishnan-Sarin, S., et al. Effects of cigarette smoking on spatial working memory and attentional deficits in schizophrenia: involvement of nicotinic receptor mechanisms. *Arch. Gen. Psychiatry* 2005;62(6):649-59.

[170] Baldeweg, T., Wong, D., Stephan, K. E. Nicotinic modulation of human auditory sensory memory: Evidence from mismatch negativity potentials. *Int. J. Psychophysiol.* 2006;59(1):49-58.
[171] George, T. P., Termine, A., Sacco, K. A., Allen, T. M., Reutenauer, E., Vessicchio, J. C., et al. A preliminary study of the effects of cigarette smoking on prepulse inhibition in schizophrenia: involvement of nicotinic receptor mechanisms. *Schizophr. Res.* 2006;87(1-3):307-15.
[172] Smith, R. C., Warner-Cohen, J., Matute, M., Butler, E., Kelly, E., Vaidhyanathaswamy, S., et al. Effects of nicotine nasal spray on cognitive function in schizophrenia. *Neuropsychopharmacology* 2006;31(3):637-43.
[173] Jacobsen, L. K., D'Souza, D. C., Mencl, W. E., Pugh, K. R., Skudlarski, P., Krystal, J. H. Nicotine effects on brain function and functional connectivity in schizophrenia. *Biol. Psychiatry* 2004;55(8):850-8.
[174] George, T. P., Vessicchio, J. C., Termine, A., Sahady, D. M., Head, C. A., Pepper, W. T., et al. Effects of smoking abstinence on visuospatial working memory function in schizophrenia. *Neuropsychopharmacology* 2002;26(1):75-85.
[175] Freedman, R., Coon, H., Myles-Worsley, M., Orr-Urtreger, A., Olincy, A., Davis, A., et al. Linkage of a neurophysiological deficit in schizophrenia to a chromosome 15 locus. *Proc. Natl. Acad. Sci. USA* 1997;94(2):587-92.
[176] Riley, B. P., Makoff, A., Mogudi-Carter, M., Jenkins, T., Williamson, R., Collier, D., et al. Haplotype transmission disequilibrium and evidence for linkage of the CHRNA7 gene region to schizophrenia in Southern African Bantu families. *Am. J. Med. Genet* 2000;96(2):196-201.
[177] Luntz-Leybman, V., Bickford, P. C., Freedman, R. Cholinergic gating of response to auditory stimuli in rat hippocampus. *Brain Res.* 1992;587(1):130-6.
[178] Adler, L. E., Pachtman, E., Franks, R. D., Pecevich, M., Waldo, M. C., Freedman, R. Neurophysiological evidence for a defect in neuronal mechanisms involved in sensory gating in schizophrenia. *Biol. Psychiatry* 1982;17(6):639-54.
[179] Freedman, R., Adler, L. E., Waldo, M. C., Pachtman, E., Franks, R. D. Neurophysiological evidence for a defect in inhibitory pathways in schizophrenia: comparison of medicated and drug-free patients. *Biol Psychiatry* 1983;18(5):537-51.
[180] Siegel, C., Waldo, M., Mizner, G., Adler, L. E., Freedman, R. Deficits in sensory gating in schizophrenic patients and their relatives. Evidence obtained with auditory evoked responses. *Arch. Gen. Psychiatry* 1984;41(6):607-12.
[181] Gottschalk, L. A., Haer, J. L., Bates, D. E. Effect of sensory overload on psychological state. Changes in social alienation-personal disorganization and cognitive-intellectual impairment. *Arch. Gen. Psychiatry* 1972;27(4):451-7.
[182] Braff, D. L. Attention, habituation and information processing in psychiatric disorders. In: Michels R., Brodie H. K., Cooper A. M., editors. Pychiatry. Philadelphia: Lippincott; 1985. p. 1-13.
[183] Braff, D. L., Geyer, M. A. Sensorimotor gating and schizophrenia. Human and animal model studies. *Arch. Gen. Psychiatry* 1990;47(2):181-8.
[184] Geyer, M. A., Braff, D. L. Startle habituation and sensorimotor gating in schizophrenia and related animal models. *Schizophr Bull* 1987;13(4):643-68.

[185] Adler, L. E., Hoffer, L. D., Wiser, A., Freedman, R. Normalization of auditory physiology by cigarette smoking in schizophrenic patients. *Am J Psychiatry* 1993;150(12):1856-61.

[186] McEvoy, J. P., Freudenreich, O., Wilson, W. H. Smoking and therapeutic response to clozapine in patients with schizophrenia. *Biol. Psychiatry* 1999;46(1):125-9.

[187] George, T. P., Sernyak, M. J., Ziedonis, D. M., Woods, S. W. Effects of clozapine on smoking in chronic schizophrenic outpatients. *J. Clin. Psychiatry* 1995;56(8):344-6.

[188] Simosky, J. K., Stevens, K. E., Adler, L. E., Freedman, R. Clozapine improves deficient inhibitory auditory processing in DBA/2 mice, via a nicotinic cholinergic mechanism. *Psychopharmacology (Berl)* 2003;165(4):386-96.

[189] Adler, L. E., Olincy, A., Cawthra, E. M., McRae, K. A., Harris, J. G., Nagamoto, H. T., et al. Varied effects of atypical neuroleptics on P50 auditory gating in schizophrenia patients. *Am. J. Psychiatry* 2004;161(10):1822-8.

[190] Kem, W. R., Mahnir, V. M., Prokai, L., Papke, R. L., Cao, X., LeFrancois, S., et al. Hydroxy metabolites of the Alzheimer's drug candidate 3-[(2,4-dimethoxy)benzylidene]-anabaseine dihydrochloride (GTS-21): their molecular properties, interactions with brain nicotinic receptors, and brain penetration. *Mol. Pharmacol.* 2004;65(1):56-67.

[191] Walker, D. P., Wishka, D. G., Piotrowski, D. W., Jia, S., Reitz, S. C., Yates, K. M., et al. Design, synthesis, structure-activity relationship, and in vivo activity of azabicyclic aryl amides as alpha7 nicotinic acetylcholine receptor agonists. *Bioorg. Med. Chem.* 2006;14(24):8219-48.

[192] de Fiebre, C. M., Meyer, E. M., Henry, J. C., Muraskin, S. I., Kem, W. R., Papke, R. L. Characterization of a series of anabaseine-derived compounds reveals that the 3-(4)-dimethylaminocinnamylidine derivative is a selective agonist at neuronal nicotinic alpha 7/125I-alpha-bungarotoxin receptor subtypes. *Mol. Pharmacol.* 1995;47(1):164-71.

[193] Woodruff-Pak, D. S., Li, Y. T., Kem, W. R. A nicotinic agonist (GTS-21), eyeblink classical conditioning, and nicotinic receptor binding in rabbit brain. *Brain Res.* 1994;645(1-2):309-17.

[194] Stevens, K. E., Kem, W. R., Mahnir, V. M., Freedman, R. Selective alpha7-nicotinic agonists normalize inhibition of auditory response in DBA mice. *Psychopharmacology (Berl)* 1998;136(4):320-7.

[195] Kitagawa, H., Takenouchi, T., Azuma, R., Wesnes, K. A., Kramer, W. G., Clody, D. E., et al. Safety, pharmacokinetics, and effects on cognitive function of multiple doses of GTS-21 in healthy, male volunteers. *Neuropsychopharmacology* 2003;28(3):542-51.

[196] Olincy, A., Harris, J. G., Johnson, L. L., Pender, V., Kongs, S., Allensworth, D., et al. Proof-of-concept trial of an alpha7 nicotinic agonist in schizophrenia. *Arch. Gen. Psychiatry* 2006;63(6):630-8.

[197] Thomsen, M. S., Mikkelsen, J. D., Timmermann, D. B., Peters, D., Hay-Schmidt, A., Martens, H., et al. The selective alpha(7) nicotinic acetylcholine receptor agonist A-582941 activates immediate early genes in limbic regions of the forebrain: Differential effects in the juvenile and adult rat. *Neuroscience* 2008.

[198] Simosky, J. K., Stevens, K. E., Freedman, R. Nicotinic agonists and psychosis. *Curr. Drug Targets CNS Neurol Disord* 2002;1(2):149-62.

[199] Allen, T., McEvoy, J. P., Keefe, R. S., D., L. E., Wilson, W. Galantamine as an adjunctive therapy in the treatment of schizphrenia. In: 11th Congress of the International Psychogeriatric Association (IPA); 2003 August 17-22; Chicago; 2003.

[200] Schreiber, R., Dalmus, M., De Vry, J. Effects of alpha 4/beta 2- and alpha 7-nicotine acetylcholine receptor agonists on prepulse inhibition of the acoustic startle response in rats and mice. *Psychopharmacology (Berl)* 2002;159(3):248-57.

[201] Bontempi, B., Whelan, K. T., Risbrough, V. B., Rao, T. S., Buccafusco, J. J., Lloyd, G. K., et al. SIB-1553A, (+/-)-4-[[2-(1-methyl-2-pyrrolidinyl)ethyl]thio]phenol hydrochloride, a subtype-selective ligand for nicotinic acetylcholine receptors with putative cognitive-enhancing properties: effects on working and reference memory performances in aged rodents and nonhuman primates. *J. Pharmacol. Exp. Ther.* 2001;299(1):297-306.

[202] Levin, E. D., McClernon, F. J., Rezvani, A. H. Nicotinic effects on cognitive function: behavioral characterization, pharmacological specification, and anatomic localization. *Psychopharmacology (Berl)* 2006;184(3-4):523-39.

[203] Lloyd, G. K., Menzaghi, F., Bontempi, B., Suto, C., Siegel, R., Akong, M., et al. The potential of subtype-selective neuronal nicotinic acetylcholine receptor agonists as therapeutic agents. *Life Sci.*1998;62(17-18):1601-6.

[204] McGurk, S. R., Levin, E. D., Butcher, L. L. Nicotinic-dopaminergic relationships and radial-arm maze performance in rats. *Behav. Neural Biol.* 1989;52(1):78-86.

[205] McGurk, S. R., Levin, E. D., Butcher, L. L. Radial-arm maze performance in rats is impaired by a combination of nicotinic-cholinergic and D2 dopaminergic antagonist drugs. *Psychopharmacology (Berl)* 1989;99(3):371-3.

[206] Levin, E. D., McGurk, S. R., Rose, J. E., Butcher, L. L. Reversal of a mecamylamine-induced cognitive deficit with the D2 agonist, LY 171555. *Pharmacol Biochem Behav* 1989;33(4):919-22.

[207] Wang, D., Noda, Y., Zhou, Y., Nitta, A., Furukawa, H., Nabeshima, T. Synergistic effect of combined treatment with risperidone and galantamine on phencyclidine-induced impairment of latent visuospatial learning and memory: Role of nAChR activation-dependent increase of dopamine D1 receptor-mediated neurotransmission. *Neuropharmacology* 2007;53(3):379-89.

[208] Shoaib, M., Schindler, C. W., Goldberg, S. R., Pauly, J. R. Behavioural and biochemical adaptations to nicotine in rats: influence of MK801, an NMDA receptor antagonist. *Psychopharmacology (Berl)* 1997;134(2):121-30.

[209] Rezvani, A. H., Levin, E. D. Nicotinic-glutamatergic interactions and attentional performance on an operant visual signal detection task in female rats. *Eur J Pharmacol* 2003;465(1-2):83-90.

[210] Levin, E. D., Bettegowda, C., Weaver, T., Christopher, N. C. Nicotine-dizocilpine interactions and working and reference memory performance of rats in the radial-arm maze. *Pharmacol. Biochem. Behav.* 1998;61(3):335-40.

[211] Aizenman, E., Tang, L. H., Reynolds, I. J. Effects of nicotinic agonists on the NMDA receptor. *Brain Res.* 1991;551(1-2):355-7.

[212] Court, J. A., Piggott, M. A., Perry, E. K. Nicotine reduces the binding of [3H]MK-801 to brain membranes, but not via the stimulation of high-affinity nicotinic receptors. *Brain Res.* 1990;524(2):319-21.

[213] Levin, E. D., Tizabi, Y., Rezvani, A. H., Caldwell, D. P., Petro, A., Getachew, B. Chronic nicotine and dizocilpine effects on regionally specific nicotinic and NMDA glutamate receptor binding. *Brain Res.* 2005;1041(2):132-42.

[214] Vige, X., Briley, M. Scopolamine induces up-regulation of nicotinic receptors in intact brain but not in nucleus basalis lesioned rats. *Neurosci. Lett.* 1988;88(3):319-24.

[215] Leblond, L., Beaufort, C., Delerue, F., Durkin, T. P. Differential roles for nicotinic and muscarinic cholinergic receptors in sustained visuo-spatial attention? A study using a 5-arm maze protocol in mice. *Behav Brain. Res.* 2002;128(1):91-102.

[216] Brown, E. N., Galligan, J. J. Muscarinic receptors couple to modulation of nicotinic ACh receptor desensitization in myenteric neurons. *Am. J. Physiol. Gastrointest. Liver Physiol.* 2003;285(1):G37-44.

[217] Erskine, F. F., Ellis, J. R., Ellis, K. A., Stuber, E., Hogan, K., Miller, V., et al. Evidence for synergistic modulation of early information processing by nicotinic and muscarinic receptors in humans. *Hum. Psychopharmacol.* 2004;19(7):503-9.

[218] Ellis, J. R., Ellis, K. A., Bartholomeusz, C. F., Harrison, B. J., Wesnes, K. A., Erskine, F. F., et al. Muscarinic and nicotinic receptors synergistically modulate working memory and attention in humans. *Int. J. Neuropsychopharmacol.* 2006;9(2):175-89.

In: Prefrontal Cortex: Roles, Interventions and Traumas ISBN 978-1-60692-415-0
Editors: Lorenzo LoGrasso and Giovanni Morretti

Chapter 3

Participation of the Prefrontal Cortex in the Processing of Sexual and Maternal Incentives

Marisela Hernández González* and Miguel Angel Guevara
Instituto de Neurociencias, Universidad de Guadalajara, México
Francisco de Quevedo 180, Col. Arcos-Vallarta
Guadalajara, Jalisco, México

Abstract

Sexual and maternal behaviors constitute motivated behaviors, the adequate manifestation of which requires an appropriate integration of external stimuli and internal states. In both is required the perception of an appropriate stimulus. For a male rat, one appropriate sexual incentive stimulus could be a receptive female, while for a female mother rat the appropriate maternal incentive could be a pup rat. The sensory clues emitted by either the potential sexual partner or the pups must be first detected and then processed in order to be perceived as incentives and as potentially rewarding. The prefrontal cortex (PFC) plays an important role both in mediating the assignation of the incentive value and in information processing. Thus, using electroencephalographic (EEG) recordings, we have characterized the prefrontal functioning during motivational states of sexual and maternal behavior in rats. In a first study, it was observed that the EEG activity of the medial (mPFC) and orbital prefrontal cortices (oPFC) was modified during the performance of male rats in a T-maze under two different conditions: sexually-motivated (with previous intromission and one receptive and one non-receptive female placed in the goal boxes of the lateral arms); and not sexually-motivated (no previous intromission and empty goal boxes). Only the sexually-motivated males showed a higher proportion in the 6-7 Hz band and a lower proportion in the 8-11 Hz band during the awake-quiet state and while walking in the maze stem. In addition, they showed an increased correlation of the 6-7 Hz band while walking in the maze stem and when remaining close to a receptive female. Similar EEG changes were obtained in

* Tel: (52) 33 38 18 07 40 ext 5860; E-mails: mariselh@cencar.udg.mx; mguevara@cencar.udg.mx

estrous female rats that were subjected to a sexually-motivated task using the same paradigm of the T-maze. In the oPFC of the sexually-motivated females and males, different EEG patterns were observed, results that suggest a different functionality of the mPFC and oPFC, which may work together in the processing of sexual incentive stimuli. Another study explored whether the mPFC of female rats shows characteristic EEG patterns during the presentation of olfactory stimuli, when (1) associated with pups (nest-bedding); and, (2) not-associated, with pups (female bedding), during the following distinct reproductive states: proestrus-estrus (P-E), diestrus (D) and lactation (L). During the smelling of nest-bedding, only the L rats showed a higher proportion in the 8-11 Hz band. This finding may represent a characteristic processing of the olfactory stimuli related to pups in the mPFC of L rats. Taken together, these data allow suggest that in rats the prefrontal cortex participates in identifying and processing sexual and maternal incentives.

Introduction

In studying the physiology of sexual and maternal behaviors it is important to gain insight into the early phases of sexual and maternal relations among animals. These phases include detection and perception of the stimuli, gender identification, motivation and arousal. Agmo (1999) has defined the term sexual motivation as the process that makes an animal search for sexual contact with another animal. It is well known that sexual motivation is activated when a suitable stimulus –e.g., a mate– is perceived. A similar definition can be applied to the maternal motivation, as the process that makes a mother search for maternal contact with a pup (her own or alien); *i.e.*, the process that promotes nurturing behaviors toward an offspring. This is activated when the suitable stimulus –e.g., a pup– is perceived. Given that the suitable stimulus generally activates approach behavior, it can be suggested that these stimuli may function as a positive incentive.

Although different neural structures have been implicated in the modulation of sexual and maternal performance, to date there are very few studies that have described which brain areas are involved in the search for sexual and maternal contact, including the processing of the sensory stimuli that are emitted from the potential partner or pup and that are fundamental in generating sexual and maternal motivation. The processing of these different stimuli with sexual and maternal meaning involves the activation of different neural systems, as well as integration with hormonal cues. In recent years, substantial evidence has been accumulated indicating the critical role of the PFC in mediating the assignation of the incentive value of the stimuli and it has been suggested that it is in this cortical region that the sensory inputs generated by distant stimuli from the potential sexual partner or pups are processed. Several techniques, such as lesions and electrical or chemical stimulation, as well as hormonal treatments, were the first ones used in attempts to understand the role of the prefrontal cortex in the motivational aspects of these behaviors. Today, more sophisticated techniques have been developed: the expression of immediate early genes, measurements of the turnover or release of neurotransmitters and descriptions of hemodynamic reactions in response to sexually-relevant stimuli have all provided relevant information concerning the role of the prefrontal cortex in the processing of such stimuli. The spontaneous brain electrical activity or electroencephalographic recording technique (EEG) has proven to be a very useful tool for studying brain functioning during specific behaviors and cognitive processes. One of its main advantages is that the EEG has an excellent temporal resolution that makes it possible to obtain recordings of brain electrical activity from milliseconds to hours, days and even months. With this in mind, the aim of the present chapter is: 1) to review the subdivisions and functions of the rat prefrontal cortex; 2) to define sexual and maternal behaviors as motivated behaviors; 3) to clarify the important role of the incentive stimuli (potential sexual partners or pups) in inducing the corresponding motivational states; and, 4) to demonstrate, by means of EEG recordings, the participation of the prefrontal cortex in the processing of incentive stimuli in relation to sexual and maternal behaviors in rats. This chapter compiles several electroencephalographic studies in which the electrical functionality of different prefrontal subregions was characterized in relation to the approach behaviors (activated by the incentive), which has been considered as a behavioral index of sexual or maternal motivation in the rat.

The Rat Prefrontal Cortex, Subdivisions and Functions

The prefrontal cortex (PFC) can be defined as the cortical region where projections from the mediodorsal nucleus of the thalamus (MD) are received (Rose and Woolsey, 1948; Uylings and Van Eden, 1990). It has been shown that the PFC directly projects to the cholinergic forebrain system and to the monoaminergic cell group in the hypothalamus and brainstem. In this way, the PFC is in a unique position to influence the transmitter systems that modulate large parts of the forebrain. Further, it has become clear that the PFC has a special relationship with the basal ganglia; not only does it project via the cortico-striatal system to the basal ganglia, but it also receives, via the thalamus, projections from these structures, an arrangement that is unique to the frontal lobe. In addition to the anterior connections, the PFC has larger and reciprocal connections with other cortical areas, so that it receives inputs predominantly from somatosensory, visual and auditory cortical association areas in the parietal, occipital and temporal lobes (for a review, see Groenewegen and Uylings, 2000). In this way, the PFC is involved in a number of largely parallel, functionally-segregated cortical-subcortical circuits that subserve sensorimotor, cognitive, emotional/motivational behaviors and visceral functions, so that the PFC is thought to be primarily involved in the cognitive and motivational/emotional processes that underlie and guide complex behavior (Passingham, 1993). Due to its special position in the circuitry of the forebrain, the PFC has been implicated in the high processing of all sensory modalities. Given that the PFC is also provided with visceral sensory input, it seems likely that it plays a role in evaluating the internal and external milieu and, based on this information, in selecting the behavioral strategy and modulating the repertoire of the corresponding autonomic adaptation accordingly.

It has been suggested that many functions are mediated by the prefrontal cortex, including the mediation of working memory for a specific domain or for attributing information, especially that involving spatial and visual object information, and also higher order relationships, such as motivation, learning and remembering complex tasks, the temporal order of events, selecting rules and strategies, and planning, monitoring and modifying sequential behavior (Shimamura et al., 1990; Goldman-Rakic, 1996; Fuster, 1997). These varieties of functions are represented in specific subregions of the PFC, so that it has been suggested that it has a functional heterogeneity based mainly on the divisions of the mediodorsal nucleus of the thalamus (MD). The concept of a functional heterogeneity in the PFC was first postulated in the 1960s (see, for example, Mishkin, 1964), when was suggested that the prefrontal subregions are functionally different. Three main regions have been determined: first, the magnocellular, medial part of the MD projects to the orbital (ventral) surface of the prefrontal cortex (which includes areas 13 and 12). This part of the PFC is called the orbitofrontal cortex, and receives information from the ventral or object-processing visual stream as well as taste, olfactory and somatosensory inputs. Second, the parvocellular, lateral part of the MD projects to the dorsolateral PFC. This part of the PFC receives inputs from the parietal cortex and is involved in tasks such as short-term spatial memory operations (Fuster, 1997; Rolls and Treves, 1998). Third, the pars paralamellaris (most lateral) part of the MD projects to the frontal eye field (area 8) in the anterior bank of the arcuate sulcus. The degree of development of these prefrontal subregions varies among species; for example, the orbitofrontal cortex is well developed in primates, including humans, but poorly developed in rodents.

It is evident from anatomical studies that the prefrontal cortex of the rat is also made up of several subregions that are functionally distinct.

In fact, it is clear from lesion studies that there are at least three distinct prefrontal regions, which include: (1) a medial prefrontal region (mPFC) made up of several subregions that are probably functionally distinct (Cg1, Cg2, Cg3 or prelimbic and infralimbic areas); (2) an orbital prefrontal region (oPFC) that is also made up of several subregions that are likely functionally distinct (ventral, lateral, ventrolateral, and medial orbital areas, and the agranular insular areas); and, (3) a region that is likely analogous to the frontal eye fields of primates (Fr2) (Kolb, 1990; Uylings and Van Eden, 1990) (Figure 1).

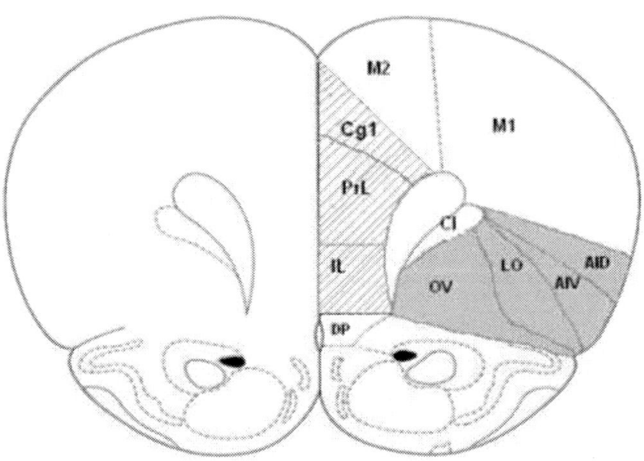

Figure 1. Schematic representation of the rat prefrontal subregions. M1, primary motor cortex; M2 secondary motor cortex; Cg1, cingulated cortex area; PrL, prelimbic cortex; IL, infralimbic cortex; OV,

ventral orbital cortex; LO, lateral orbital cortex; AIV, agranular insular cortex ventral; AID, agranular insular cortex dorsal; Cl, claustrum; DP, dorsal peduncular cortex.With shadow is indicated the medial prefrontal subregion, whereas in gray color is indicated the orbital prefrontal subregion. Anterior-posterior coordinates are given with respect to Bregma (Paxinos and Watson, stereotaxic atlas, 1997).

The mPFC is involved in various functions, such as the temporal ordering of sequential events, mnemonic tasks and motive-emotional processes, while the oPFC is mainly involved in the processing of higher levels of somatosensory, visual, auditory, olfactory and gustatory sensory information, participating actively in the performance of high-order olfactory processing. Moreover, it plays a pivotal role in goal-directed behaviors and in guiding behaviors based on reward (for reviews, see Kolb, 1990; Uylings and Van Eden, 1990; Yonemori et al., 2000; Uylings et al., 2003).

The participation of the PFC in reward processing has been demonstrated in various studies. The PFC is part of the mesocorticolimbic dopaminergic system and receives prominent dopaminergic input from the VTA and inputs from other subcortical basal ganglia structures via the mediodorsal thalamus. In turn, it projects back to the VTA and the nucleus accumbens septi (Acc), which are generally considered to be the main components of the brain reward system. Evidence for the involvement of the mPFC in the reward-related mechanism comes primarily from three types of studies: conditioned place preference, intracranial self-stimulation, and self-administration of drugs (Tzschentke, 2000), so that available data strongly suggests that the mPFC forms part of the brain reward circuitry.

Various studies have demonstrated that both sexual (Sheffield et al., 1951, 1954; Denniston, 1954; Kagan, 1955; Beach and Jordan, 1956; Whalen 1961; Whalen et al., 1961; Jowaisas et al., 1971; Hetta and Meyerson, 1978; Everitt and Stacey, 1987; Agmo, 1999; López and Ettenberg, 2001) and maternal behaviors (Fleming and Luebke, 1981; Fleming, 1986; Fleming et al., 1989, 1994; Stern, 1996) are intrinsically rewarding or reinforcing motivated behaviors. Their execution is associated with the activation of several brain regions in the reward circuitry.

The Motivated Behaviors

Biological evolution is characterized by an increase in the integrative capacity of the nervous system accompanied by the expression of more complex behavior patterns. At the same time, however, the basic requirements for life must be met. Thus, during the course of evolution a variety of digestive, respiratory and cardiovascular mechanisms must be coordinated with behavioral responses that assure biological adaptation and survival. The neural integration of visceral responses, which are modulated by the autonomic nervous system and the endocrine system, tends to maintain a relatively constant internal environment, while adaptive behavioral responses involve the somatomotor control system, sensory mechanisms and also sensory-motor interaction. Behavioral responses can be triggered by both internal and external signals and, because they contribute to homeostasis and survival, this is also the case of the primary motivated behaviors: eating, drinking and thermoregulation. However, there are other motivated behaviors that are also very important for the reproduction and survival of the species though they do not result from a deficit in the organism but, rather, mainly from an adequate hormonal medium and the perception of external stimuli that turn out to be relevant for them. This is the case of sexual and maternal behaviors, which have been considered as secondary motivated behaviors. Sexual behavior in both sexes comprises a complex series of motoric events that ensure the successful transfer of sperm from the male to the female's reproductive tract, whereas maternal behavior comprises another complex series of motoric events designed to ensure the growth and survival of the offspring (one's own or alien young). In both cases of motivated behaviors the nervous system must detect and process a series of sensory stimuli, a task in which, as has been clearly shown, the prefrontal cortex plays a pivotal role.

Before examining sexual and maternal behaviors in detail, however, it will be useful to outline the sequential stages that are common to a variety of adaptive or goal-oriented behaviors, in order to place the problem of the underlying neural mechanism in perspective. For descriptive purposes, such behavioral responses can be divided into initiation, procurement and consummatory phases. Current evidence suggests that the initiation phase may involve: 1) the detection of peripheral and central signals; 2) sensory information from the external environment; and, 3) cognitive factors. The procurement phase is characterized by a general state of behavioral arousal and by searching behavior, which involves locomotor activity, sensory information and previous experience. The final, consummatory, phase relies to a considerable degree on preprogrammed motor responses, that are stereotyped and species-typical (Swanson and Mogenson, 1981). Another useful classification of goal-oriented behaviors that has been used for many years, is one in which motivated behaviors are divided into appetitive and consummatory components (Everitt, 1990; Pryce et al., 1993; Timberlake and Silva, 1995). The appetitive component is made up of those behaviors that bring the organism into contact with an attractive or desired stimulus object or goal, while the consummatory component is composed of the ones that are performed once the goal is achieved. Wallen (1990) has made an analogous distinction by referring to these categories as desire *vs*. ability: appetitive behavior reflects an underlying motivation, appetite, drive or desire to engage in a behavioral interaction with a specific goal or object, while consummatory behavior reflects the ability to perform specific behavioral responses once the goal object is attained.

Thus, the term motivation can refer to a variety of neuronal and physiological factors that initiate, sustain and direct behavior. In the case of sexual and maternal behaviors, voluntary movements are initiated to approach a specific goal (a potential sexual partner or a pup), so that the motivated state impels the individual to perform sexual and/or maternal acts. The sexual and maternal activities of the rat are naturally occurring behavior patterns with a well-organized behavioral sequence and a specific temporal and spatial order, where voluntary goal-directed movements, automatic stereotyped responses and consummatory acts can all be distinguished. The prefrontal cortex is involved in the motivational processing of relevant goals and various studies have demonstrated that lesions in this cortical area alter the sequential organization, sensory processing and mnemonic aspects of motivated behaviors (Kolb, 1984; 1990). The medial prefrontal cortex receives highly processed sensory information from visual, auditory and somatosensory regions (Groenewegen and Uylings, 2000) and, like the ventral tegmental area (VTA), has been implicated in integrating motor action with sensory information (Mogenson et al., 1980; Kolb and Cioe, 2004).

Traditionally, the occurrence of the appetitive component of a species-typical behavior has been taken as evidence of increased motivation: that is, if an organism acts on its environment to obtain a particular stimulus (pups, mate, food), then that stimulus is attractive and thus reflects an underlying increase in motivation.

There are two classes of external stimuli or events: hedonically-potent and hedonically-neutral. The first may be further divided into hedonically-positive and hedonically-negative stimuli or events. Hedonically-positive stimuli or events are associated with approach behavior and may be called positive incentives. Hedonically-negative stimuli –*i.e.*, those associated with withdrawal or escape behaviors– can be called negative incentives. Based on this classification, Agmo (1999) has proposed that the motivation aroused by stimuli with rewarding properties be called incentive motivation. Under this proposition, an appropriate sexual incentive for a male rat would be a sexually-receptive female, for a female receptive rat a sexually active-male, and for a female mother rat, a pup rat. As these suitable stimuli activate approach behaviors it is possible to consider that they may function as positive incentives.

One of the main animal models that have been used to study the neurophysiological and hormonal bases of sexual and maternal behaviors is the rat. Recent research has shown that the rat serves as an excellent animal model of PFC functions (Kesner, 2000; Brown and Bowman, 2002; Uylings et al., 2003), and several studies have demonstrated the differential functioning of the prefrontal subregions in this animal. Taking into account these considerations, the next section discusses a series of experiments that evaluated the possible participation of the PFC in the motivational and performance aspects of sexual and maternal behaviors. However, before examining these different experiments, it is necessary to explain the appetitive and consummatory components of each one of these motivated behaviors in the rat.

Male Rat Sexual Behavior

Two processes can be distinguished in the sexual behavior of the male rat: first, a series of arbitrary responses that lead to the male approaching the female (orientation, smelling, persecution of the female and latency to initiate mating), that together constitute the appetitive component; and, second, a subsequent series of stereotyped motor activities that make up the act of copulation itself (mounting, intromission and ejaculation responses) and constitute the consummatory component of the male rat's sexual behavior (Agmo, 1999; 2002; Pfaff and Agmo, 2002).

Sexual behavior occurs spontaneously when specific external sensory stimuli are present (those emitted by a potential sexual partner); however, to detect a stimuli as sexually attractive an adequate internal state of the subject is necessary (*i.e.*, adequate levels of circulating hormones and neurotransmitters, adequate neural functionality, etc.), that makes it more alert to incentive stimuli from the potential partner. However, simple detection of the sensory stimuli is not sufficient. Also required is an adequate processing of the stimuli that contain sexual meaning that permits the assignation of the incentive value as well as its perception as rewarding. It has been suggested that the processing that entails acquiring the incentive value of the stimuli is mediated by limbic-prefrontal circuits, including mainly the reciprocal projections between the oPFC and the amygdala (Armony et al., 1997; Balkenius and Morén, 2001; Hall et al., 2001). Moreover, Rolls and Treves (1998) have proposed that the oPFC may contribute to the acquisition of the reward value of the stimulus through its connections with the amygdala.

The force that drives the subject to search for sexual interaction with a mate –*i.e.*, the appetitive component or sexual motivation– has been measured under different experimental paradigms. Several studies have confirmed the fact that sex is an efficient incentive (Sheffield et al., 1951, 1954; Denniston, 1954; Kagan, 1955; López and Ettenberg, 2001) and have used sex as a reward in classical operant tasks such as mazes and Skinner boxes (Jowaisas et al., 1971; Everitt and Stacey, 1987). Both, Beach and Jordan (1956) and Whalen (1961) have shown that male rats readily learn to run through a runway when access to a receptive female is used as an incentive, and access to a female can also be used to reinforce other responses; e.g., bar-pressing (Jowaisas et al., 1971; Everitt and Stacey, 1987; Everitt et al., 1987;), or the search for proximity to a female (Hetta and Meyerson, 1978). However, it has also been shown that it is not necessary for the male to work or to perform an operant task in order to gain access to a female and hence demonstrate his sexual motivation. Agmo (2002) has proposed that an adequate and easy measure of the sexual incentive motivation could be approach behavior and the time that a male remains near an inaccessible receptive female. Using this paradigm, the effectiveness of the stimuli emitted by a receptive female in terms of functioning as a positive incentive for male rats has been demonstrated.

Female Rat Sexual Behavior

The female rat's sexual behavior comprises three basic elements: attractivity, proceptivity and receptivity. Attractivity can be defined as a "female's value as a sexual incentive stimulus" and includes both behavioral and non-behavioral components, such as olfactory cues that stimulate the male to engage in sexual behavior with her. Proceptivity includes a number of solicitational behaviors that are followed by increases in the number of sexual mounts by males. These behaviors are exhibited spontaneously by estrous female rats during the normal course of mating and include hopping, darting and ear-wiggling (Beach, 1976; Madlafousek and Hlinak, 1977), a posing or presenting posture (Emery and Moss, 1984a,b), a rapid sequence of approaches toward, orientation to, and withdrawal from, proximity to a sexually-active male (McClintock and Adler, 1978), and the emitting of ultrasonic vocalizations known to stimulate mating by males (White and Barfield, 1989). These behaviors reflect in some way the appetitive aspect of sexual behavior and implied a motivation to mate. Receptivity is indicated by the reflex response of the female to sexual contact with the male and consists in adopting a posture that positions her genitalia to allow penile intromission by the male, dorsiflexion of the spine, elevation of the head, deviation of the tail and extension of the rear legs.

The several solicitational behaviors displayed by the female have been used to ascertain an overall level of sexual readiness as an estimate of the female's motivation to mate, and are considered as appetitive components. On the other hand, the receptivity or lordosis response that results from sexual contact with the male constitutes the consummatory component of the female's sexual behavior.

As in the male's sexual interaction, other behaviors expressed under several experimental conditions have furnished measures of female sexual motivation. Among the different paradigms that have been used to measure female sexual motivation we can mention the following: sexual preference and proximity (Meyerson and Lindstrom, 1973; Clark et al., 1981; Edward and Pfeifle, 1983; Broekman et al., 1988); the female´s willingness to cross an electrified grid to approach a sexually-active male (Meyerson and Lindstrom, 1973); operant tasks such as bar pressing by males (Bermant, 1961; French et al., 1972) and conditioned place preference (Oldenburger et al., 1992; Paredes and Alonso, 1997; Matthews et al., 1997).

Maternal Behavior in the Rat

Parental behavior can be defined as any behavior by a member of a species toward a reproductively-immature conspecific that increases the probability that the recipient will survive to maturity. Since in mammals it is the female that lactates, the mother is the primary caregiver of her offspring; we refer to such behavior as maternal.

Rodents offer good examples of maternal care patterns in species with altricial young (immobile at birth). Since most rodent young are helpless, essentially immobile and incapable of temperature regulation at birth, they are kept in a secluded nest that the mother builds prior to parturition, which also serves to insulate the young in the mother's absence. When the female is in the nest area, she crouches over the young in order to warm and nurse them. The female also licks her young, particularly in their anogenital region, to stimulate urination and defecation. If the nest site is disturbed, or if pups are displaced from it, the rodent mother will engage in transport or retrieval behavior in which she carries pups (one at a time) in her mouth to a new nest site or back to the original one. Another aspect of maternal care in rodents is the occurrence of maternal aggression toward intruders at the nest site, presumably to protect the young. In describing maternal care in rodents, one can therefore refer to pup-directed patterns (retrieving, licking, nursing) and non-pup-directed patterns (nest-building, maternal aggression), all of which contribute to the successful rearing of the offspring. Thus, those behaviors that a female performs in order to gain access to her pups have been classified as appetitive (pup retrieval, pup licking), while nursing (low and high crouching) behaviors are considered as consummatory responses.

Like male and female sexual behaviors, maternal behavior also has an implicit and strong rewarding or reinforcing component. For example, it has been shown that postpartum females and hormone-induced maternal virgins are much more likely than virgin females to retrieve pups under stressful conditions, such as in a T-maze (Stern and Mackinnon., 1976), open-field or in elevated plus maze (Fleming and Luebke, 1981; Bitran et al., 1991). Therefore, a marked reduction in the duration of the freezing reaction in lactating females was found when compared to virgin females who had not been exposed to pups (Hard and Hansen, 1985; Hansen and Ferreira, 1986). Ferreira et al. (1989) examined the punished drinking response in virgin and postpartum females using a test in which licking from a water spout is punished by electric shocks. It was found that lactating females drank more than virgins. Various paradigms, such as place preference (Fleming et al., 1994; Magnusson and Fleming, 1995; Mattson et al., 2001) and pressing a bar in an operant chamber at a high rate in order to obtain access to rat pups as a reward (Lee et al., 2000) have clearly shown that pups can serve as strong reinforcers for postpartum females.

Neural and Hormonal Regulation of Sexual and Maternal Behaviors

It is quite evident that hormones need to act on specific neurons somewhere in the brain or the peripheral nervous system in order to exercise their stimulatory effect on the structures involved in the motivational and execution aspects of sexual and maternal behaviors. The brain needs to be exposed to some hormones in order to react to internal and external stimuli with sexual and/or maternal responses. Thus, it is well known that the testicular and ovarian hormones are necessary for sexual and maternal behaviors in all mammals, including humans. Castration (Bremer, 1958; Rossenblat and Aronson, 1958; Davidson, 1966; Heim and Hursch, 1979; Larsson, 1979; Willie and Beler, 1989), ovariectomy (Boling and Blandau, 1939; Dempsey et al., 1939; Robinson, 1954) and other means of reducing testicular and ovarian hormone concentrations (Bradford and Pawlack, 1993; Reilly et al., 2000) always lead to a reduced motivation or intensity of sexual behavior and altered maternal behavior, at least immediately after parturition (for a review, see Hull et al., 2002; Blaustein and Erskine, 2002; González-Mariscal and Poindron, 2002).

Hormones have no effect unless they are bound to the appropriate receptor. The gonadal hormone receptors are widely distributed in the brain. Among the sites expressing androgen receptors are the medial preoptic area, the medial amygdale, the ventromedial nucleus of the hypothalamus, the bed nucleus of the stria terminalis and the prefrontal cortex. Estrogen receptors are found in the medial preoptic area, the ventromedial nucleus of the hypothalamus, the olfactory bulbs and many other sites (for a review, see Genazzani et al., 1996).

Though the neural structures involved in the regulation of sexual and maternal behaviors are similar, there are certain differences. In the case of *male sexual behavior*, there is evidence of the participation of the olfactory bulb, the amygdala, the bed nucleus of the stria terminalis, the medial preoptic area, several nuclei of the hypothalamus (paraventricular, ventromedial and lateral), the midbrain periaqueductal gray, the nucleus paragigantocellularis of the medulla, among others, with the medial preoptic area playing an essential role in the motivational and performance aspects of that behavior. With respect to *feminine sexual behavior*, the ventromedial nucleus of the hypothalamus, the medial preoptic area, the amygdala, the bed nucleus of the stria terminalis, the ventral tegmental area and the midbrain central gray, among others, have been implicated, with the ventromedial nucleus of the hypothalamus playing a crucial role. In terms of *maternal behavior,* a traditional view has been that in non-primate mammals such behavior is hormonally-regulated by the endocrine events of late pregnancy, parturition and lactation, while the maternal behavior of primates is emancipated from endocrine control and instead is influenced by a variety of social experiences (see Numan and Insel, 2003). In general terms, structures such as the cortex, the trigeminal complex and olfactory circuit, the septum and the bed nucleus of the stria terminalis, the medial preoptic area, the paraventricular nucleus and the habenular complex have all been implicated in the modulation of maternal behavior. In an insightful review, Newman (1999; 2002) has emphasized the large amount of overlap in the neural circuits that regulate a variety of social behavior in mammals. These social behaviors included male and female sexual behavior, offensive aggression and parental behavior, and the neural regions she referred to included the medial preoptic area/bed nucleus of the stria terminalis, the medial amygdala, and the lateral septum. This author speculates that there may be a common central network that regulates a variety of social behaviors, and that the precise behavior that occurs may be determined by the stimuli that have access to this social circuit. In this chapter, we will not describe the specific hormonal and neural regulation of each one of these motivated behaviors, we should not lose sight of the important role that hormones play in the neural substrates involved in the motivational and execution aspects of these reproductive behaviors.

In Which Brain Structures Is the Incentive Value of Sexual and Maternal Stimuli Processed?

Although different neural structures have been implicated in the modulation of sexual and maternal performance, there are as yet very few studies that describe which brain areas are involved in the search for sexual and maternal contacts, including the processing of the sensory stimuli emitted by a potential partner or pup, which is fundamental in generating sexual and maternal motivation. The processing of these different stimuli with sexual and maternal meanings involves the activation of different neural systems, as well as integration with hormonal cues.

In males, among the few structures that have been proposed as participants in the processing of incentive stimuli is the medial preoptic area. Studies by Everitt (Everitt and Stacey, 1987; Everitt, 1999) after preoptic lesions showed that while males ceased to copulate with females, they still performed operant responses to gain access to them. Similarly, the pursuit of receptive females, or approaches to inaccessible ones, also ceased (Paredes et al, 1993; Hurtazo et al., 2003), as did the males' interest in odors from receptive females, all of which disappeared after preoptic lesions in male rats and ferrets (Paredes and Baum, 1995; Paredes et al., 1998). Taken together, these data show that reactions to sexual incentives are reduced or abolished by preoptic lesions, thus supporting the idea that this cerebral area is crucial for sexual motivation.

Other brain structures, such as the medial amygdala (ME), have been proposed as one important site for integrating chemosensory and hormonal cues (Wood, 1998). A specific distribution of their functioning has been described, in which the posteromedial amygdalar region (MEpd) is more involved in processing stimuli with sexual meaning (Kollack-Walker and Neuman, 1992, 1995). For example, Maras and Petrulis (2006) demonstrated that MEpd-lesioned male hamsters showed deficits in opposite-sex odor preference that appear to be a result of their decreased attraction to female odors.

Another brain structure that has been involved in the processing of sexual incentive stimuli in males is the prefrontal cortex. For example, Bunnell et al. (1996) showed that the ablation of the cingulated and retrosplenial cortices in hamsters caused an increase in the threshold for reaching sexual arousal. Similarly, Agmo (1995) demonstrated that extensive ablations of the medial and dorsal prefrontal cortex in male rats significantly increased (up to two hours or more) the onset of sexual interaction, despite continued exposure to a receptive female.

In females, the preoptic area is also important in the capacity of distant sexual incentive stimuli to activate approach behaviors. Lesions in this area reduce the intensity of approaches both to an inaccessible male and to a male in a situation where copulatory interactions were possible (Guarraci and Clark, 2006). Moreover, the sexual incentive properties of the odor of a male are abolished by radiofrequency lesions of the medial preoptic area (Xiao et al., 2005). These interesting data show that, in female rats, this area is crucial for the distant sexual incentive properties of a male. Another structure that has been shown to participate in female proceptive and receptive behaviors is the ventromedial nucleus of the hypothalamus (Pfaff and Sakuma, 1979; Floody, 2002); and it has been suggested that it is the combined action of the preoptic area and the ventromedial nucleus that controls all aspects of female sexual behavior, from the approach to a mate to the execution of copulatory reflexes (Agmo, 2007).

Moncho-Bogani et al. (2005) demonstrated that attraction to sexual pheromones and associated odorants in female mice involves the activation of cerebral structures such as the basolateral amygdala. They studied the chemoinvestigatory behavior of female mice towards volatile and non-volatile chemicals contained in male-soiled bedding, in combination with analyses of c-fos expressions induced by such behavior. The cerebral structures were differentially activated by the primary pheromones and secondarily by attractive odorants: the primary attractive pheromone activates the basolateral amygdala and the shell of the nucleus accumbens, but neither the ventral tegmental area nor the orbitofrontal cortex. In contrast, the secondarily attractive male-derived odorants involve activation of a circuit that includes the basolateral amygdala, the prefrontal cortex and the ventral tegmental area.

In maternal behavior: as in male and female sexual behavior, it has been recognized that the medial preoptic area plays a crucial role in the appetitive aspects of maternal behavior and, hence, in the detection and processing of the incentive stimuli emitted by pups. Electrolytic or radiofrequency lesions of this region disrupt retrieving, nest-building and nursing in lactating rats (Numan, 1974; Numan et al, 1977; Jacobson et al., 1980; Gray and Brooks, 1984). Moreover, virgin females (ovariectomized or intact) lesioned in the MPOA do not show maternal behavior, even after many days of exposure to pups (Numan et al., 1977; Miceli et al., 1983; Gray and Brooks, 1984). Therefore, by applying "kindling"-type electrical stimulation to the MPOA, maternal responsiveness to foster pups is promoted in both experienced mothers and virgins (Morgan et al., 1999); so these findings and others (Lee et al., 2000) support the idea that the activity of this brain structure is critical not only for the performance of maternal behavior but also in mediating the reinforcing properties of young pups in postpartum and "sensitized" virgin rats.

Participation of the Prefrontal Cortex in the Processing of Incentive Stimuli with Sexual or Maternal Meaning

The first studies designed to investigate the neural control of sexual behavior in male mammals used lesion techniques, mainly the gross removal of large areas of the brain. Using these techniques, after removal of the neocortex it became clear that the greatest deficits in the copulatory interaction of male rats (Beach, 1940; Larsson, 1962, 1964) and cats (Beach et al., 1955, Beach and Jordan, 1956; Zitrin et al., 1956) were associated with the removal of the frontal cortex. Bunnell et al. (1966) showed in hamsters with ablation of the cingulated and retrosplenial cortices, that the threshold to reach sexual arousal increased; and similar results were reported in rats by Soulairac and Soulairac (1972). These were the first attempts to investigate the possible role of the frontal cortex in sexual behavior. Since then, other studies have been performed to determine the exact role that this cortical region plays in sexual behavior. Studies such as those by Lubar et al. (1973), Michal (1973) and Kolb (1984, 1990) have demonstrated that lesions in this cortical area alter the sequential organization, sensory processing and memory of motivated behaviors, such as sexual interaction. Moreover, prefrontal lesions in male rats increase intromission and ejaculation latencies as well as the duration of the postejaculatory interval, thus rendering them less likely to mate successfully (Fernández-Guasti et al., 1994). As mentioned above, it was not until 1995 that Agmo and collaborators made an interesting study in which extensive ablations of the medial and dorsal prefrontal cortex increased the time required to begin copulatory performance (two hours or more) in males that were in continual exposure to a receptive female. However, as soon as copulation began the sexual behavior of the lesioned animals became completely normal (Agmo et al., 1995). The authors suggested that these data indicated a difficulty for males to identify the female as a sexual incentive.

In the case of incentive stimuli with maternal meaning, there are also several studies that have demonstrated the activation of prefrontal regions in relation to the processing of stimuli emitted by pups in dams. For example, some have described a high activation of the mPFC in human mothers who listen to an infant crying (Lorberbaum et al., 2002), a selective activation of this brain area in dam rats during their first experience with pups (Walsh et al., 1996), and an enhanced c-fos expression in the mPFC of ewes when exposed to lambs (Kendrick et al., 1997). Similar increases in the c-fos mRNA expression have been demonstrated in the mPFC of ewes exposed to odors from their own or strange lambs, although the inactivation of this cortical area only prevents ewes from responding with motor aggression to odor cues from strange lambs and has no effect on the formation of an olfactory recognition memory for their own offspring (Broad et al., 2002). Similarly, an enhanced metabolic activation of the mPFC in response to the presentation of emotionally-relevant maternal nursing calls has also been shown in *Octodon degus* pups (Braun and Poeggel, 2001).

In recent years, substantial evidence has been accumulated indicating the critical role of the PFC in mediating the assignation of the incentive value of the stimuli. For example, it has been shown that many prefrontal neurons encode a representation of olfactory stimuli that is dependent on their association with a reward (Rolls, et al., 2000) and that the medial PFC neurons show different responses to conditioned sensory stimuli (auditory or visual) when associated, or not, with a reward (Takenouchi et al., 1999; Jodo et al., 2000). In more specific studies, it has been suggested that this processing, which implies the acquisition of the incentive value of the stimuli, is mediated by limbic-prefrontal circuits, including mainly the reciprocal projections between the oPFC and the amygdala. These models propose that the oPFC may contribute to acquiring the reward value of the stimulus through its connections with the amygdala (Armony et al., 1997; Rolls and Treves, 1998; Balkenius and Morén, 2001; Hall et al., 2001), where the AMG increases the incentive value of a novel stimulus and the OFC confirms or –in the case of known stimuli– updates this value (Rolls 2000; 2004; Rolls and Treeves, 1998).

Functionality of the Prefrontal Cortex during the Processing of Incentive Stimuli: Electrophysiological Studies

A Brief Introduction to Electrophysiological Techniques

The first studies to investigate the different neuroanatomical areas involved in regulating sexual and maternal behaviors used lesion or electrical stimulation techniques. These techniques tended to be either relatively crude or too invasive. Today, sophisticated techniques have been developed that allow us to determine with greater precision the different cerebral areas that function during the reproductive behaviors that interest us and how they operate. Techniques such as determinations of the expression of immediate early genes and measurements of the turnover or release of neurotransmitters during exposure to incentive stimuli have been used in several studies. Similarly, descriptions of hemodynamic reactions in response to sexually-relevant stimuli have become popular and various imaging studies performed in humans have been published that use, for example, positron emission tomography (Stoléru et al., 1999; Leon-Carrion et al., 2007). Although modern techniques have been developed that allow researchers to obtain instantaneous images from different brain structures with high spatial definition, they have poor temporal definition. Despite its limitation in spatial definition, the electroencephalographic technique (EEG) has an excellent temporal resolution that allows us to obtain recordings of brain electrical activity from milliseconds to hours, days and even months. It is probably due to this advantage that the EEG is still used in numerous laboratories around the world.

The electroencephalogram (EEG) is defined as a mixture of rhythmic sinusoidal-like fluctuations in voltage generated by the brain that, it has been suggested, represent the global activity from the pyramidal cells of the cortex and the activity of neurons in the subcortical structures. Another more specific technique that has been used to study the functioning of brain structures is multiple unit activity (MUA), which is a general index of the net activity within a certain neuronal population. It represents a relatively large and mixed sample of local activity in which different kinds of neurons may be present. The net increase or decrease of MUA may reflect both the involvement of a given brain structure in the neuronal mechanisms of specific behaviors and the predominant response (increase or decrease of firing) of its neuronal components (Buchwald et al., 1973; Olds, 1973; Horio et al, 1986). Finally, the most detailed and specific electrophysiological technique involves the single unit activity recordings of neurons in a particular cerebral region that, it has been suggested, represents the action potentials fired by a certain neuron.

The quantitative analysis of EEG is a useful tool that has allowed researchers to relate changes in brain electrical activity to specific behavioral situations and/or experimental manipulations. Several studies in animals related to sexual and maternal behaviors have been published (Schwartz and Whalen, 1965; Kurtz and Adler, 1973; Holmes and Egan, 1973; Kurtz, 1975; Michael et al., 1977; Lincoln et al., 1980; Bennet et al., 1982; McIntosh et al., 1984; Mead and Vanderwolf, 1992). In contrast, very few studies have been done on humans to correlate the EEG of different cortical areas with the motivational and performance aspects of sexual and maternal behaviors (Mosovich and Tallaferro, 1954; Heath, 1972; Cohen et al., 1976, 1985; Tucker and Dawson, 1984; Graber et al., 1985; Rosen et al., 1986; Cervantes et al., 1992).

Taking into account that behavior results from the simultaneous and coordinated functioning of various cerebral structures, and considering that EEG recordings are a useful tool for investigating the simultaneous functioning of several brain structures in a precise temporal relation with the performance of specific behaviors, several of the studies conducted in our laboratory have been designed to characterize the functioning of the prefrontal cortex and other limbic structures during the motivational states and motor activities involved in the sexual and maternal behaviors of rats. Thus, we have developed different techniques of quantitative analysis to examine EEG recordings, and this has allowed us to obtain information that simple visual observation cannot (Hernández-González et al., 1977a, 1997b; Guevara et al., 2003; Guevara et al., 2005).

The methodology used in all such experiments was similar. Electrodes made of stainless-steel wire (0.2 mm in diameter), insulated with epoxy resin except for a small recording area left exposed at the tip, were implanted in specific cortical and subcortical structures of male or female rats, following the stereotaxic coordinates of Paxinos and Watson atlas (1997). The cable connecting the electrodes implanted in the rat was then connected to a slip-ring. This arrangement allowed the rats free movement and during this time the EEGs from the brain structures were recorded continuously. The cables were connected to the AC preamplifiers of a Grass 7B polygraph (band pass 3-30 Hz) and their outputs plugged into a PCL-812 analog-to-digital converter (Advantech, Co.), which operated as an interface to a microcomputer (PC-compatible). The EEG signals were recorded at a sampling rate of 256 Hz and calibrated with a pulse of 50 microvolts (μV), produced by the preamplifiers and delivered to a PC as a reference to convert the output of the analog-to-digital converter into μV. The capturing of the EEG signals that corresponded to each one of the different conditions was performed using a board unit with eight on/off buttons connected to the digital input lines of the PCL-812. Thus, capturing of 2-sec segments of EEG corresponding to the different behavioral situation began when a specific button on the board unit was pressed; while a different button was pushed to terminate signal input. Absolute power (AP) between 4 and 21 Hz was calculated by means of a Fast Fourier Transformation (FFT) and power densities were obtained for each Hz value. The raw EEG signals were digitally filtered according to the new boundaries using a rectangular window, and relative power (RP) (the proportional contribution of each band expressed as a percentage of total power between 4 and 21 Hz) was calculated for each band of frequencies. It has been suggested that the degree of correlation (r) between two neural regions is indicated by the degree of similarity between the EEG activity at the two sites (López da Silva, 1991), which in turn is the outcome of the functional state of the neuronal networks (Shaw, 1984). Low r reflects higher functional differences and vice versa; higher r reflects a more homogeneous functioning between structures. Thus, the inter- and intra-hemispheric correlation was obtained in the time domain for the same bands by means of Pearson product-moment correlation coefficients between successive amplitude values of EEG segments from the left and right cortical and subcortical regions.

Prefrontal EEG Activity in Relation to Male Sexual Motivation

At the beginning of this chapter, we described that the prefrontal cortex of rats is divided into two main functionally-distinct subregions: the medial (mPFC) and orbital (oPFC) prefrontal cortices (Yonemori, 2000; Kesner, 2000; Uylings et al., 2003). Lesions in these prefrontal areas induce different alterations in the male rat's sexual behavior; however, no one has yet investigated whether or not the subregions of the PFC play different roles in the motivational aspects and, more specifically, in the approach phase during which the detection and processing of the stimuli emitted by the female occur. Hence, to explore the functionality of the mPFC and oPFC in the sexual motivation of the male rat, an experiment was designed (Hernández-González, et al., 2007) to examine the characteristic EEG patterns during approach behavior in a T-maze, and to determine whether these EEG patterns vary through the different behaviors performed by sexually-motivated or non-sexually-motivated male rats.

Brown and colleagues (1974) have reported that every sexual intromission (used as reinforcers) increases sexual arousal considerably until the male reaches ejaculation. Thus, the sexually-motivated condition was generated in the male such that before recording in the T maze he had 1 or 2 intromissions with a receptive female rat and was then immediately placed in the start box, with one receptive and one non-receptive female in the goal-boxes of the T maze (Figure 2). In the non-motivated condition, the male rats were placed in the start box without previous intromission and the goal boxes in the lateral arms were empty.

One group of male rats was bilaterally implanted in the mPFC and the other group in the oPFC. The experiment was conducted on a T-shaped apparatus made of polyurethane-sealed wood that consisted of a brown wood start alley with a start box at one end and two lateral arms with goal boxes at the other. The start box was separated from the start alley by a wooden, guillotine door. At the end of each arm was a small goal box with an opening covered with wire mesh. This meant that the male could hear, see and smell the females, but no copulatory interaction was possible, though some limited physical contact through the wire mesh could occur (Figure 2).

The procedure followed for resolving the T maze in the sexually- and non-sexually motivated task was as follows. Briefly, each rat was placed in the start box for about 5 min, during which time the basal EEG in the awake-quiet condition was recorded. Immediately after this, the guillotine door was raised and the EEG was recorded during the walk through the maze stem and during the time they remained anywhere near the goal boxes of the lateral arms. The EEG from the left and right mPFC and oPFC was recorded simultaneously under different conditions in the T maze, as described previously.

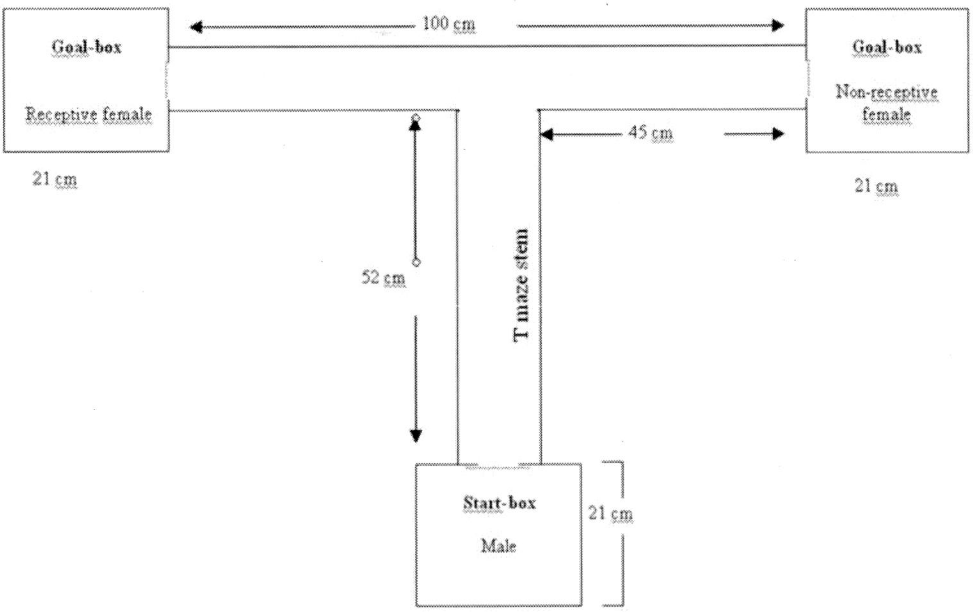

Figure 2. Schematic representation of the wood T-maze used to recording the EEG of male rats during the sexually-motivated (with previous intromission and one receptive and one non-receptive females placed in the goal boxes of the lateral arms); and not sexually-motivated (no previous intromission and empty goal boxes) conditions. For a description of details, see text.

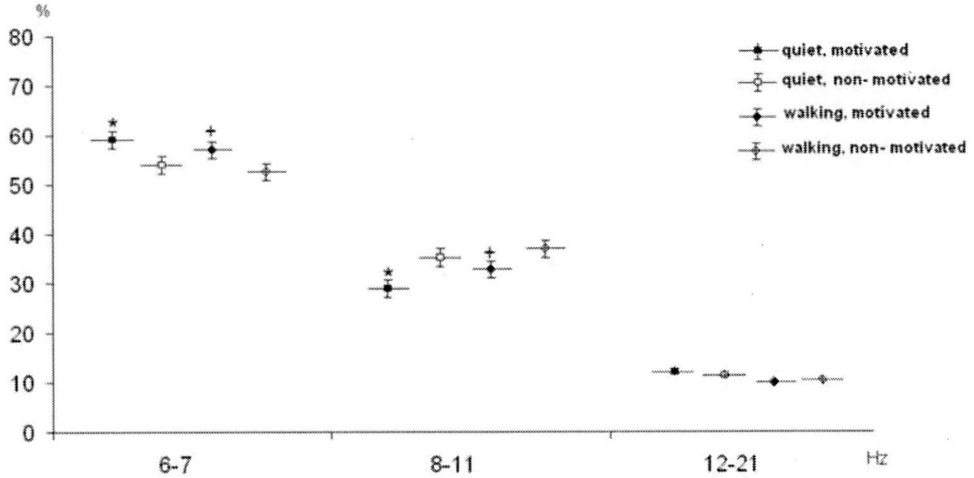

* $p < 0.05$ as compared to awake-quiet condition in the non-motivated male rats.
+ $p < 0.05$ as compared to walking condition in the non-motivated male rats.

Figure 3, Mean and standard error of Relative power (%) of three frequency bands in the left medial prefrontal cortex (mPFC) during the awake-quiet condition and walking of the sexually and non-sexually motivated male rats. Two way ANOVA for repeated measurements and Tukey tests.

In general terms, the sexually-motivated male rats showed a higher motivation for engaging in sexual behavior compared to the non-sexually motivated ones, as has been demonstrated in other studies (Pfaff and Agmo, 2002; López and Ettenberg, 2001).

An increased relative power (RP) of the low frequencies (6-7 Hz) and a decrease in the 8-11 Hz band was observed in the mPFC during the awake-quiet state in the start box and during the walk in the maze only in the sexually-motivated males (Figure 3). This increase in the RP of the 6-7 Hz band may be associated with the arousal or general activation that characterizes the motivated state, as well as with the orientation of the male's movements, as has been shown in other studies (Gemmel and O´Mara, 1999).

Only the sexually-motivated males presented a higher interprefrontal correlation of the 6-7 Hz band during the walk in the maze stem and during the time they remained near the goal box that contained a receptive female (Figure 4).

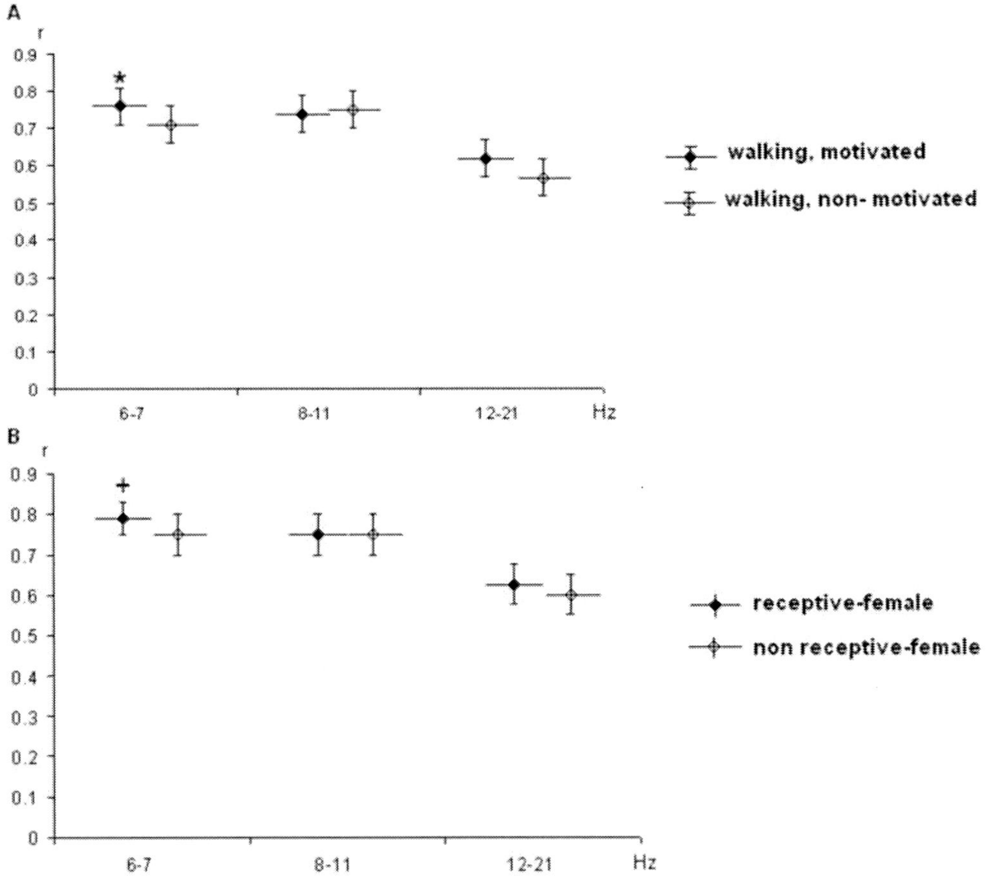

* $p \leq 0.01$ as compared to walking in the non-motivated male rats.

+ $p \leq 0.05$ as compared to sexually motivated rats when remained near to goal boxes with a non-receptive female.

Figure 4. Mean and standard error of Interprefrontal correlation transformed to Fisher´s Z scores of three frequency bands in motivated and non-motivated rats during the walking in the T maze (A) and during the time they remained near to goal boxes with receptive or non-receptive females (B).

In the oPFC, only the RP of the 6-7 Hz band increased whereas the RP of the 8-11 Hz band was decreased as the motivated males walked through the maze stem (Figure 5). Various studies have demonstrated that distal stimuli from a receptive female function primarily to arouse and orient males, so that it is possible that the higher RP values in the 6-7 Hz band in both the mPFC and the oPFC among the sexually-motivated males during the walk in the maze stem may be associated with various processes: the "motivated state" that results from intromission with the female before entering the maze; spatial orientation and selection of the goal; and the processing of the odors and sounds received from the female. It would not be unfounded, then, to suggest that both subregions of the prefrontal cortex manifest a similar functionality during the walk in the maze stem, given the extensive series of anatomical interconnections they possess.

This data suggests that in sexually-motivated males the mPFC is involved in the anticipatory processes *–i.e.*, sensory processing and assigning the incentive value– and in motor execution during the performance of the T maze task, whereas the oPFC is only involved in the motor execution of the T maze (Hernández-González, et al., 2007).

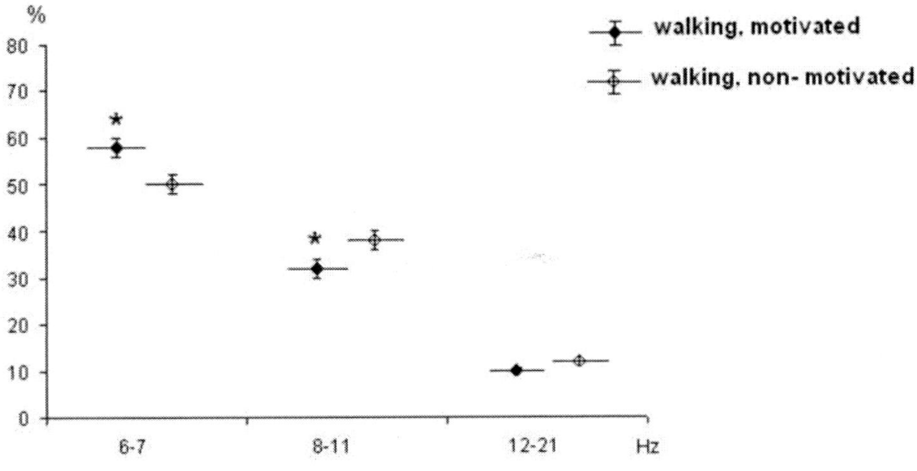

* $p \leq 0.01$ as compared to walking in the non-motivated male rats.

Figure 5, Mean and standard error of Relative power (%) of three frequency bands in the left orbital prefrontal cortex (oPFC) during the walking of the sexually and non-sexually motivated rats. Two way ANOVA for repeated measurements and Tukey tests.

Another study showed that the different frequency bands of the prefrontal EEG were precisely correlated in time with well-defined motor components of the male rat's copulatory activity, as well as with the behaviors related to the motivational or approach phase. The copulatory pelvic movements of the male rats were recorded by means of an accelerometric technique described elsewhere (Contreras and Beyer, 1979; Hernández-González, et al., 1993). A cloth harness was adapted to the rat without causing it any discomfort. At the level of the pelvis, the harness carried a strain gauge transducer (Entran EGB-125-50DC miniature accelerometer) that measures acceleration on a plane. The accelerometer was connected to a DC preamplifier coupled to a Grass 7B polygraph and the output was plugged into a PCL-812 analog-to-digital converter (Advantech, Co.) that operated as an interface to a microcomputer. Electrical signals generated by the accelerometer during pelvic thrusting were continuously recorded at a sampling rate of 128 Hz on the microcomputer for further correlation with EEGs from the prefrontal cortex and the MUA activity from the ventral tegmental area (VTA) and the pedunculopontine nucleus (PPN) (Figure 6).

In the prefrontal cortex, the absolute power (AP) of the different frequency bands (4-16, 18-24 and 26-32 Hz) showed characteristic changes in relation to the execution of pelvic thrusting during mounting, intromission and the ejaculation responses. The approach behaviors, such as orientation and persecution of the female rat that, it has been suggested, are an index of sexual motivation, were correlated with a decreased AP of the fast frequencies and a increases of the low frequencies. Thus, these results confirmed that the electroencephalographic activity of the prefrontal cortex of the male rat is related to the motivation and performance of its sexual behavior (Hernández-González, et al., 1998). The average MUA firing rate in the VTA and PPN increased during pursuit of the female, further augmented during the execution of the pelvic thrusting trains of mounting, intromission and ejaculation responses, and decreased immediately after the pelvic thrusting ended.

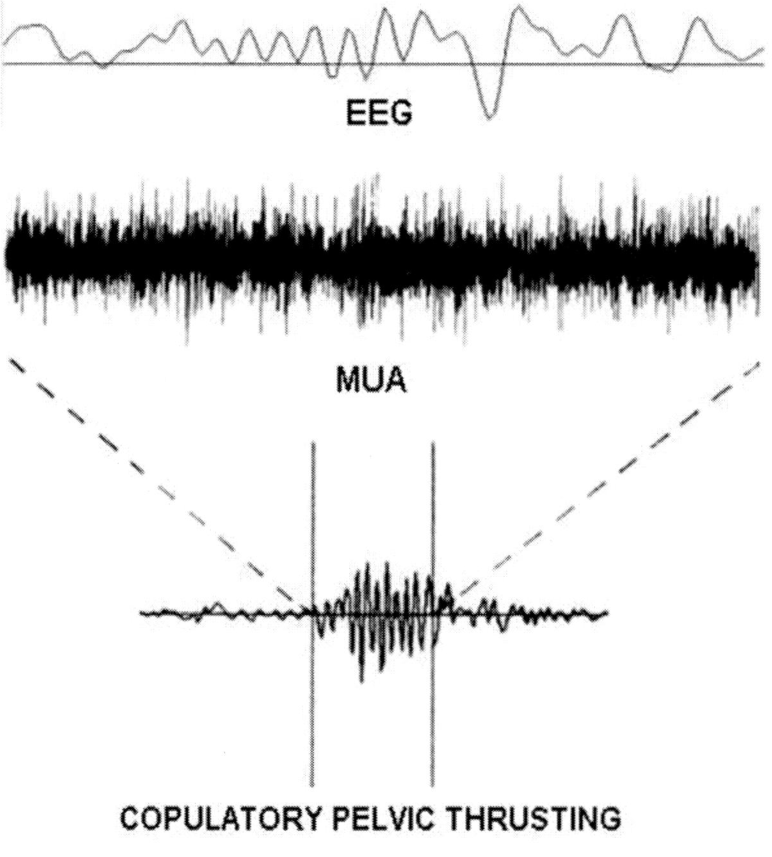

Figure 6. Tracings corresponding to the simultaneous recording of EEG from mPFC and MUA from VTA in relation to the accelerometric recording of pelvic thrusting performed during a 500-msec period corresponding to a ejaculation response.

Similar changes in the MUA firing rate of the medial preoptic area (mPOA) were found by Horio et al. (1986) during both pursuit and pelvic thrusting. It has been suggested that the VTA is involved in the motivational and/or motor aspects of male copulatory behavior (Eibergen and Caggiula, 1973; Hull et al., 1990; Hull et al., 1991), whereas the PPN, located in the caudal mesencephalic tegmentum, is a major component of the mesencephalic locomotor region (MLR) (Grillner and Shik, 1973). Thus, it can be suggested that the VTA and PPN are involved in the motor aspects of the male rat's copulatory activity, though implications in the motivational process could also be proposed.

It is clear, then, that according to the above description of the EEG and MUA studies, the PFC manifests a characteristic functionality in relation to the motivational and motor components of sexual behavior.

Prefrontal EEG Activity in Relation to Female Sexual Motivation

Various reports have shown that the estrous cycle of the rat is a process modulated by hormonal changes that, in turn, are associated with changes of the attraction or sensitivity with which females perceive different sensory stimuli (Pietras and Moulton, 1974; Guevara-Guzman et al., 1997). It is known that during the estrous phase the female rat shows typical receptive and proceptive behaviors associated with the emission of specific vocalizations and odors that together constitute the essential signals with sexual meaning emitted by a receptive female. Moreover, it has been demonstrated that when estrous female rats receive 2-5 intromissions their behavioral proceptivity is increased (Erskine et al., 1989; Rowe and Erskine, 1993; Coopersmith et al., 1996). Thus, in an effort to determine whether the functionality of the oPFC and mPFC prefrontal subregions in female rats is different from that seen in sexually-motivated males, another study was carried out in our laboratory. There, female rats chronically implanted in the oPFC and mPFC were submitted to a sexually-motivated task using the same paradigm of the T maze (Guevara et al., 2004). In this experiment, female rats in the estrous phase received 1 or 2 intromissions in order to increase their sexual proceptivity (and probably sexual motivation to engage in sexual interaction). The procedure for the performance in the T maze test was similar to that used in the previous study, except that in the sexually-motivated test a sexually-active male was placed in one of the goal boxes, whereas in the non-motivated test, the goal boxes remained empty.

The sexually-motivated female rats showed clear behavioral indices of a high motivation to engage in sexual behavior.

During the walk in the T maze stem, the sexually-motivated females showed in the mPFC an increased RP of the low frequencies (4-7 Hz), a decrease in the 8-11 Hz band (Figure 7), and an increased interprefrontal correlation between the left and right mPFC of the 4-7 Hz band; whereas during the awake-quiet state, the mPFC of the sexually-motivated females showed a decreased RP of the low frequencies and an increased RP of the 8-11 Hz band.

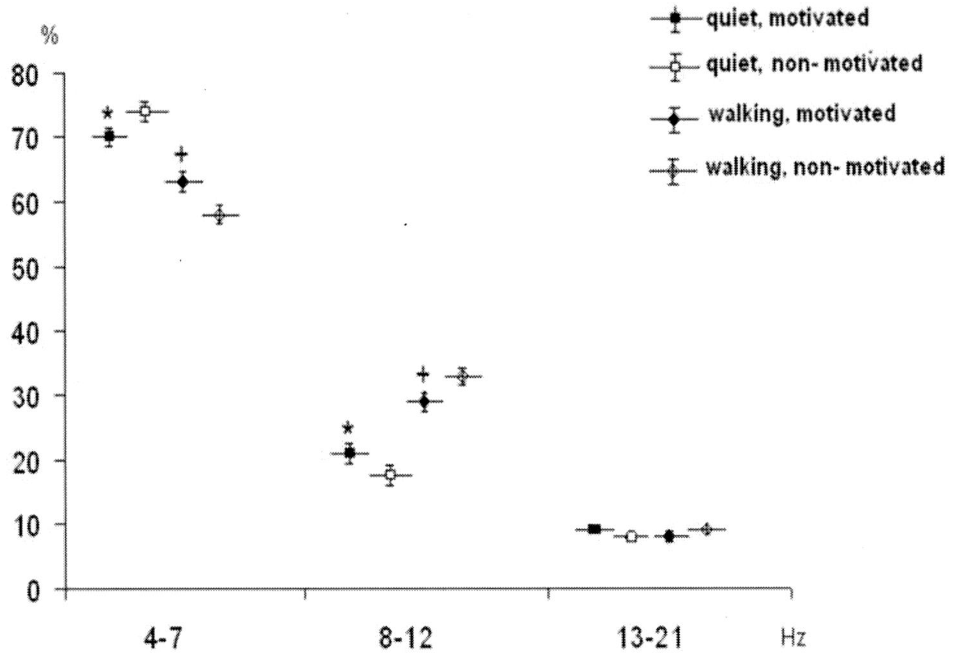

* $p < 0.05$ as compared to awake-quiet condition in the non-motivated female rats.
+ $p < 0.05$ as compared to walking condition in the non-motivated female rats.

Figure 7. Mean and standard error of Relative power (%) of three frequency bands in the left medial prefrontal cortex (mPFC) during the awake-quiet condition and walking of the sexually and non-sexually motivated female rats. Two way ANOVA for repeated measurements and Tukey tests.

These EEG data suggest that in sexually-motivated male and female rats the functionality of the mPFC is similar during the processing of signals that allow the orientation of the subject's movements in the T maze, as well as with the "aroused state" that results from penile or vagino-cervical stimulation (by intromission) before entering the maze. This similar functioning of the mPFC could also be associated with the processing of odors and sounds that are received from the sexual partner. In contrast, during the awake-quiet state, the EEG of the mPFC in sexually-motivated female rats was different from those observed in the sexually-motivated males.

The electroencephalographic functioning of the oPFC in sexually-motivated females was characterized by an increased RP of the low frequencies during the awake-quiet state. A similar EEG pattern in the oPFC of sexually-motivated males was observed during the walk in the maze stem. It is probable that this high proportion of the low frequencies in the oPFC is associated with the general motivated state of the subjects without taking into account the behavior that the male or female rat performs.

The results of this study concord with the data obtained in males, and show that when rats of both sexes are sexually motivated the functioning of the prefrontal subregions is different compared to that of the prefrontal subregions in non-sexually-motivated subjects. Taken together, these data support the idea that the functioning of the prefrontal subregions varies according to the sexually-motivated state of male and female rats.

Prefrontal EEG Activity in Relation to Maternal Motivation

Maternal behavior is also a motivated behavior, which in rats consists of motorically active behaviors (appetitive behaviors) such as nest repair, pup retrieval, mouthing, licking, and inactive nursing behaviors (consummatory behaviors) that involve a series of postural adjustments and limb immobility that leads to crouching and suckling behaviors (Stern, 1996).

Some lesion and pharmacological studies support the possible involvement of the PFC in maternal behavior. Lesions of the VTA and PFC induce a permanent behavioral syndrome in rats, characterized by locomotor hyperactivity and hypoexploration in an open field (Lemoal et al., 1976; Gaffori and Le Moal, 1979). Lesions of the PFC resulted in alterations such as the disruption of goal-directed behaviors (Kolb, 1984, 1990) and disorganized and persistent retrieving (Stamm, 1955; Slotnick, 1967). A high activation of the mPFC of human mothers while listening to an infant's cries (Lorberbaum et al., 2002), a selective activation of this brain area in dam rats during their first experience with pups (Fleming and Korsmit, 1996; Walsh et al., 1996) and an enhanced c-fos expression in the mPFC of ewes exposed to lambs have all been reported (Kendrik et al., 1997; Broad et al., 2002).

Very few attempts have been made to study brain electrical activity related to maternal behaviors, but the studies that do exist have centered on the hippocampus (Mead and Vanderwolf (1992) or the cortical areas (Lincoln et al., 1980; Cervantes et al., 1992). However, electrical changes in the mPFC in relation to maternal behaviors have not been elucidated; hence, we conducted an experiment to investigate the functioning of the PFC and of the ventral tegmental area (VTA, a subcortical structure that sends the main dopaminergic innervation to PFC) during the motivational (pup retrieval, pup licking) and consummatory (low and high crouching) acts of rat maternal behavior (Hernández-González et al., 2005).

Lactating rats implanted bilaterally in the PFC and VTA were submitted to one or two tests of maternal behavior and EEG recordings were taken between 3 and 10 days post-partum. An EEG baseline was recorded during non-maternal, motorically similar behaviors: 1) walking, recorded during spontaneous horizontal locomotion; 2) forepaw licking, recorded when the female licked her own forepaws; and, 3) awake-quiet condition, recorded when the undisturbed rat, outside the nest, held its head up against gravity with its eyes open and made no movements or only slight vibrissae movements. All baseline recordings were obtained while pups were with their mothers (to eliminate stress in dams due to pup separation). At the start of the 60-min test, the pups were briefly removed and scattered around the opposite side of the nest (to stimulate retrieval) and the EEG was recording during the following maternal behaviors: 1) pup retrieval, recorded when the female picked up a pup in her mouth and carried it to her nest site; 2) pup licking, recorded when the dam picked up a pup with her forepaws and licked the pup's genital region while sitting, but without considering licking or grooming of the head or any other part of the pup's body; 3) low crouching, recorded when the female arched her back over the pups, with the pups underneath, usually with the dam immobile; and, 4) high crouching, recorded when the female positioned herself over the pups, arched her back with all four legs rigidly extended, typically in a splayed position to accommodate the litter mass and allow the pups to suckle. The EEG session was terminated once all behaviors had been performed by the mother or after 1 h.

In both structures, the mPFC and the VTA, a significant increase was obtained in the absolute power of the 8–11 Hz band during pup retrieval compared with basal walking behavior (Figure 8).

During pup licking, the AP of the three frequency bands in the mPFC showed a significant increase compared to forepaw licking, a non-maternal behavior with equivalent postural adjustments and motor elements to those of pup licking. In the VTA, the AP of the 6–7, 8–11 and 12–21 Hz bands also increased during pup licking in relation to forepaw licking (Figure 9).

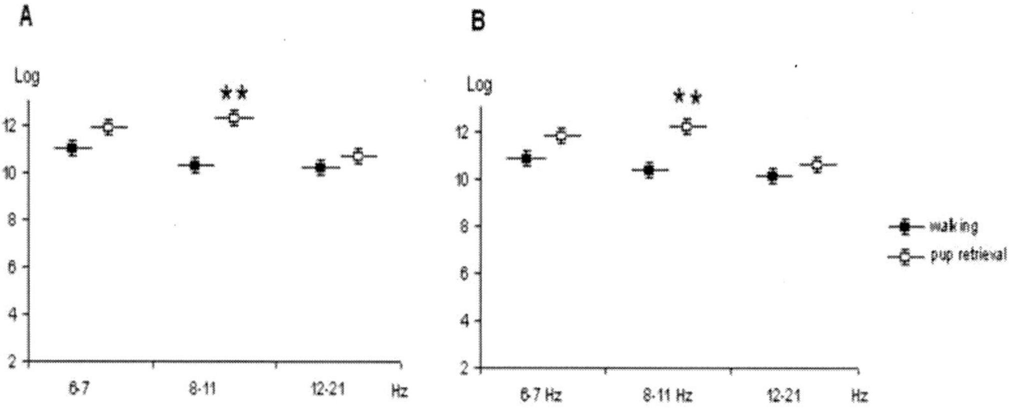

** $p < 0.01$ as compared to walking.

Figure 8. Mean and standard error of absolute power (log) of three frequency bands in medial prefrontal cortex (A) and ventral tegmental area (B) during walking and pup retrieval of dam rats. One-way ANOVA for repeated measurements and Tukey tests.

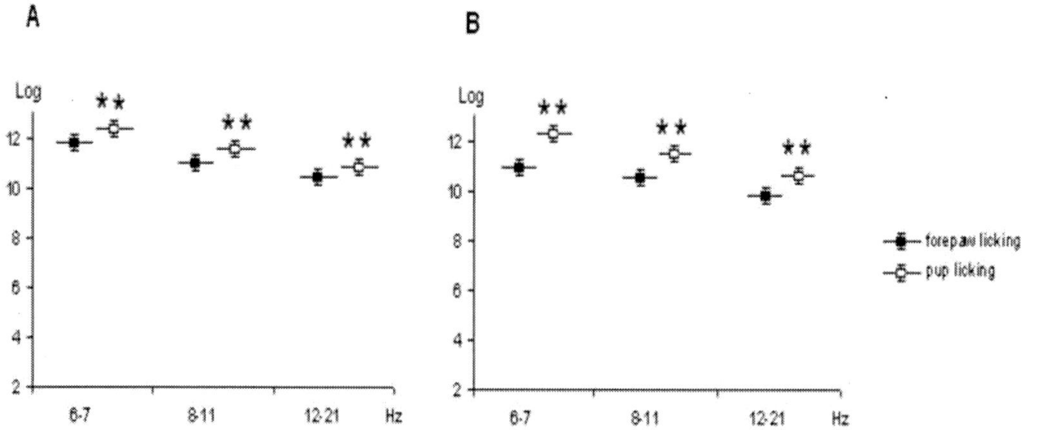

** $p < 0.01$ as compared to forepaw licking.

Figure 9. Mean and standard error of absolute power (log) of three frequency bands in medial prefrontal cortex (A) and ventral tegmental area (B) during forepaw licking and pup licking of dam rats. One-way ANOVA for repeated measurements and Tukey tests.

Various studies have suggested a major role for the medial prefrontal cortex in modulating sequential behaviors and in the spatial orientation of motivated behaviors (Kolb et al., 1983, 1989; Kolb, 1990; Kolb and Cioe, 2004;); thus, one possible explanation is that the increase in the AP of the 8–11 Hz band in mPFC is related to spatial orientation or sequential organization processing performed in this cortical area during pup retrieval acts.

The medial prefrontal cortex receives highly processed sensory information from visual, auditory and somatosensory regions (Groenewegen and Uylings, 2000) and, like the VTA, has been implicated in the integration of motor action with sensory information (Mogenson et al., 1980; Kolb and Cioe, 2004;). Therefore, one possible explanation of the increased AP of the 8–11 Hz band in the mPFC and the VTA during pup retrieval is that this cortical functioning reflects a motivational state and/or sensory processing in these brain structures while the dam is engaged in this activity.

In the left and right mPFC and VTA a clear increment of AP was found in the three bands during pup licking compared to forepaw licking. According to Stern's classification (1996), pup retrieval and pup licking are motorically active behaviors that precede and contribute to the success of dam-initiated nursing and hence form part of the appetitive aspects of maternal behaviors. The VTA has been considered a critical structure in the integration of multimodal stimuli and their transmission to the performance systems (Mogenson et al., 1980; Mirenowicz and Schultz, 1996). Moreover, it has been found that the unit activity of the VTA increases during appetitive behaviors but decreases during consummatory acts (Nishino et al., 1986). Hence, the higher potency of the three bands that appears in the mPFC and the VTA during pup licking is probably associated with the performance of this appetitive behavior and could reflect the particular functioning of these structures in the global neural circuit responsible for pup licking behavior.

An interesting observation based on the present results is that during inactive maternal behaviors –low and high crouching– the mPFC and VTA showed no EEG changes compared to the awake-quiet basal state. Given that these inactive maternal behaviors constitute the consummatory components of maternal care, it is probable that the lack of EEG changes during low and high crouching could be associated with the low participation of the PFC and the VTA in the manifestation of these behaviors, as well as with the consummatory aspects characteristic of the maternal behaviors. Present results demonstrate that both motorically active maternal behaviors are related to a different neural processing in the mPFC and VTA, which could support the suggestion that the mPFC and VTA are involved in processing sensory stimuli to promote adequate motivational and motor responses concerned with maternal behavior.

It is well known that the perception of sensory stimuli, particularly olfactory and somatosensory ones (Pietras and Moulton, 1974; Guevara-Guzman et al., 1997), the willingness of cycling female rats to show maternal behavior or sexual behavior (González and Deis 1986), and the excitability and electrical activity of several brain structures (Corsí-Cabrera et al., 1992; Guevara-Guzman et al., 1997; Contreras et al., 2000) vary through the estrous cycle. Gonadal hormones affect the sensitivity at which the sensory stimuli are perceived and processed by the subjects, and throughout the different reproductive states of the female rat evident changes in hormonal levels appear. Maternal behavior is a motivated behavior that, like sexual interaction, requires an appropriate integration between external stimuli and internal states for its adequate manifestation. There are reports that sensory clues from the pups are important reinforcers for mother rats (Oley and Slotnick., 1970; Stern and Mackinnon, 1976).

Thus, with the aim of investigating the importance of gonadal hormones for the impact of olfactory stimuli on the brain functionality of female rats, in another study we explored whether the PFC and VTA show characteristic EEG patterns during the presentation of olfactory stimuli either associated or not-associated with pups, and whether these EEG patterns vary across the different reproductive states of the female rat (proestrus-estrus, diestrus and lactation).

Virgin female rats were bilaterally implanted in both hemispheres, specifically into the mPFC and the VTA. EEG recordings were obtained in the proestrous-estrous (P-E) and diestrous (D) states (determined through analyses of vaginal smears), and the female rats were then mated with a sexually-active male until they received three ejaculations. During the gestation period, they were housed individually and the first day on which a litter was found was counted as post-partum day 1. The EEG recordings of the lactating female rats (L) were performed during the first 8 days postpartum. The procedure followed for olfactory stimulation was the same as that previously used by Bressler and Baum (1996). Briefly, each rat was placed in the recording cage (with clean sawdust bedding) where it remained at least 5 min before the test. A glass recipient with either nest bedding (obtained from a plexiglas cage where a lactating female rat and its pups had been housed at least 6 h before) or female bedding (obtained from a plexiglas cage where 4-5 virgin female rats, at least two in proestrus-estrus and two in diestrus, had been housed at least 6 h earlier) was placed in a corner of the recording cage, opposite from where the female rat stayed. The EEG from the left and right mPFC and VTA was recorded simultaneously during three different conditions: 1) awake-quiet (no olfactory stimulus present); 2) smelling of nest bedding; and, 3) smelling of female bedding. In all conditions, the EEG was recorded while the undisturbed rat held its eyes open and while the female´s four paws were beneath her, without making any movement with the exception of slight vibrissae movements. The presentation of both olfactory stimuli was randomly counterbalanced and the interval between the presentations of each stimulus was 15 min.

Lactating rats presented the highest frequency of smelling the nest material as compared to P-E and D rats and also remained a longer time smelling the nest bedding compared to P-E rats. When the females were exposed to female bedding, no significant differences were observed in any of these parameters among the different reproductive states, suggesting that the lactating rats showed the highest motivation to approach to the olfactory stimuli associated with pups.

During the awake-quiet condition, which was considered as the basal EEG recording, the lactating rats showed an increased RP of the 12-21 Hz band in the mPFC (Figure 10) and VTA compared to both the P-E and D rats. In L rats, in which estrogen levels are decreased, the EEG activity of mPFC and VTA was characterized by a predominance of fast frequencies that may represent a possible increased arousal state similar to an anxiety state that could result from pup separation (Hard and Hansen, 1985; Ferreira et al., 1989), or could be result from the diminished levels of estrogens as has been reported in other studies (Fernandez-Guasti and Picazzo, 1992; Picazo and Fernández-Guasti, 1993; Guevara-Guzmán et al., 1997;

Contreras et al., 2000; Morgan and Paff., 2002). Thus, it is possible that in the present study the increased proportion of fast frequencies in L rats could be associated with a moderate level of anxiety or alertness that presumably optimizes the motivational state of the L rats to search for their pups.

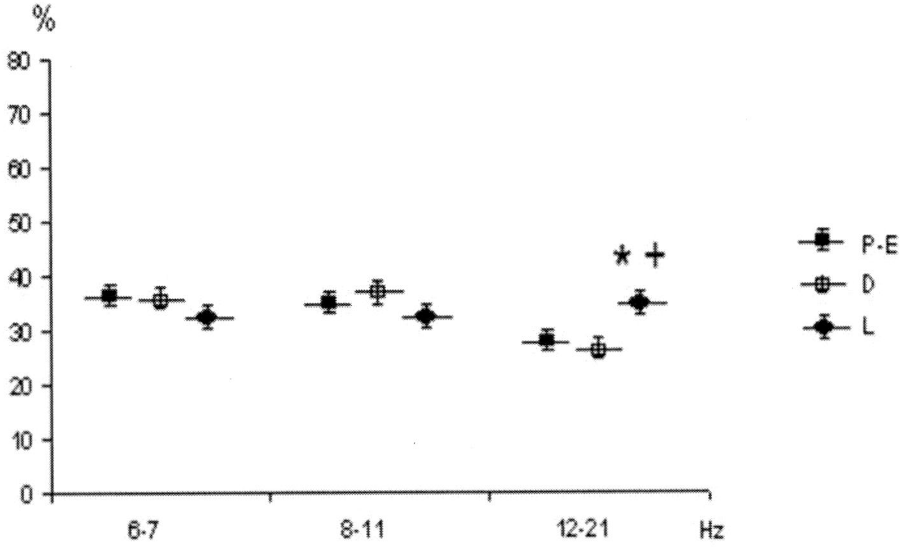

* $p < 0.05$ as compared to P-E rats.
\+ $p < 0.05$ as compared to D rats.

Figure 10. Mean and standard error of Relative power (%) of the three frequency bands in the medial prefrontal cortex during the awake-quiet condition of female rats in different reproductive states: Proestrus-estrus (P-E), diestrus (D), and lactation (L). Two way ANOVA for repeated measurements and Tukey tests.

During the smelling of nest bedding, the RP of the 8-11 Hz band in the mPFC of L rats became increased while that of the 6-7 and 12-21 Hz bands decreased as compared to the P-E and D rats (Figure 11).

In the VTA, this phenomenon was observed mainly in the lactating rats. Moreover, the interprefrontal r values of the three frequency bands, mainly those of the 8-11 Hz band, was increased in the D and L rats during the smelling of nest bedding, so that only the olfactory stimuli associated with pups resulted in a higher degree of similarity between the EEG activity of the two cortices (Figure 12).

During the smelling of female bedding, no significant differences were observed between reproductive states. The fact that in both structures of the L rats the slow rhythmical activity showed the main changes in relation to the smelling of nest bedding could be associated with the "relaxed behavior" that L rats showed upon finding pup-associated odors, the higher attraction of the dams for the odor of pups, or both processes. Various L rats showed a behavioral pattern that could be associated with "relaxed behavior"; *i.e.*, they remained on the nest bedding for some time in a sleep-like state. Because these EEG changes characterized by slow rhythmical waves in these structures, is manifested in association to relevant olfactory odors from the nest bedding, which could be associated with a "relaxed state" only in L rats.

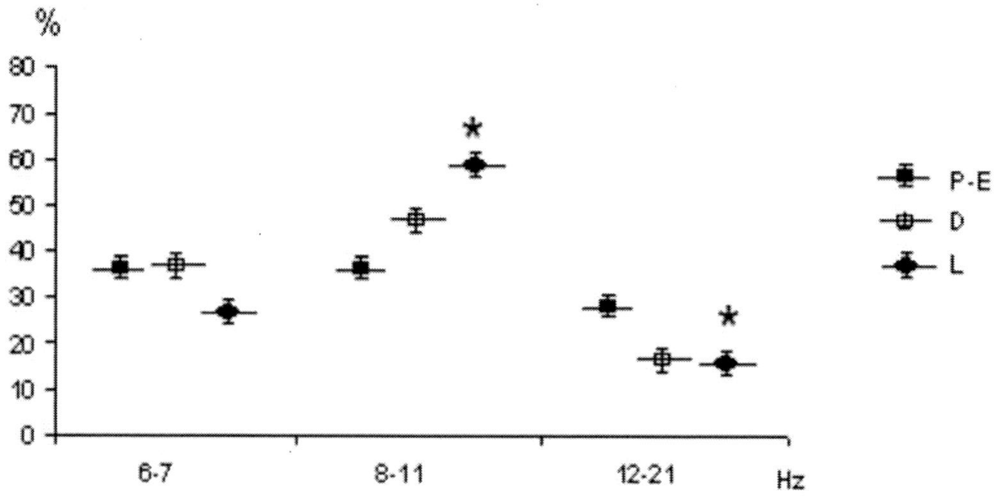

* $p < 0.05$ as compared to P-E and D rats.

Figure 11. Mean and standard error of Relative power (%) of the three frequency bands in the medial prefrontal cortex during the smelling of nest bedding in female rats under different reproductive states: Proestrus-estrus (P-E), diestrus (D), lactation (L). Two way ANOVA for repeated measurements and Tukey tests.

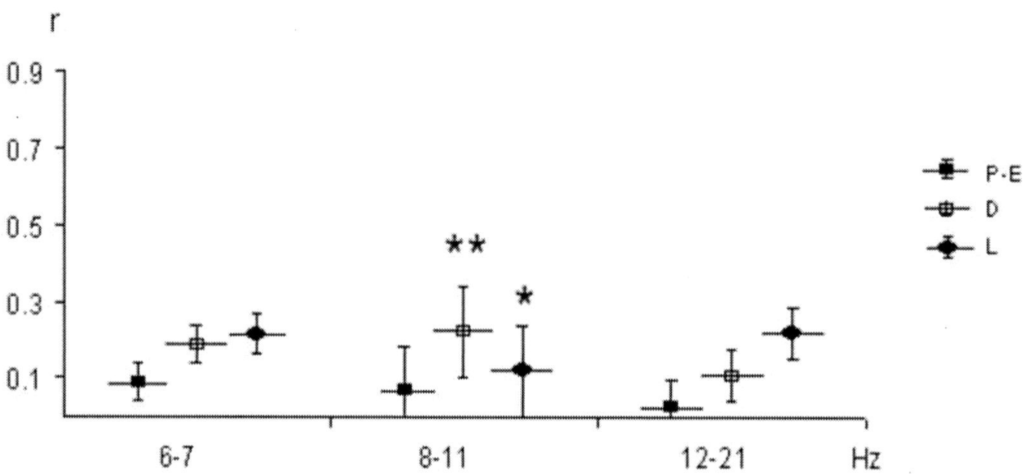

** $p \leq 0.01$ as compared to P-E rats.
+ $p \leq 0.05$ as compared to P-E rats.

Figure 12. Mean and standard error of Interprefrontal correlation transformed to Fisher´s Z scores of the three frequency bands in female rats under different reproductive states: proestrus-estrus (P-E), diestrus (D) and lactation (L) during the smelling of nest bedding.

Although the mPFC and VTA are not directly implicated in olfactory perception, various studies have suggested an important role for these structures in sensory information processing. For example, it has been found that the mPFC neurons show different responses to conditioned sensory stimuli (auditory or visual) when associated, or not, with a reward (Takenouchi et al., 1999; Jodo et al., 2000), and that the mPFC shows an enhanced metabolic activation in response to the presentation of emotionally-relevant maternal nursing calls (Braun and Poegel., 2001). The VTA has also been shown to present a discriminated response of the neurons in association to rewarded and non-rewarded stimuli (Mirenowicz and Schultz., 1996), and in various studies the VTA has been considered as a critical structure in the integration of multimodal stimuli and their transmission to the performance systems (Mogenson et al., 1980). Thus, it is possible that the higher proportion of slow frequency bands in the mPFC and VTA of L rats in association to smelling of nest bedding could represent a characteristic processing of the olfactory stimuli related to pups, so that, as other studies have suggested (Thompson and Kristal, 1996), these structures may participate in the adequate integration of olfactory stimuli to modulate the motivational and performance aspects of maternal behavior.

It has been suggested that distal stimuli from the pups function primarily to arouse and orient the dams (Stern, 1989), so it is possible that the higher r values of the 8-11 Hz band in L rats during the olfaction of nest bedding is associated with various processes: the “relaxed behavior” that L rats showed when they smelled pup-associated odors, the higher attraction of the dams for pup odor, or the processing of olfactory mediated responses (as was proposed by Fleming and Korsmith (1996). It should be noted that all of these events will contribute to reinforcing dams with respect to pups and hence to maternal motivation. Thus, it is possible to suggest that the mPFC and VTA participate in the adequate integration of olfactory stimuli associated with pups in L rats and so modulate the reinforcement and motivational processes that play a crucial role in the expression of maternal behavior.

Conclusion

Since the pioneering work of Beach (1940) on the participation of the cortex in the male rat’s sexual behavior, a few studies have been carried out in relation to this topic. One possible reason for the limited interest in studies of the prefrontal cortex and sexual behavior is Beach’s proposal that the cerebral cortex is of little importance for such behaviors. However, that view was challenged in a few reports that showed that some cortical areas were indeed important for copulation, while others were less so. More recent studies have found that the selective destruction of the prefrontal cortex has deleterious effects on many aspects of copulatory and maternal behavior, including the processing of incentive stimuli and, therefore, motivational aspects. One of the crucial elements in inducing subjects to engage in a motivated behavior is the adequate processing of the incentive stimuli. The prefrontal cortex is one of the neural substrates that participate in the processing of the stimuli necessary to induce and maintain a motivated state, and this chapter has reviewed several EEG studies of the PFC that show how characteristic changes in the functionality of the mPFC and oPFC, manifested in a predominance of rhythmical slow waves, were observed in association with the presentation of incentive stimuli with sexual or maternal meaning in male and female rats. It seems, therefore, possible to conclude that the PFC does indeed play an important role in the motivated conditions of the subjects. To what degree this different prefrontal functionality could be an index of the processing of the sensory stimuli that induce the motivated state or the general arousal state related to sexual or maternal behaviors is a difficult question to resolve, but taken together, these results constitute a good approximation to knowledge of the neural basis involved in the processing of incentive stimuli and hence, in sexual and maternal motivation.

In the section on the neural bases of sexual and maternal behavior, the pivotal role that the medial preoptic area plays in the three motivated behaviors discussed here was specified. In relation to this aspect Agmo, in his recent book (2007), has suggested an interesting proposition with respect to female sexual behavior "*The sensory input generated by distant stimuli needs to be elaborated somewhere else and given sexual significance before it is directed to the preoptic area. I have suggested that the medial prefrontal cortex may be the site where this stimulus elaboration occurs*." Considering the anatomical similarities in the neural substrates and the large amount of overlap in the cerebral circuits that regulate male and female sexual behaviors and maternal behavior, it would not be illogical to think that this proposal could be applied to these three motivated behaviors. In this context, Newman (1999) has suggested that it is possible that a common central network exists, and that the exact behavior that occurs may be determined by the stimuli that have access to this neural circuit. Therefore, it is possible that the prefrontal cortex has an important involvement in the processing and assignation of the incentive value of the specific stimuli for sexual and maternal behavior.

Motivated states such as sexual and maternal behaviors are temporal processes that have a beginning and an end, whose intensity varies through the time and –depending on the feasibility of reaching the goal and the consequences of doing so– the willingness of the subjects to engage again in these motivated behaviors may change. In the case of sexual and maternal motivation, this changes during sexual and maternal interaction. It has been suggested that the ordered sequence of events within a specific behavior can be understood as an interplay between reciprocal short-term excitatory and inhibitory influences (Agmo, 1999), so it is probable that this excitatory-inhibitory interplay could be associated with brief periods of high and low motivation that are intercalated in the temporal sequence of the motivated behavior, which may then be associated with specific changes in cerebral functioning. In light of these considerations, the EEG technique has an important advantage in that it allows the researcher to obtain data with a high temporal resolution, a critical point indeed in investigating the functioning of several brain structures along the entire sequence of events from the moment that the animal discovers a potential goal (sexual partner or pup) until the successful performance of the sexual or maternal interaction. Thus, although various reports have described a role for the prefrontal cortex in these motivated behaviors, the use of the EEG technique made it possible to obtain a precise temporal correlation of the PFC functionality with the motivated states of male and female rats, as well as with the performance of sexual and maternal behaviors. Taken together, the EEG data demonstrate that the prefrontal cortex in rats participates in identifying and processing sexual and maternal incentives.

Acknowledgments

The various research projects discussed herein were supported by a grant to M.H.G. from the "Consejo Nacional de Ciencia y Tecnología" (CONACYT), Grant No. 28592N.

References

Ågmo, A. (1999). Sexual motivation – an inquiry into events determining the occurrence of sexual behavior. *Behav Brain Res*, 105,129-150.

Ågmo, A. (2002). Copulation-contingent aversive conditioning and sexual incentive motivation in male rats: evidence for a two-stage process of sexual behavior. *Physiol Behav*, 77,425-435.

Ågmo, A. (2007). Functional and dysfunctional sexual behavior. A synthesis of neuroscience and comparative psychology. Academic Press, San Diego.

Ågmo, A., Villalpando, A., Picker, Z. and Fernández, H. (1995). Lesions of the medial prefrontal cortex and sexual behavior in the male rat. *Brain Res*, 696, 177-186.

Armony, J, Servan-Schreiber, D.J. and LeDoux, J.E. (1997). Computational modeling of emotion, explorations through the anatomy and physiology of fear conditioning. *Psychol. Rev.,* 81, 199-213.

Balkenius, C. and Morén, J. (2001). Emotional Learning, A computational model of the amygdale. *Cybernet Systems,* 32, 611-636.

Beach F.A. (1940). Effects of cortical lesions upon the copulatory behavior of male rats. *J. Comp. Psychol.*, 29,193-245.

Beach F.A., Zitrin A. and Jaynes J. (1955). Neural mediation of mating in male cats. II. Contributions of the frontal cortex. *J. Exp. Zool.*, 130,381-402.

Beach, F.A. and Jordan, L. (1956). Effects of sexual reinforcement upon the performance of male rats in a straight runway. *J. Comp. Physiol. Psychol.*, 49,105-111.

Beach, F.A. (1976). Sexual attractivity, proceptivity, and receptivity in female mammals. *Horm. Behav.,* 7, 105–138.

Bennet, T., Hill P. and French J. (1982). Biotelemetry recording of the electrical activity of the hippocampus and amygdale during sexual behavior in the cat. *Bull Psychom. Soc.*, 20(1),57-60.

Bermant, G. (1961). Response latencies of female rats during sexual intercourse. *Science,* 133, 1771–1773.

Bitran, D., Hilvers, R.J. and Kellogg, C.K. (1991). Ovarian endocrine status modulates the anxiolytic potency of diazepam and the efficacy of γ-aminobutyric acid-benzodiazepine receptor-mediated chloride ion transport. *Behav. Neurosci.,* 105, 653-662.

Blaustein, J.D. and Erskine, M.S. (2002). Feminine sexual behavior: Cellular integration of hormonal and afferent information in the rodent brain. In: In: DW Pfaff., AP Arnold., AM Etgen., SE Fahrbach., and RT Rubin, (eds.) *Hormones, brain and behavior*. Academic Press, Elsevier Science, USA., Vol. 1, pp. 139-214.

Boling, J.L. and Blandau, R.J. (1939). The estrogen-progesterone induction of mating responses in the spayed female rat. *Endocrinology*, 25(582),6.

Bradford, J.M.W. and Pawlaka, A. (1993). Double-blind placebo crossover study of cyproterone-acetate in the treatment of the paraphilias. *Arch. Sex Behav.*, 22, 629-641.

Braun, K. and Poeggel, G. (2001). Recognition of mother's voice evokes metabolic activation in the medial prefrontal cortex and lateral thalamus of *Octodon degus* pups. *Neuroscience*, 103, 861-864.

Bremer, P. (1958). Asexualization: a follow-up study of 244 cases. Oslo University Press: Oslo Briken, P., Berner, W., Noldus, J., Nika, E. and Michl, U. (2000). Therapie mit dem LHRH-agonisten Leuprolinacetat bei Paraphilien und sexuell aggressiven Impulshandlungen. *Nervenarzt* 71, 380-385.

Bressler, S.C. and Baum, M.J. (1996). Sex comparison of neuronal Fos immunoreactivity in the rat vomeronasal projection circuit after chemosensory stimulation. *Neuroscience*, 71, 1063-1072.

Broad, K.D., Hinton, M.R., Keverne, E.B. and Kendrick, K.M. (2002). Involvement of the medial prefrontal cortex in mediating behavioural responses to odour cues rather than olfactory recognition memory. *Neuroscience*, 114, 715-729.

Broekman, M., de Bruin, M., Smeenk, J., Slob, A.K., and Vander Schoot, P. (1988). Partner preference behavior of estrous female rats affected by castration of tethered male incentives. *Horm. Behav.*, 22, 324–337.

Brown, V.J. and Bowman, E.M. (2002). Rodent models of prefrontal cortical function. *Trends Neurosci.*, 25, 340-343.

Buchwald, J.S., Holstein, S.B. and Weber, D.S. (1973). Multiple unit recording technique, interpretation and experimental application. In RF Thompson., MM Patterson, (eds). *Bioelectric recording techniques*. Vol. 1A. Academic Press, New York. pp. 201-242.

Bunnel, B.N., Friel, J. and Flesher, C.K. (1966). Effects of median cortical lesions on the sexual behaviour of the male hamster. *J. Comp. Physiol. Psychol.*, 61, 492-495.

Cervantes, M., Ruelas, R. and Alcalá, V. (1992). EEG signs of "relaxation behavior" during breast feeding in a nursing woman. *Arch. Med. Res.*, 23, 123-127.

Clark, A.S., Pfeifle, J.K., and Edwards, D.A. (1981). Ventromedial hypothalamic damage and sexual proceptivity in female rats. *Physiol. Behav.*, 27, 597–602.

Cohen H., Rosen R. and Goldstein, L. (1976). Electroencephalographic laterality changes during human sexual orgasm *Arch. Sex Behav.*, 5, 189-199.

Cohen, A.S., Rosen, R.C. and Goldstein, L. (1985). EEG hemispheric asymmetry during sexual arousal: Psyshophysiological patterns in responsive, unresponsive, dysfunctional men. *J. Abnorm. Psychol.*, 94, 580-590.

Contreras, C.M., Molina, M., Saavedra, M. and Martínez-Mota, L. (2000). Lateral septal neuronal firing rate increase during proestrus-estrus in the rat. *Physiol. Behav.*, 68, 279-284.

Contreras, J.L. and Beyer, C.A. (1979). Polygraphic analysis of mounting and ejaculation in the New Zeland white rabbit. *Physiol. Behav.*, 23, 939-943.

Coopersmith C., Candura C., and Erskine M.S. (1996). Effects of paced mating and intromissive stimulation on feminine sexual behavior and estrus termination in the cycling rat. *J. Comp. Psychol.*, 110. 176-186.

Corsi-Cabrera, M., Juárez, J., Ponce-de-Leon, M., Ramos, J. and Velásquez, P.N. (1992). EEG activity during estral cycle in the rat. *Electroenceph Clin Neurophysiol*, 83, 265-269.

Davidson, J.M. (1966). Activation of the male rat´s sexual behavior by intracerebral implantation of androgen. *Endocrinology*, 79, 783-794.

Dempsey, E.W., Hertz, R. and Young, W.C. (1939). The experimental induction of oestrus (sexual receptivity) in the normal and ovariectomized guinea pig. *Am. J. Physiol.*, 116, 201-209.

Denniston, R.H. (1954). Quantification and comparation of sex drives under various conditions in terms of learned responses. *J. Comp. Physiol. Psychol.*, 47, 437-440.

Edwards, D.A., and Pfeifle, J.K. (1983). Hormonal control of receptivity, proceptivity and sexual motivation. *Physiol. Behav.*, 30, 437–443.

Emery, D.E., and Moss, R.L. (1984a). Lesions confined to the ventromedial hypothalamus decrease the frequency of coital contacts in female rats. *Horm. Behav.*, 18, 313–329.

Emery, D.E., and Moss, R.L. (1984b). p-Chlorophenylalanine alters pacing of copulation in female rats. *Pharmacol. Biochem. Behav.*, 20, 337–341.

Eibergen, R.D. and Caggiula, A.R. (1973). Ventral midbrain involvement in copulatory behavior of the male rat. *Physiol. Behav.*, 10, 435-441.

Erskine M.S., Kornberg E., and Cherry J.A. (1989). Paced copulation in rats: Effects of intromission frequency and duration on luteal activation and estrus length. *Physiol. Behav.*, 45, 33-39.

Everitt, B.J. and Stacey, P. (1987). Studies of instrumental behavior with sexual reinforcement in male rats (Rattus norvegicus): II. Effects of preoptic area lesions, castration, and testosterone. *J Comp Psychol,* 101,407-419.

Everitt, B.J., Fray, P., Kostarczyk, E., Taylor, S. and Stacey, P. (1987). Studies of instrumental behavior with sexual reinforcement in male rats (Rattus norvegicus): I. Control by brief visual stimuli paired with a receptive female. *J. Comp. Psychol.*, 101, 395-406.

Everitt, B.J. (1990). Sexual motivation: a neural and behavioral analysis of the mechanisms underlying appetitive and copulatory responses of male rats. *Neurosci. Biobehav. Rev.*, 14, 214-232.

Fernandez-Guasti, A. and Picazo, O. (1992). Changes in burying behavior during the estrous cycle: effect of estrogen and progesterone. *Psychoneuroendocrinology,* 17, 681-689.

Fernández-Guasti, A., Omana-Zapata, I., Luján, M. and Condés-Lara, M. (1994). Actions of sciatic nerve ligature on sexual behavior of sexually experienced and inexperienced male rats: effects of frontal pole decortication. *Physiol. Behav.*, 55, 577-581.

Ferreira, A., Hansen, S., Nielsen, M., Archer, T. and Minor, B.G. (1989). Behavior of mother rats in conflict tests sensitive to anti-anxiety agents. *Behav. Neurosci.,* 103, 193-201.

Fleming, A.S. and Luebke, C. (1981). Timidity prevents the nulliparous female from being a good mother. *Physiol. Behav.,* 27, 863-868.

Fleming, A.S. (1986). Psychobiology of rat maternal behavior. How and where hormones act to promote maternal behavior at parturition. *NY Acad. Sci.*, 474, 234-251.

Fleming, A.S., Cheung, U.S., Myhal, N. and Kessler, Z. (1989). Effects of maternal hormones on "timidity" and attraction to pup-related odors in females. *Physiol. Behav.*, 46, 449-453.

Fleming, A.S., Korsmit, M. and Deller, M. (1994). Rat pups are potent reinforcers to the maternal behavior animal: effects of experience, parity, hormones, and dopamine function. *Psychobiology,* 22, 44-53.

Fleming, A.S. and Korsmith, M. (1996). Plasticity in the maternal circuit: Effects of maternal experience on Fos-Lir in hypothalamic, limbic, and cortical structures in the postpartum rat. *Behav. Neurosci.,* 110, 567-582.

Floody, O.R. (2002). Time course of VMN lesion effects on lordosis and proceptive behavior in female hamsters. *Horm. Behav.*, 41, 366-376.

French, D., Fitzpatrick, D., and Law, O.T. (1972). Operant investigation of mating preference in female rats. *J. Comp. Physiol. Psychol.,* 81, 226–232.

Fuster, J.M. (1997).*The prefrontal cortex: Anatomy, physiology, and neuropsychology of the frontal lobe.* 3rd ed. Lipincott-Raven, New York.

Gaffori, O. and Le Moal, M. (1979). Disruption of maternal behavior and appearance of cannibalism after ventral mesencephalic tegmentum lesions. *Physiol. Behav.*, 23, 317-323.

Gemmel, C. and O´Mara, S.M. (1999). Medial prefrontal cortex lesions cause deficits in a variable-goal location task but not in object exploration. *Behav. Neurosci.*, 113, 465-475.

Genazzani, A.R., Peytaglia F. and Purdy R.H. (1996). *The brain: source and target for sex steroid hormones*. The Parthenon Publishing Group Limited, New York.

Goldman-Rakic, P.S. (1996). The prefrontal landscape: Implications of functional architecture for understanding human mentation and the central executive. *Philos Trans. R Soc London*, 351, 1445-1453.

Gonzalez, D.E. and Deis, R.P. (1986). Maternal behavior in cyclic and androgenized female rats. Role of ovarian hormones. *Physiol. Behav.*, 38, 789-793.

González-Mariscal, G. and Poindron, P. Parental care in mammals:immediate internal and sensory factors of control. (2002). In DW Pfaff., AP Arnold., AM Etgen., SE Fahrbach., and RT Rubin (eds). *Hormones, brain and behavior*. Academic Press, Elsevier Science, USA., Vol. 1, pp. 215-298.

Graber B., Rohrbaugh J., Newlin, D., Varner J. and Ellingson R. (1985). EEG during masturbation and ejaculation orgasm *Arch. Sex Behav.*, 14, 491-503.

Gray, P. and Brooks, P.J. (1984). Effect of lesion location within the medial preoptic-anterior hypothalamic continuum on maternal and male sexual behaviors in female rats. *Behav. Neurosci.*, 98, 703-711.

Grillner, S. and Shik, M.I. (1973). On the descending control of the lumbosacral spinal cord from the mesencephalic locomotor region. *Acta Physiol. Scand*, 87, 320-333.

Groenewegen, H.J. and Uylings, H.B.M., (2000). The prefrontal cortex and the integration of sensory, limbic, and autonomic information. In: HBM Uylings., CG Van Eden., JPC de Bruin., MGP Feenstra., CMA Pennartz. (eds). Cognition, Emotion and autonomic responses: The integrative role of the prefrontal cortex and limbic structures. *Progress in Brain Research,* vol 126, Elsevier, Amsterdam., pp. 3-28.

Guarraci, F.A. and Clark, A.S. (2006). Ibotenic acid lesions of the medial preoptic area disrupt the expression of parter preference in sexually receptive female rats. *Brain Res,* 1076, 163-170.

Guevara, M.A., Hernández-González, M. and Ramos-Guevara, J.P. (2004). Especialización subregional de la corteza prefrontal en la rata: diferente actividad durante una tarea sexualmente motivada. In MA Guevara., M Hernández-González., P Durán-Hernández., (eds.) *Aproximaciones al estudio de la corteza prefrontal.* Universidad de Guadalajara, México. pp.151-178.

Guevara M. A., Hernández González M., Zarabozo D. and Corsi Cabrera M. (2003). POTENCOR: A program to calculate power and correlation spectra of EEG signals. *Comp. Meth. Prog. Biomed.*, 72, 241-250.

Guevara, M.A., Ramos, J., Hernández-González, M. and Corsi-Cabrera, M. (2005). FILDIG: a program to filter brain electrical signals in the frequency domain. *Comp. Meth Prog. Biomed.* 80, 93-186.

Guevara-Guzmán, R., Barrera-Mera, B. and Weiss, M.L. (1997). Effect of the estrous cycle on olfactory bulb response to vaginocervical stimulation in the rat: Results from electrophysiology and Fos immunicytochemistry experiments. *Brain Res. Bull.,* 44, 141-149.

Hall, J, Parkinson, J, Connor, T, Dickinson, A, and Everrit B.J. (2001). Involvement of the central nucleus of the amygdala and nucleus accumbens core in mediating pavlovian influences on instrumental behavior. *Eur. J. Neurosci.*, 13, 1984-1192.

Hansen, S. and Ferreira, A. (1986). Food intake, aggression, and fear in the mother rat: control by neural systems concerned with milk ejection and maternal behavior. *Behav. Neurosci.*, 100, 64-70.

Hard, E. and Hansen, S. (1985). Reduced fearfulness in the lactating rat. *Physiol. Behav.*, 35, 641-643.

Heath R. (1972). Pleasure and brain activity in man *The Journal of Nervous and Mental Disease,* 154(1),3-18.

Heim, N. and Hursch, C.J. (1979). Castration of sex offenders: treatment or punishment? A review and critique of recent European literature. *Arch. Sex Behav.,* 8, 281-306.

Hernández-González, M., Guevara, M.A., Oropeza, M.V. and Moralí, G. (1993). Male rat pelvic copulatory movements: computarized analysis of accelerometric data. *Arch. Med. Res.*, 24, 155-160.

Hernández-González, M., Guevara, M.A., Moralí, G. and Cervantes, M. (1997). Computer programs to analyze brain electrical activity during copulatory pelvic thrusting in male rats. *Physiol. Behav.*, 62,701-708.

Hernández-González M., Guevara M. A., Moralí G., and Cervantes M (1997). Subcortical multiple unit activity changes during male sexual behavior of the rat. *Physiol. Behav.*, 61(2), 285-291.

Hernández-González, M., Guevara, M.A., Cervantes, M., Moralí, G. and Corsi-Cabrera, M. (1998). Characteristic frequency bands of the cortico-frontal EEG during the sexual interaction of the male rat as a result of factorial analysis. *J. Physiol. (Paris),* 92, 43-50.

Hernández-González, M., Prieto-Beracoechea, C.A., Navarro-Meza, M. and Guevara, M.A. (2005). Prefrontal and tegmental electrical activity during olfactory stimulation in virgin and lactating rats. *Physiol. Behav.,* 83, 749–758.

Hernández-González M., Prieto-Beracoechea C.A., Arteaga-Silva M. and Guevara M.A. (2007). Different functionality of the medial and orbital prefrontal cortex during a sexually motivated task in rats. *Physiol. Behav.*, 90, 450-458.

Hetta, J. and Meyerson, B.J. (1978). Sexual motivation in the male rat: a methodological study of sex-specific orientation and the effects of gonadal hormones. *Acta Physiol. Scand Suppl.*, 453, 1-67.

Holmes, J. and Egan, K. (1973). Electrical activity of the cat amygdale during sexual behavior. *Physiol. Behav.*, 10, 863-867.

Horio, T., Shimura, T., Hanada, M. and Shikochi, M. (1986). Multiple unit activities recorded from the medial preoptic area during copulatory behavior in freely moving male rats. *Neurosci. Res.,* 3, 311-320.

Hull, E.M., Meisel, R.L. and Sachs, B.D. Male sexual behavior. (2002). In DW Pfaff., AP Arnold., AM Etgen., SE Fahrbach., and RT Rubin (eds). *Hormones, brain and behavior*. Academic Press, Elsevier Science, USA., Vol. 1, pp: 1-138.

Hull, E.M., Bazzet, T.J., Warner, R.K., Eaton, R.C. and Thompson, J.T. (1990). Dopamine receptors in the ventral tegmental area modulate male sexual behavior in rats. *Brain Res.*, 512, 1-6.

Hull, E.M., Weber, M.S., Eaton, R.C., Dua, R., Markowski, V.P., Lumley, L., and Moses, J. (1991). Dopamine receptors in the ventral tegmental area affect motor, but not motivational or reflexive components of copulation in male rats. *Brain Res.*, 554, 72-76.

Hurtazo, H.A., Paredes, R.G. and Ågmo, A. (2003). Inactivation of the medial preoptic area/anterior hypothalamus (MPOA/AH) reduces sexual incentive motivation in male rats. *Soc. Neurosci. Abstr.,* 404,6.

Jacobson, C.D., Terkel, J., Gorski, R.A. and Sawyer, C.H. (1980). Effects of small medial preoptic area lesions on maternal behavior: retrieving and nest building in the rat. *Brain Res.*, 194, 471-478.

Jodo, E., Suzuki, Y. and Kayama, Y. (2000). Selective responsiveness of medial prefrontal cortex neurons to the meaningful stimulus with a low probability of occurrence in rats. *Brain Res.*, 856, 68-74.

Jowaisas, D., Taylor, J., Dewsbury, D.A. and Malagodi, E.F. (1971). Copulatory behavior of male rats under an imposed operant requirement. *Psychonom. Sci.*, 25,287-290.

Kagan, J. (1955). Differential reward value of incomplete and complete sexual behavior. *J. Comp. Physiol. Psychol.*, 48,59-64.

Kendrick, K.M., Da Costa, A.P.C., Broad, K.D., Okhura, S., Guevara, R., Levy, F. and Keverne, E.B. (1997). Neural control of maternal behavior and olfactory recognition of offspring. *Brain Res. Bull.*, 44, 383-395.

Kesner, R.P. (2000). Neural mediation of memory for time: role of the hippocampus and medial prefrontal cortex. *Psychol. Bull Rev.*, 5,585-596.

Kollack-Walker, S. and Neuman, S.W. (1992). Mating behavior induces selective expression of Fos protein within the chemosensory pathways of the male Syrian hamster brain. *Neurosci. Lett,* 143, 223-228.

Kollack-Walker, S. and Newman, S.W. (1995). Mating and agonistic behavior produce different patterns of Fos immunolabeling in the male Syrian hamster brain. *Neuroscience,* 66, 721-736.

Kolb, B., Sutherland, R.J. and Whishaw, I.Q., (1983). A comparison of the contribution of the frontal and parietal association cortex to spatial localization in rats. *Behav. Neurosci.,* 97, 13-27.

Kolb, B. (1984). Functions of the frontal cortex of the rat. A comparative review. *Brain Res. Rev.*, 8, 65-98.

Kolb, B., Buhrmann, K. and McDonald, R., (1989). Dissociation of prefrontal, posterior parietal, and temporal cortical regions to spatial navigation and recognition memory in the rat. *Soc. Neurosci.,* Abstract 15, 607.

Kolb, B. (1990). Prefrontal cortex. In B Kolb., RC Tees. (eds). *The Cerebral Cortex of the Rat*. MA: The MIT Press, Cambridge. pp. 437-58.

Kolb, B. and Cioe, J., (2004). Organization and plasticity of the prefrontal cortex of the rat. In S Otani. (ed). *Prefrontal Cortex: From synaptic plasticity to cognition*. Kluwer Academic Publishers, France. pp. 1-32.

Kurtz, R. and Adler N. (1973). Electrophysiological correlates of copulatory behavior in the male rat *J. Comp Physiol. Psychol.*, 84, 225-239.

Kurtz, R. (1975). Hippocampal and cortical activity during sexual behavior in the female rat *J Comp. Physiol Psychol.*, 89(2),158-169.

Larsson, K. (1962). Mating behaviour in male rats after cerebral cortex ablation. I. Effects of lesions in the dorsolateral and the median cortex. *J. Exp. Zool.,* 151, 167-176.

Larsson, K. (1964). Mating behaviour in male rats after cerebral cortex ablation. II. Effects of lesions oh the frontal lobes compared to lesions un the posterior half of the hemispheres. *J. Exp. Zool.,* 155, 203-214.

Larsson, K. (1979). Features of the neuroendocrine regulation of masculine sexual behavior. In C. Beyer, (ed). *Endocrine control of sexual behavior*. Raven Press, New York. pp. 77-163.

Lee, A., Clancy, S. and Fleming, A.S. (2000). Mother rats bar-press for pups: effects of lesions of the MPOA and limbic sites on maternal behavior and operant responding for pup-reinforcement. *Behav. Brain Res.*, 108, 215-231.

Lemoal, M., Stinus, L. and Galey, D., (1976). Radiofrequency lesion of the ventral mesencephalic tegmentum: Neurological and behavioral considerations. *Exp. Neurol.*, 50, 521-535.

Leon-Carrion, J., Martín-Rodriguez, J.F., Damas-López, J., Pourrezai, K., Izzetoglu, K., Barroso, J.M. y Martin, M. and Dominguez- Morales, R. (2007). Does dorsolateral prefrontal cortex (DLPFC) activation return to baseline when sexual stimuli cease? The role of DLPFC in visual sexual stimulation. *Neurosci. Let*, 416, 55-60.

Lincoln, D.W., Hentzen, K., Hin, T., Van der Schoot, P., Clarke, G. and Summerlee, A.J.S. (1980). Sleep: A prerequisite for reflex milk ejection in the rat. *Exp. Brain Res.*, 38, 151-162.

Lorberbaum, J.P., Newman, J.D., Horwitz, A.R., Dubno, J.R., Bruce Lydiard, R., Hamner, M.B., Bohning, D.E. and George, M.S. (2002). A potential role for thalamocingulate circuitry in human maternal behavior. *Biol. Psychiatry,* 51, 431-445.

López da Silva, F.H. (1991). Neural mechanisms underlying brain waves from neural membranes to networks. *Electroenceph. Clin. Neurophysiol.,* 79, 81-93.

López, H.H. and Ettenberg, A. (2001). Dopamine antagonism attenuates the unconditioned incentive value of estrous female cues. *Pharmacol. Biochem. Behav.,* 68, 411-416.

Lubar, J.F., Herrman, T.J., Moore, D.R. and Shouse, M.N. (1973). Effect of septal and frontal ablations on species typical behavior in the rat. *J. Comp. Physiol. Psychol.,* 83, 260-270.

Madlafousek, J., and Hlinak, Z. (1977). Sexual behavior of the female laboratory rat: Inventory, patterning, and measurement. *Behaviour,* 63, 129–174.

Magnusson, J.E. and Fleming, A.S. (1995). Rat pups are reinforcing to the maternal rat: role of sensory cues. *Psychobiology*, 23, 69-75.

Maras, P.M. and Petrulis, A. (2006). Chemosensory and steroid-responsive regions of the medial amygdala regulate distinct aspects of opposite-sex odor preference in male Syrian hamsters. *Eur. J. Neurosci.,* 24, 3541-3552.

Matthews, T.J., Grigore,M., Tang, L., Doat, M., Kow, L.M. and Pfaff, D.W. (1997). Sexual reinforcement in the female rat. *J. Exp. Anal. Behav.*, 68, 399-410.

Mattson, B.J., Williams, S., Rosenblatt, J.S. and Morrell, J.I. (2001). Comparison of two positive reinforcing stimuli: pups and cocaine throughout the postpartum period. *Behav. Neurosci.*, 115, 683-694.

McClintock, M.K. and Adler, N.T. (1978). The role of the female during copulation in wild and domestic norway rats *(Rattus norvegicus). Behaviour*, 67, 67–96.

Mclntosh R., Barfield R. and Thomas D. (1984). Electrophysiological and ultrasonic correlates of reproductive behavior in the male rat. *Behav. Neurosci.*, 98,1100-1103.

Mead, L.A. and Vanderwolf, C.H. (1992). Hippocampal electrical activity in the female rat: The estrous cycle, copulation, parturition, and pup retrieval. *Behav. Brain Res.*, 50, 105-113.

Meyerson, B.J. and Lindstrom, L.H. (1973). Sexual motivation in the female rat. A methodological study applied to the investigation of the effect of estradiol benzoate. *Acta Physiol. Scand Suppl.*, 389, 1-80.

Michal, E.K. (1973). Effects of limbic lesions on behavior sequences and courtship behavior of male rats (Rattus norvergicus). *Behavior*, 44:264-285.

Michael R., Holbrooke C., and Weller. C. (1977). Telemetry and continuous energy analysis of hypothalamic EEG changes in female cats during intromission by the male. *Psychoneuroendocrinology*, 2, 287-301.

Miceli, M.O., Fleming, A.S. and Malsbury, C.W. (1983). Disruption of maternal behavior in virgin and postparturient rats following sagittal plane knife cuts in the preoptic area-hypothalamus. *Behav. Brain Res.*, 9,337-360.

Mirenowicz, J. and Schultz, W. (1996). Preferential activation of midbrain dopamine neurons by appetitive rather than aversive stimuli. *Nature,* 379, 449-451.

Mishkin, M. (1964). Perseveration of central sets after frontal lesions in monkeys. In JM Warren., K. Akert, (eds). *The frontal granular cortex and behavior*. McGraw-hill, New York. pp. 219-241.

Mogenson, G.J., Jones, D.L. and Yim, C.Y., (1980). From motivation to action: Functional interface between the limbic system and the motor system. *Prog. Neurobiol.,* 14, 69-97.

Moncho-Bogani, J., Martinez-Garcia, F., Novejarque, A. and Lanuza, E. (2005). Attraction to sexual pheromones and associated odorants in female mice involves activation of the reward system and basolateral amygdala. *Eur. J. Neurosci.,* 21, 2186-2189.

Morgan, H.D., Watchus, J.A., Milgram, N.W. and Fleming, A.S. (1999). The long lasting effects of electrical stimulation of the medial preoptic area and medial amygdala on maternal behavior in female rats. *Behav. Brain Res.*, 99, 61-73.

Morgan, M.A. and Pfaff, D.W. (2002). Estrogen´s effects on activity, anxiety, and fear in two mouse strains. *Behav. Brain Res.,* 132, 85-93.

Mosovich A. and Tallaferro A. (1954). Studies on EEG and sex function orgasm. *Diseases of the Nervous System*, 15,218-220.

Newman, S.W. (1999). The medial extended amygdale in male. *Ann. NY Acad Sci.,* 877, 242-257.

Newman, S.W. (2002). Pheromonal signals access the medial extended amygdale: one node in a proposed social nehabior network. In DW Pfaff., AP Arnold., AM Etgen., SE Fahrbach., and Rubin, R.T. (eds.) *Hormones, brain and behavior.* Vol. 2, Academic Press, San Diego. pp. 17-32.

Nishino, H., Ono, T., Muramoto, K., Fukuda, M. and Sasaki, K. (1986). Neuronal activity in the ventral tegmental area (VTA) during motivated bar press feeding in the monkey. *Brain Res.*, 413, 302-313.

Numan, M. (1974). Medial preoptic area and maternal behavior in the female rat. *J. Comp. Physiol. Psychol.*, 87, 746-759.

Numan, M., Rosenblatt, J.S. and Komisaruk, B.R. (1977). Medial preoptic area and onset of maternal behavior in the rat. *J. Comp. Physiol. Psychol.*, 91, 146-164.

Numan, M. and Insel, T.R. (2003).The neurobiology of parental behavior. *Hormones Brain and behavior.* Springer-Verlag, New York.

Oldenburger, W.P., Everitte B.J., and DeJonge, F.H. (1992). Conditioned place preference induced by sexual interactionin female rats. *Horm. Behav.*, 26, 214–228.

Olds, J. (1973). Multiple unit recording from behaving rats. In RF Thompson., MM Patterson, (eds). *Bioelectric recording techniques*. Vol. 1A. Academic Press, New York. pp. 165-198.

Oley, N.N. and Slotnick, B.M. (1970). Nesting material as a reinforcement for operant behavior in the rat. *Psychonom. Sci.,* 21, 41-43.

Paredes, R.G., and Alonso, A. (1997). Sexual behavior regulated (paced) by the female induces conditioned place preference. *Behav. Neurosci.*, 111, 123–128.

Paredes, .R.G, and Baum, M.J. (1995). Altered sexual parter preference in male ferrets given excitotoxic lesions of the preoptic area antrerior hypothalamus. *J. Neurosci.,* 15, 6630.

Paredes, R.G., Highland, L. and Karam, P. (1993). Socio-Sexual behaviour in male rats after lesions of the medial preoptic area: evidence of reduced sexual motivation. *Brain Res.,* 618, 271-276.

Paredes, R.G., Tzschentke, T. and Nakach, N. (1998). Lesions of the medial preoptic area/anterior hypothalamus (MPOA/AH) modify partner preference in male rats. *Brain Res.,* 813, 1-8.

Passingham, R. (1993). *The frontal lobes and voluntary action.* Oxford Psychology Series, Vol. 21, Oxford University Press, Oxford U.K. pp. 299.

Paxinos, G. and Watson, C. (1997) *The rat brain in stereotaxic coordinates*. Academic Press, New York.

Pfaff, D.W. and Sakuma, Y. (1979). Facilitation of the lordosis reflex of female rats from the ventromedial nucleus of the hypothalamus. *J. Physiol.*, 288, 189-202.

Pfaff, D.W. and Agmo, A. (2002). Reproductive motivation. In R Gakkistel., H Pashler, (eds). *Steven's Handbook of Experimental Psychology, Learning, Motivation and Emotion*. Wiley, (chapter 17).

Picazo, O. and Fernandez-Guasti, A. (1993). Changes in experimental anxiety during pregnancy and lactation. *Physiol. Behav.*, 54, 295-299.

Pietras, J.R. and Moulton, G.D. (1974). Hormonal influences on odor detection in rats: Changes associated with the estrous cycle, pseudopregnancy, ovariectomy, and administration of testosterone propionate. *Physiol. Behav.*, 12, 475-491.

Pryce, C.R., Dobeli, M. and Martin, R.D. (1993). Effects of sex steroids on maternal motivation in the common marmoset (*Callithrix jacchus*): development and application of na operant system with maternal reinforcement. *J. Comp. Psychol.,* 107, 99-115.

Reilly, D.R., Delva, N.J., and Hudson, R.W. (2000). Protocols for the use of cyproterone, medroxyprogesterone, and lwuprolide in the treatment of paraphilia. *Can. J. Psychiat.,* 45, 559-563.

Robinson, J.T. (1954). The necessity of progesterone with estrogen for the induction of recurent estrus in the ovariectomixed ewe. *Endocrinology,* 55, 403-408.

Rolls, E.T. (2000). The orbitofrontal cortex and reward. *Cereb. Cortex*. 10, 284-294.

Rolls, E.T. (2004). The functions of the orbitofrontal cortex. *Brain and Cognition,* 55, 11-29.

Rolls, E.T., Treves, A. (1998). *Neural networks and brain functions*. Oxford, Oxford University Press.

Rose, J.E. and Woolsey, C.N. (1948). The orbitofrontal cortex and its connections with the mediodorsal nucleus in rabbit, sheep and cat. *Res. Publ. Assn. Nerv. Dis.,* 27, 210-232.

Rosen, R.C., Goldstein, L., Scoles, V. and Lazarus, C. (1986). Psychophysiologic correlates of nocturnal penile tumescence in normal males. *Psychosom Med.*, 48, 423-429.

Rosenblatt, J.S. and Aronson, L.R. (1958). The decline of sexual behavior in male cats after castration with special reference to the role of prior sexual experience. *Behavior*, 12, 285-338.

Rowe D.W., and Erskine M.S. (1993). c-fos Proto-oncogene activity induced by mating in the preoptic area, hypothalamus and amygdala in the female rat: role of afferent input via the pelvic nerve. *Brain Research,* 621. 25-34.

Shaw, J.C. (1984). Correlation and coherence analysis of the EEG. *A tutorial review Int. J. Psychophysiol*, 1,255-266.

Shwartz, A. and Whalen R. (1965). Amygdala activity during sexual behavior in the male cat. *Life Sciences*, 4, 1359-1365.

Sheffield, F.D., Wulff, J.J. and Backer, R. (1951) Reward value of copulation without sexual drive reduction. *J. Comp. Physiol. Psychol.,* 44, 3-8.

Sheffield, F.D., Roby, T.B. and Campbell, B.A. (1954). Drive reduction versus consummatory behavior as determinants of reinforcement. *J. Comp. Physiol. Psychol,* 47, 349-354.

Shimamura, A.P., Janowski, J.S. and Squire, L.R. (1990) Memory for the temporal order of events in patients with frontal lobe lesions and amnesic patients. *Neuropsychologia*, 28, 803-813.

Slotnick, B.M., (1967). Disturbances of maternal behavior in the rat following lesions of the cingulated cortex. *Behavior* 29, 204-236.

Soulairac, A. and Soulairac, M.L. (1972). Action des substances neurostimulantes sur le comportement sexual du rat mậle après lésions du cortex cérébral. *J. Physiol.,* 65, Suppl. 3, 504.

Stamm, J.S., (1955). The function of the medial cerebral cortex in maternal behavior in rats. *J. Comp. Physiol. Psychol.,* 48, 347-356.

Stern, J.M. (1989). Maternal behavior: sensory, hormonal and neural determinants. In FR Brush., S Levine, (eds). *Psychoendocrinology.* Academic Press, New York. pp. 103-226.

Stern, J. M., (1996). Somatosensation and maternal care in Norway rats. In JS Rosenblatt., CT Snowdon, (eds). Parental care, evolution, mechanisms and adaptative significance. *Advances in the study of behavior*. vol. 25, Academic Press, New York. pp. 243-294.

Stern, J.M. and MacKinnon, D.A. (1976). Postpartum, hormonal, and non-hormonal induction of maternal behavior in rats: effects on T-maze retrieval of pups. *Horm. Behav.*, 7: 305-316.

Stoléru Serge, M.D., Grégoire, M.C., Gerard, D., Decety, J., Lafarge, E., Cinotti, L., Lavenne, F., Le Bars, D., Vernet-Maury, E., Rada, H., Collet, C., Mazoyer, B., Forest, M.G., Magnin, F., Spira, A. and Comar, D. (1999). Neuroanatomical correlates of visually evoked sexual arousal in human males. *Arch. Sex Behav.*, 28(1), 1-21.

Swanson, L.W. and Mogenson, J. (1981). Neural mechanisms for the functional coupling of autonomic, endocrine and somatomotor responses in adaptative behavior. *Brain Res. Rev.*, 3: 1-34.

Takenouchi, K., Nishijo, H., Uwano, T., Tamura, R., Takigawa, M. and Ono, T. (1999). Emotional and behavioral correlates of the anterior cingulated cortex during associative learning in rats. *Neuroscience*, 93: 1271-1287.

Timberlake, W. and Silva, K.M. (1995). Appetitive behavior in ethology, psychology, and behavior systems. In NS Thompson, (ed). *Perspectives in ethology*, Vol. 11. Behavioral design Plenum Press, New York. pp 211-253.

Thompson, A.C. and Kristal, M.B. (1996). Opioid stimulation in the ventral tegmental area facilitates the onset of maternal behavior in rats. *Brain Res.*, 743, 184-201.

Tucker, D.M. and Dawson S.L. (1984). Asymmetric EEG changes as method actors generated emotions. *Biol. Psychol.*, 19, 63-75.

Tzschentke, T.M. (2000). The medial prefrontal cortex as a part of the brain reward system. *Amino Acids*, 19, 211-219.

Uylings, H.B.M. and Van Eden, C.G. (1990). Qualitative and quantitative comparison of the prefrontal cortex in rat and in primates, including humans. In HBM Uylings., CG Van Eden., JPC de Bruin., MA Corner., and MPG Feenstra (eds). *The prefrontal cortex: Its structure, function and pathology*. Prog Brain Res Elsevier, Amsterdam. 85: 31-62.

Uylings, H.B.M., Groenewegen, H.J. and Kolb, B. (2003). Do rats have a prefrontal cortex? *Behav. Brain Res.,* 146, 3-17.

Wallen, K. (1990). Desire and ability: hormones and the regulation of female sexual behavior. *Neurosci. Biobehav. Rev.*, 14, 233-241.

Walsh, C., Fleming, A.S., Lee, A. and Magnusson, J (1996). The effects of olfactory and somatosensory desensitization on fos-like immunoreactivity in the brains of pup-exposed postpartum rats. *Behav. Neurosc.*, 110, 1-20.

Whalen, R.E. (1961). Effects of mounting without intromission and intromission without ejaculation on sexual behavior and maze learning. *J. Comp. Physiol. Psychol.*, 54, 409-415.

Whalen, R.E., Beach, F.A. and Kuehn, R.E. (1961). Effects of exogenous androgen on sexually responsive and unresponsive male rats. *Endocrinology,* 68, 373-380.

Willie, R. and Beler, K.M. (1989). Castration in Germany. *Annual Sex Research* 2, 103-133.

White, N.R., and Barfield, R.J. (1989). Playback of female rat ultrasonic vocalizations during sexual behavior. *Physiol. Behav.*, 45, 229–233.

Wood , R.I. (1998). Integration of chemosensory and hormonal input in the male Syrian hamster brain. *Ann. NY Acad. Sci.*, 855, 362-372.

Xiao, K., Kondo, Y. and Sakuma, Y. (2005). Differencial regulation of female rat olfactory preference and copulatory pacing by the lateral septum and medial preoptic area. *Neuroendocrinology,* 81, 56-62.

Yonemori, M., Nishijo, H., Uwano, T., Tamura, R., Furuta, I., Kawasaki, M., Takashima, Y. and Ono, T. (2000). Orbital cortex neuronal responses during an odor-based conditioned associative task in rats. *Neuroscience*, 95,691-703.

Zitrin A., Jaynes, J. and Beach, F.A. (1956) Neural mediation of mating in male cats. III. Contributions of occipital, parietal and temporal cortex. *J. Comp. Neurol.*, 105, 111-122.

In: Prefrontal Cortex: Roles, Interventions and Traumas
Editors: Lorenzo LoGrasso and Giovanni Morretti
ISBN 978-1-60692-415-0

Chapter 4

From Conflict to Problem Solution: The Role of the Medial Prefrontal Cortex in the Learning of Memory-Guided and Context-Adequate Behavioral Strategies for Problem-Solving in Gerbils

Holger Stark
Leibniz Institute for Neurobiology,
Brenneckestr. 6, D-39118 Magdeburg, Germany

Abstract

We conducted an investigation of the way in which animals acquire problem-solving behavioral strategies. The focus was on the search for sequential feedback rules that guide an individual along the stepwise learning process from the initial conflict generated by a novel situation to the context-adequate, problem-solving and, therewith, successful behavioral strategy.

The medial prefrontal cortex plays a complex role in acquisition and storage of behavioral strategies. It is an important part of the internal reward system, inducing a motivational drive for the development of a memory-guided, goal-directed behavioral strategy. This view is also strongly supported by our work on the learning-related dynamics of prefrontal dopamine release.

Using Mongolian gerbils (Meriones unguiculatus) as an animal model, we found that the formation of an avoidance strategy in a shuttle-box during the stage of avoidance learning is accompanied by a strong increase of the activity in the prefrontal dopamine system. Cortical theta activation was found to be, overall, negatively correlated with the formation of avoidance strategy during learning. In learning stages preceding the stage of avoidance learning we found different decreases of theta activity. However, when the animals entered the stage of avoidance learning, i.e., the phase when prefrontal dopamine release increases, theta activity increased again as well. A detailed analysis of theta activation revealed unique events in single trials marking the transition between behaviorally-defined learning stages and reflecting the actual change of the task-context for the animal.

Based on the correlation between behavioral data and data of learning-relevant physiological parameters, i.e., prefrontal dopamine and theta activation, we discuss cognitive processes like feedback learning, error processing, planning, decision making, and short-term memory as components of working memory functions during stepwise learning. The detailed analysis of learning processes in simple avoidance conditioning paradigms is a prerequisite for a deeper understanding of information processing during the goal-directed formation of behavioral strategies.

Introduction

The tremendous capability of living creatures to individually acquire and store information ensures their survival by fast and adequate adaptation to their environment. Therefore, learning and memory have multiple facets and involve a complex and distributed network in the brain [Eichenbaum, 2008]. Our contribution in the field of cognition will be limited to observations on cortical and prefrontal dopamine as well as cortical theta activity during aversive learning and retrieval. Our hypotheses are derived from correlations between the behavior of learning animals and the aforementioned physiological learning-dependent observables. Nevertheless, we are dealing here with fundamental processes of individual acquisition and storage of information. The discussion will focus on two points: (1) how the learning process is initiated, and (2) the way in which the learner forms a goal for guiding the learning process.

This chapter is composed in the form of a lab report to illustrate that the sequence of experiments and discussions presents a learning process itself driven by steadily arising scientific questions.

Animal Model

The animal model we used allows a stringent formation of both simple and more complex behavioral strategies by the individuals. Parallel to the conditioning procedure, we recorded physiological, learning-relevant parameters like prefrontal dopamine release and theta activation to interpret our behavioral observations. We chose Mongolian gerbils because the natural abilities, i.e., attention, cognitive flexibility, and consciousness of that small desert rodents make them appropriate for fast conditioning in learning models like the shuttle-box., one-year-old male animals were trained to develop aversively-motivated avoidance and discrimination strategies over several days and were subjected to parallel long-term brain microdialysis or recording of electroencephalograms over the right prefrontal cortex as a learning-relevant brain area.

Both avoidance and discrimination learning in the shuttle-box represent operant conditioning paradigms including aversively-motivated classical conditioning [Riess, 1972; Wasserman and Miller, 1997]. Conditioned tone stimuli (CS) were paired with footshock punishment as an unconditioned stimulus (UCS). In the individual animal, the footshock initiates a conflict. It can either simply tolerate this punishment or find a strategy to escape from it. Thus, as a first important issue (1) the origin of the learning process is a conflict realized by the individual, which represents an actual detraction from familiar existence conditions in the present surroundings. The general goal of the learning individual is then to re-establish convenient environmental life conditions. This delivers, so to speak, the "potential energy" for the learning process in which the individual adapts to the changed environmental situation. In the present experiments the strength of the conflict is related to the individual's inability to tolerate the punishment. It thus depends on the strength of the footshock and on its stringency in the behavioral context, but also on a subjective evaluation of the conflict by the animal. Furthermore, the animal has no chance to flee from the uncomfortable situation of footshock punishment during shuttle-box learning. Therefore, the only way to minimize the conflict strength is to acquire an adequate behavioral strategy related to the shuttle-box context. The animal creates coordinated associations making use of the formerly indifferent, meaningless tone stimuli paired with the unconditioned footshock. During learning, the tones become conditioned stimuli carrying after learning the matured conditioned avoidance response, or containing the information for the immediately following decision making in the case of acquired discrimination strategy, respectively. The stepwise formation of essential associations requires cognitive performances such as comparing of facts, reasoning, comprehension, planning, error processing and decision making, and feedback processing.

At the beginning of learning the animal does not know the concrete behavioral strategy that solves the conflict. Therefore, the question remains in which way an individual can find out by itself how to direct its behavior towards the concrete goal, in order to cope with the conflicting situation. We hypothesize that during stepwise learning the gerbil evaluates trial outcome by trial outcome for conflict attenuation caused by its own successful actions in the shuttle-box. Any realized conflict reduction will be perceived as a useful step in the direction of conflict solving. Hence, the second important issue of this report (2) concerns the realization of useful actions with respect to conflict reduction by an internal emotional reward percept that provides the key information to reinforce and to rule the development of a behavioral strategy for the solution of the problem. Therefore, we propose that the internal reinforcement as the motivational side of learning essentially contributes to the goal-directed formation of a behavioral strategy.

Transient increase of activity in cortical and prefrontal dopamine systems indicate the formation of relevant associations underlying a successful behavioral strategy

Differential Activation of the Dopamine System in Auditory Cortex in Trained, Pseudotrained, and Auditory Control Animals during Avoidance Conditioning

The first idea about the learning stage-dependent involvement of cortical dopamine systems in the formation of behavioral strategies in gerbils we derived from investigations of the auditory cortex of gerbils [Stark et al., 1997]. This brain area has been shown to be a site of widespread neuronal learning processes especially in the context of auditory conditioning behavior with behavioral and motivational relevance of incoming information [Scheich and Zuschratter, 1995; Zuschratter et al., 1995; Ohl and Scheich, 1996].

We investigated whether the dopaminergic and serotonergic systems are involved in auditory cortex learning. Chronic microdialysis from the auditory cortex was obtained before, during and after daily footshock avoidance training. Levels of extracellular homovanillic acid (HVA) as metabolite of the dopaminergic transmission as well as 5-hydroxyindoleacetic acid (5-HIAA) as metabolite of the serotonergic transmission were analyzed as estimates of the responses of both systems in the auditory cortex during acoustic learning in the shuttle-box. The basal levels of dopamine and serotonin in the microdialysis samples of most cases were below the reliable detection limit [Stark et al., 1997].

In the group of trained animals subjected to paired tone-footshock combinations, the values of the dopamine metabolite HVA revealed a transient strong increase of the activity of cortical dopamine system shortly after the start of the first training session, i.e. in the stage of strong increase of conditioned avoidance responses (Figure 1).

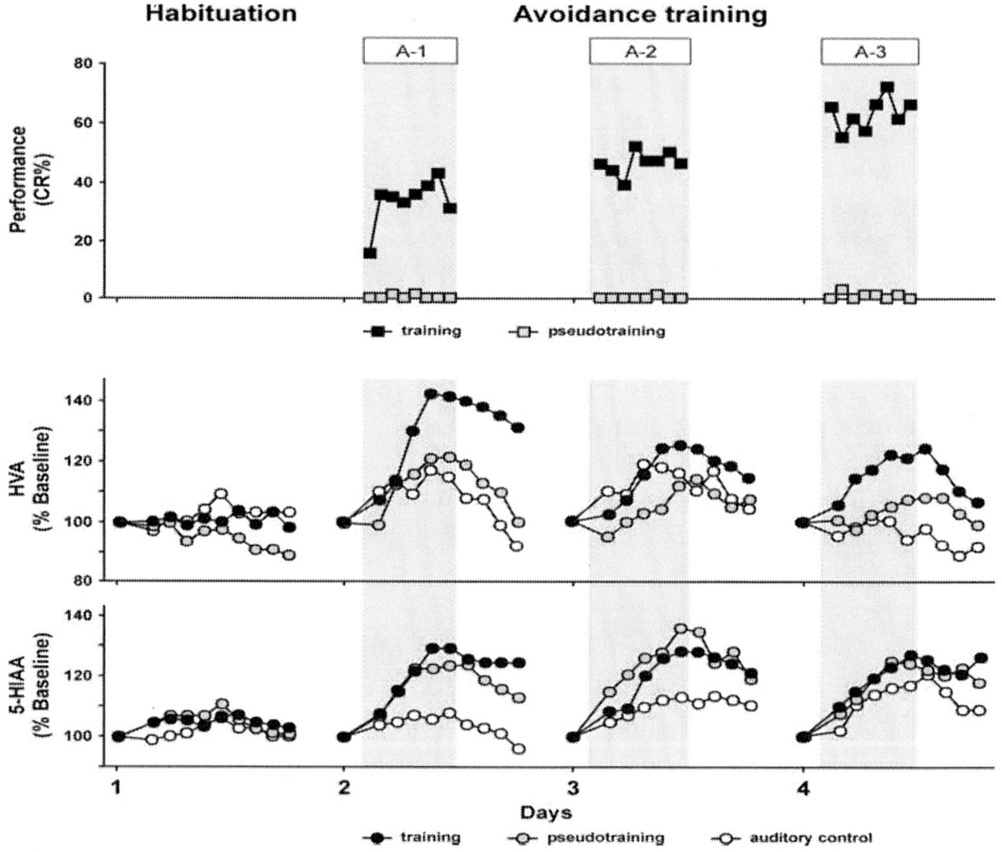

Figure 1. Temporal profiles of averaged learning curves (above) during the first day (unstimulated habituation), the first avoidance training session A-1 on the second day and the following two training sessions A-2 and A-3 on days 3 and 4 (retrieval), and of the relative content of HVA (middle) and 5-HIAA (bottom) in 15-min microdialysis samples from auditory cortex of trained, pseudotrained (no contingency between tones and footshocks), and auditory control animals (only tones without footshock).

The response of the dopaminergic system appeared to reflect the initial formation of behaviorally relevant associations exclusively during the first training day. In comparison, only a moderate increase in cortical dopamine was found in pseudotrained and in auditory control animals in the first training session. Whereas auditory controls received only the tones, footshocks were presented randomly within the next intertrial interval in the pseudotrained animal group. The duration of the footshock used thereby matched the footshock duration applied to the trained animals. In training sessions 2 and 3 all three animal groups showed only a moderate increase in the dopamine metabolite HVA.

The serotonergic response appeared to be correlated with the stress level of animals. The 5-HIAA values were increased in trained and pseudotrained animals in comparison to auditory controls without footshock punishment (Figure 1). The serotonin system seems to be rather involved in the stressful aspect of the situation by participating in the regulation of anxiety and defensive behavior [Deakin and Graeff, 1991; Graeff, 1993; Glass et al., 1993; Young, 1993]. From the HVA data we conclude that (1) the strong increase of cortical dopamine activity is correlated only with the formation of the relevant associations between tone stimulus and footshock connected with further associations like instrumental responses required for a context-adequate, conflict-solving behavioral strategy [Sawaguchi et al., 1990; Imperato et al., 1992; Goldman-Rakic, 1992; Young, 1993]. Supporting this assumption, it was previously shown in gerbil primary auditory cortex that pairing of a tone with an aversive stimulus led within minutes to specific changes of frequency receptive fields of about 60 % of excited neurons [Ohl and Scheich, 1996]. Suggestions that dopamine is acting as an "internal reinforcer" necessary only as long as the initiation of an appropriate behavioral strategy is in progress came previously from results in medial prefrontal cortex [Brozoski et al., 1979; Sawaguchi and Goldman-Rakic, 1991; Sokolowski et al., 1994], nucleus accumbens [Salamone, 1994], and parietal cortex [Schultz et al., 1993]. After the formation of a matured behavioral strategy, the activity of the dopamine system is only moderately increased in further avoidance training sessions. Therefore, the retrieval of the avoidance strategy in a shuttle-box (2) seems to be limited to the detection of the conditioned tone stimulus with a lower demand on the cognitive system. A strong increase of prefrontal dopamine was missing in pseudotrained animals with unpaired tone–footshock presentations. We found in gerbils subjected to an escape conditioning with a gap between a 5-s tone offset and the footshock onset of 20 s no increase of the prefrontal dopamine release (unpublished results). So we conclude that the animals had no possibility to associate the key stimuli due to a lacking temporal contiguity [Bischof et al., 2000]. (3) Non-specific stress like footshock punishment does not strongly increase the activity of dopamine system [Herman et al., 1982; Abercrombie et al., 1989; Hernandez and Hoebel, 1990; Imperato et al., 1992]. The moderate increases of cortical dopamine in pseudotrained animals receiving the same number of auditory and electric stimuli as trained animals, and in auditory control animals subjected exclusively to tone stimuli reflects presumably the initial novelty of the applied stimuli and, in the course of training sessions, a readiness for possible associative tasks. Thus, the dopamine system of the sensory auditory cortex is responsive to associative learning, i.e. (4) the function of this brain area seems not to be limited to perception of incoming auditory stimuli. Rather, the sensory field of auditory cortex and the medial prefrontal cortex with its central executive functions [Atkinson and Shiffrin, 1968, Baddeley, 1998] seem to be functionally linked by their dopamine systems during information processing.

Selective Activation of the Prefrontal Dopamine System in the Stage of Strong Increase of Performance during Avoidance Conditioning

From investigations in the auditory cortex the question arose whether a transient increase in dopamine system also occurred in medial prefrontal cortex during formation of key associations in avoidance conditioning. Microdialysis from right medial prefrontal cortex and recordings of learning behavior in the shuttle-box from gerbils subjected to avoidance training sessions were performed. Thereby, individual learning progress was monitored and related to dopamine levels [Stark et al., 1999]. It was of particular interest, whether prefrontal dopamine increase was correlated with the establishment or with the retrieval of the avoidance strategy.

Three behavioral parameters, the attention responses in terms of movement arrest of animals after CS onset as indication of auditory signal detection, the reaction time from tone onset to change of shuttle-box compartment, and the avoidance performance as percent conditioned responses to the conditioned tone stimulus, were used to divide post hoc individual performances into three behavioral stages: (1) low improvement of performance, (2) strong improvement of performance, and (3) constant high performance.

In the stage of low improvement of performance, there was a steep increase in the number of attention responses from initially low levels, a moderate decrease of reaction times, and a moderate increase of avoidance responses to less than 20% (Figure 2). During this stage, the initially indifferent tone became a meaningful tone signal, announcing the footshock, although the tone-dependent avoidance strategy was still undeveloped. There was no increase in prefrontal dopamine at this stage (Figure 2).

During strong improvement of performance the percentage of attention responses was already between 75 and 100%. The reaction times became shorter and jittered around the critical limit of 5 s, i.e. the jumps occurred frequently already during the presentation of the conditioned stimulus leading to footshock avoidance. Animals in this stage relevant for formation of the avoidance strategy showed now a stronger increase in performance (Figure 2). During association of the tone signal with the unconditioned footshock resulting in the avoidance response, prefrontal dopamine steadily and significantly increased until the middle of the training session and dropped before the session was finished (Figure 2).

In the last stage of constant high performance, animals always showed attention responses, reaction times before footshock onset, and a stable high level of avoidance responses (Figure 2). This behavioral stage characterized by the recall of the avoidance strategy showed basal dopamine levels again (Figure 2). The results confirm our hypothesis that the strong increase of dopamine due to the formation of relevant associations for strategy formation was also found in prefrontal cortex.

The temporal requirement in the acquisition of the avoidance strategy appeared to be highly individual. Aiming at a better time resolution for the correlation between individual behavior and dopamine content in dialysates, we exemplary collected dialysates from the right medial prefrontal cortex during the avoidance training session over 30 trials from trial to trial at 2-min intervals in a single experiment [Stark et al., 2000] (Figure 3).

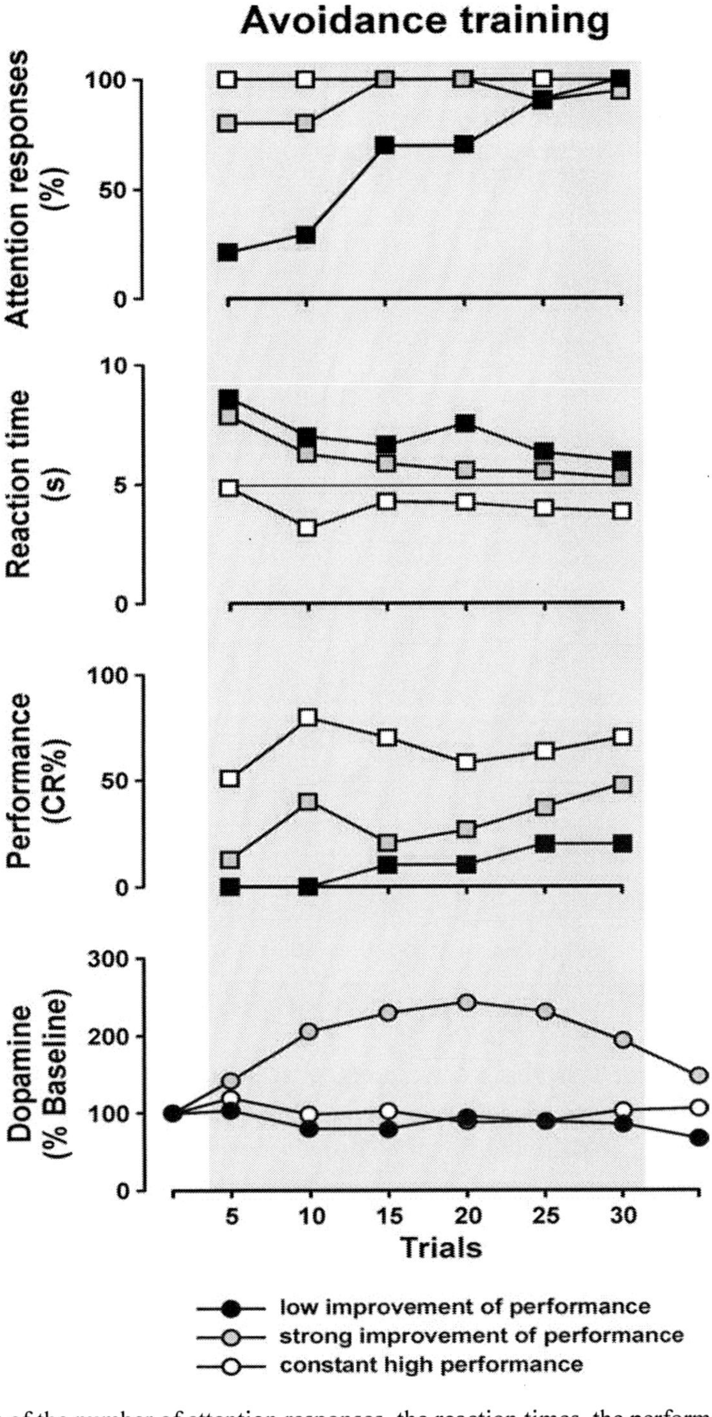

Figure 2. Profiles of the number of attention responses, the reaction times, the performances, and of the relative content of dopamine in dialysates from medial prefrontal cortex of gerbils subjected to avoidance training in the shuttle-box during the behavioral stages of low improvement of performance, of strong improvement of performance, as well as of constant high performance. During the stage of strong improvement of performance a transient strong increase of dopamine values was evident.

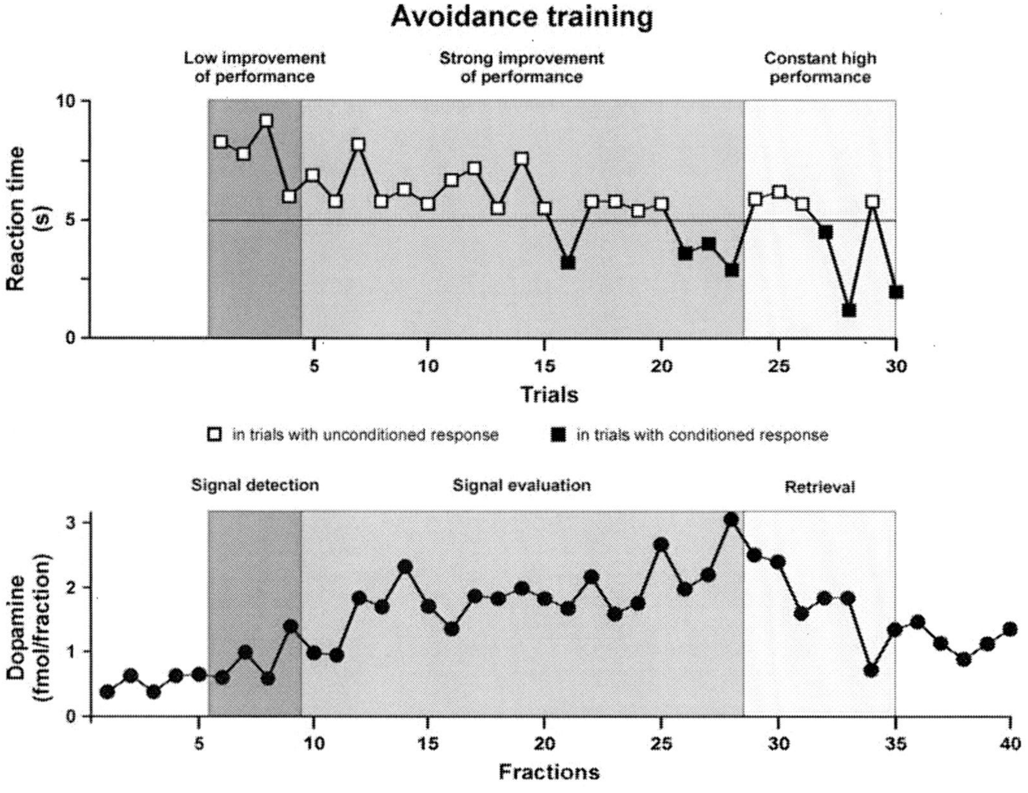

Figure 3. Individual temporal profiles of reaction times and dopamine values of microdialysis samples from prefrontal cortex in the course of avoidance conditioning in the shuttle-box. A reaction time longer than 4.9 s indicates an unconditioned escape response and shorter than 5.0 s a conditioned avoidance response, respectively. Correlation between reaction times and dopamine values from 2-min trial to the next 2-min trial converge into the division of avoidance strategy formation into three learning stages (1) "signal detection", (2) "signal evaluation", and (3) "retrieval of avoidance strategy".

For dopamine measurement in the 2-min dialysate fractions a highly sensitive HPLC analysis was developed. This closer correlation between individual behavioral measures and the learning relevant prefrontal dopamine release in single learning animals enabled us to interpret the cognitive background of the defined behavioral stages. From the first trial to about trial 4 of the avoidance training session we found reaction times far from the 5-s footshock onset time without avoidance responses as well as dopamine values close to the basal level. This first behavioral stage of "Low improvement of performance" [Stark et al., 1999] from trial 1 to 4 was probably characterized by promotion of the initially indifferent tone stimulus to a meaningful signal which announced the following unconditioned footshock. However, this essential key association as prerequisite for further learning still lacks information about the temporal contingency between tone onset and footshock onset, the clear direction for the escape response, namely the change into the contralateral shuttle-box compartment, as well as many instrumental requirements for avoidance behavior. This information, however, is crucial for the animal to build up a successful behavioral strategy to cope with the footshock. Accordingly, the behavioral stage of "Low improvement of performance" was defined as the cognitive stage of (1) "Signal detection". From trial 5 the reaction times became continuously shorter up to trial 23 including reaction times lower than 5 s. In contrast, the dopamine values steadily increased until trial 23. At the end of the second behavioral stage of "Strong improvement of performance" the frequency of responses with a reaction time lower than 5.0 s was already high and the increasing dopamine values reached their maximum. We assume that by about trial 24 the gerbil had acquired the essence of the behavioral strategy which includes the acquisition of further key associations.

The individual first learned to escape into the safe contralateral shuttle-box compartment after footshock onset. At the same time, the animal had started to test the temporal contingency between tone and footshock onset to recognize the possibility to avoid the footshock up to 4.9 s after tone onset. Thereby, the perception of a conditioned avoidance response after the execution of a trial with a reaction time lower than 5.0 s presumably was the most important association for the animal to acquire the avoidance strategy. At this point the individual was qualified to realize that the conflict could be solved by own goal-directed behavior. The behavior in the stage of "Strong improvement of performance" comprises the cognitive side of (2) "Signal evaluation", i.e. the tone signal was attributed with the new meaning signaling the possible escape from or avoidance of the footshock. Note that a clear separation of the stage of "escape learning" from the stage of "avoidance learning" was impossible at that time, due to the fact that a close correlation between behavioral measures and reliable prefrontal dopamine values from dialysates was very limited in this respect. For this distinction, another experimental approach was necessary (see below). From trial 24 in the stage of "Constant high performance" the gerbil started to retrieve the avoidance strategy, and the dopamine values started to attenuate. Presumably, there was no further need of forming additional key associations. Now the behavioral strategy was matured and stored in the memory. The cognitive reflection of this stage of "Constant high performance" may be described best as cognitive stage of (3) "Retrieval of avoidance strategy".

The Role of the Cortical Dopamine System in Cognition

Many aspects of adaptive behavior such as emotional states and motivational and cognitive functions interact with the dopamine system of medial prefrontal cortex. Prefrontal dopamine efflux was increased in response to arousal, stressful situations and appetitive stimuli [Abercrombie et al., 1989; Hernandez and Hoebel, 1990; Broersen et al., 1995; Feenstra and Botterblom, 1996; Spanagel and Weiss, 1999; Feenstra, 2000; Wightman and Robinson, 2002]. Electrophysiological studies of midbrain dopamine neurons terminating in the medial prefrontal cortex revealed that dopamine is integrated in functions of prediction and reward [Fibiger and Phillips, 1986; Koob, 1992; Schultz et al., 1993; Schultz et al., 1997; Schultz, 2002]. Cognitive aspects like attention, cognitive flexibility and consciousness as well as working memory functions are also mediated by dopamine in medial prefrontal cortex [Atkinson and Shiffrin, 1968; Goldman-Rakic, 1992; Goldman-Rakic, 1995; Watanabe et al., 1997; Baddeley, 1998]. Cognitive functions are disturbed by dopamine depletion or D1-receptor blockade [Brozoski et al., 1979; Sawaguchi et al., 1990; Sawaguchi and Goldman-Rakic, 1994; Sokolowski et al., 1994; Seamans et al., 1998]. Dopamine agonists can improve attention and impaired working memory [Arnsten et al., 1994; Granon et al., 2000].

The working memory based on short-term memory principles is vulnerable to dopamine loss [Goldman-Rakic, 1992]. The hypothesis of working memory implies that a recent cognitive information is temporarily kept in such a way that it can be related to the total experience stored in the long term memory as well as to the succeeding input of information [Atkinson and Shiffrin, 1968; Baddeley, 1998]. Presumably, the significance of the working memory system extends far beyond the involvement in specialized working memory tasks like matching or non-matching to sample tasks. It is assumed that this system is used for the performance of many cognitively demanding processes involved in comprehension and problem solving [Eysenck et al., 1997].

Obviously, in the stage of "Signal evaluation" animals acquired the most important information for the formation of the shuttle-box avoidance strategy, i.e. they learned to avoid the punishment by the unconditioned stimulus changing the compartment within the period between onset of the conditioned stimulus and onset of the unconditioned footshock [Fuster, 1989]. We assume that hereby the previously accumulated experience with respect to the developing avoidance strategy is repeatedly compared, combined and completed by continuing feedback information from recent trials. After execution of the recent trial the animal extracts the actual information about an executed unconditioned escape response with footshock punishment or a conditioned avoidance response [Sternberg, 1969] leading to „memory-guided performance" [Goldman-Rakic, 1992] stepwise structured by single trials [Rescorla, 1988]. We assume further that during "Signal evaluation" short-term memory mechanisms could be utilized as proposed for working memory tasks [Atkinson and Shiffrin, 1968; Eysenck et al., 1997; Baddeley, 1998], i.e. to hold the feedback information of recent trials for adequate association with stored experience about shuttle-box learning. This feedback is necessary for comparing the outcome of conditioned compartment changes without footshock with compartment change triggered by footshock. It is further involved in making decisions like "jump before 4.9 s" or "wait for footshock", in planning, and in error processing. All these different sub-processes play an important role in experiments designed as delayed alternation tasks accompanied by strong prefrontal dopamine release. During such a delayed alternation task a prominent prefrontal dopamine increase in monkeys indicating the involvement of working memory was also observed [Watanabe et al., 1997]. The effective learning of an operant discrimination task was accompanied by a significantly increased prefrontal dopamine efflux in rats [Yamamuro et al., 1994; Izaki et al., 1998]. The prominent prefrontal dopamine increase in certain stages of avoidance conditioning in gerbils corresponded to prefrontal dopamine increase in monkeys during a delayed alternation task indicating the involvement of working memory principles [Watanabe et al., 1997]. During retrieval of the established shuttle-box avoidance strategy, the activity of prefrontal dopamine system was strongly attenuated. Therefore, we conclude that working memory principles are presumably not required anymore, i.e. in the stage of retrieval the tone signal implements the full behavioral strategy, and the tone onset triggers a procedure related to reference memory. However, the retrieval of a strategy implicating the "delayed alternation task" including decision making requires also working memory processes [Watanabe et al., 1997].

Thus, the working memory is considered as a tool for memory-guided information processing, i.e. with respect to avoidance learning the correct association between the incoming information of recent trials with information stored in long-term memory.

Moreover, the stepwise formation of a behavioral strategy implicates that the animal rules its behavior to direct it towards the goal of learning.

Findings that the activity of prefrontal and further dopamine systems are increased by appetitive stimuli [Hernandez and Hoebel, 1990; Schultz, 1992; Feenstra and Botterblom, 1996] and that dopamine could play a role in internal reinforcement for optimization of learning processes [Schultz et al., 1997; Schultz, 2002; Fiorillo et al., 2003] may lead to the assumption that working memory principles in medial prefrontal cortex are presumably involved in the interaction with dopamine systems of limbic system signaling the individual a correct compartment change before footshock onset as a conflict-solving „internal reward" and in this way as conditioned response [Koob, 1992; Young, 1993]. The question remains in which areas of the brain these signals are initiated that direct the development of a behavioral strategy towards a goal by reward related reinforcement of correct responses.

Activation of Prefrontal Dopamine System during Behavioral Strategy Changes from Avoidance to Discrimination

In summary, what we can learn from the described experiments is that (1) the prefrontal dopamine system is mainly activated presumably in a stage of the formation of key associations related to the recognition of the temporal contingency between the conditioned tone stimulus and the following unconditioned footshock as well as to the recognition of a conditioned avoidance response. Assumingly, working memory principles are markedly involved in this type of information processing indicated by transient nevertheless strong increase of activity of prefrontal dopamine system. (2) During retrieval of the matured avoidance strategy a remarkable activation of prefrontal dopamine system was lacking. Presumably, the retrieval of the avoidance strategy as a signal-coded procedure does not extensively require working memory principles. We hypothesized that the acquisition of a new behavioral strategy is generally accompanied by this extra prefrontal dopamine release.

A further experiment aimed at testing this hypothesis. For the acquisition of a pre-experience, gerbils were trained in the shuttle-box to generalize two conditioned tone stimuli a1 and a2 associated with the GO-condition. Relearning was induced with discrimination training (GO- vs. NO-GO-trials) [Wetzel et al., 1998] by changing the condition of tone a2 from GO to NO-GO. Using microdialysis, medial prefrontal dopamine efflux was compared between the retrieval of the accomplished avoidance response to the two tone stimuli and the relearning requiring discrimination behavior.

After avoidance pre-training the animals were familiar with the complete shuttle-box context including conditioned tone and unconditioned footshock stimuli. By this, arousal and stress as possible sources of dopamine increase [Abercrombie et al., 1989; Feenstra and Botterblom, 1996; Feenstra, 2000] were minimized in the relearning part of the experiment. Thus, any strong prefrontal dopamine increase should relate to the relearning, i.e. to the formation of associations for the new discrimination behavior. Compared to the avoidance learning the rather difficult relearning of discrimination behavior is assumed to be cognitively more demanding. Accumulation of partial experiences, comparing of events, comprehension of their relationships, reasoning, decision making, error processing, and planning could be again performed by working memory principles [Stark et al., 2004]. The reversal of GO-condition associated to tone stimulus a2 entailed important consequences for the animals.

Gerbils were subjected to an initial misguidance and concurrently to a loss of successful avoidance of punishment. The question arose in which way an animal could develop by itself the goal-directed behavioral strategy for successful discrimination.

After extensive avoidance pre-training and insertion of microdialysis probe into medial prefrontal cortex the gerbils showed an avoidance performance of about 80 $CR^{GO}\%$ to both tone stimuli considered as sufficient pre-experience with the stimuli and the paradigm. Both tone signals a1 and a2 were generalized by the animals as verified by randomized application. No significant differences in dopamine profiles between post hoc divided strongly and weakly relearning animals were found. Prefrontal dopamine increased moderately during retrieval of avoidance response in sessions A1-5 and A2-5 [Stark et al., 2004] (Figure 4).

In discrimination training session D-1 all gerbils responded incorrectly to tone a2 by crossing the hurdle as expected from their avoidance pre-experience and were unexpectedly subjected to a footshock punishment. Therefore, any increase of $CR^{NO\text{-}GO}\%$ started from a low level of performance. But also the GO-performance $CR^{GO}\%$ of both strongly and weakly relearning animals was strongly reduced in the first discrimination training session D-1 compared with the last avoidance training session A2-5 indicating that the meaning of GO-response of an avoidance strategy is completely different from the meaning of GO-response of a discrimination strategy from the cognitive point of view. Presumably, the recent experiences from NO-GO-trial outcomes to tone a2 induced wrong associations in planning of actions concerning the next GO-trials to tone a1. Consequently, the gerbils did not change the shuttle-box compartment to tone a1 and were, therefore, punished again. The formerly high GO-performance of strongly and weakly relearning individuals during the last avoidance training sessions A1-5 and A2-5 collapsed although the GO-condition associated with tone a1 was formally retained.

However, strongly relearning individuals increased significantly their GO-performance during discrimination training sessions D-2 and D-3 resulting in an increased discrimination performance in contrast to weakly relearning animals (Figure 4 top). Obviously, weakly relearning animals could not differentiate between the conditions of the two tone signals, and changed the shuttle-box compartment in the GO-trials mainly on footshock onset. Presumably, weakly relearning animals regressed to an escape strategy from footshock, an initial behavior that had been overcome during avoidance training in the pre-experience period. Consequently, they missed important components of discrimination learning by passively staying in the start compartment of the shuttle-box. Therefore, we assume that they kept inflexibly the generalized GO-condition associated to tone a2 and were not able to substitute it for the NO-GO-condition.

Despite similar behavior of all animals in session D-1 the strongly relearning individuals were obviously able to start instantly a complex relearning process based on an effective recombination of the signal tones a1 and a2 as well as their associated GO- and NO-GO-conditions to establish the essential associations for goal-directed learning. Probably, the rapid abolishment of the generalized GO-condition associated to both tone stimuli was the prerequisite for the following differential re-evaluation with respect to the tones a1 and a2 which were now differentially associated with GO- or NO-GO-conditions.

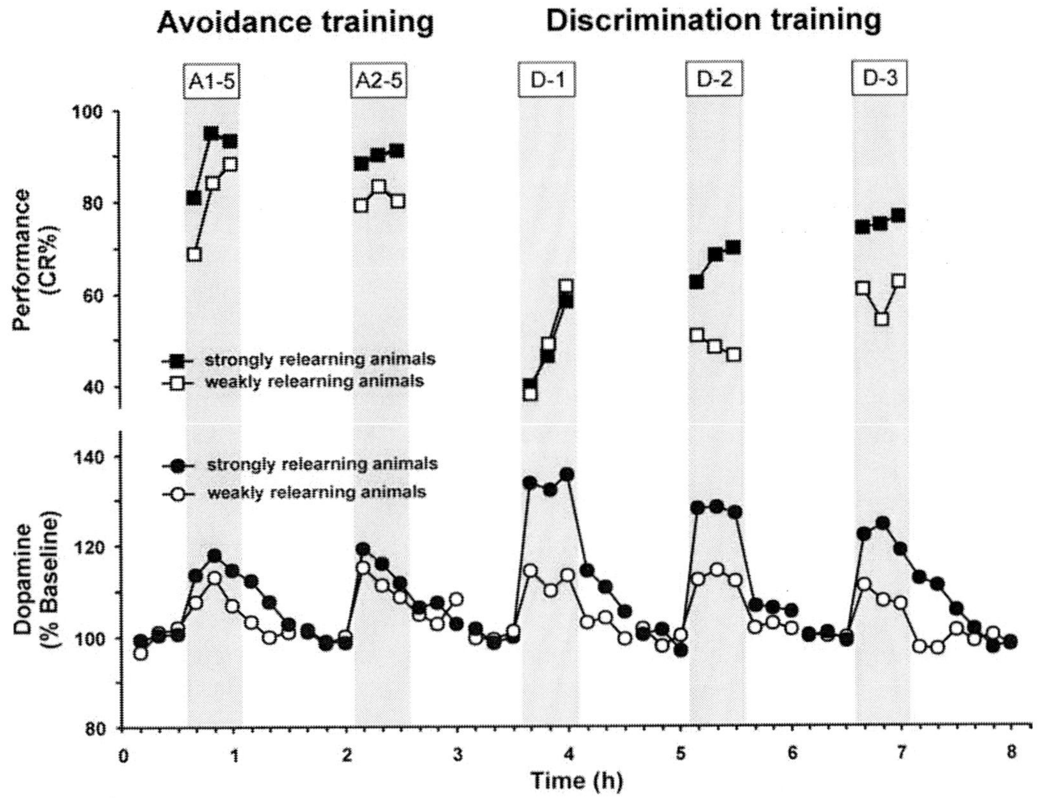

Figure 4. Temporal profiles of avoidance performances ($CR^{GO}\%$) and discrimination performances ($CR^{GO}\% + CR^{NO\text{-}GO}\%$) parallel to dopamine values in post hoc divided strongly relearning and weakly relearning animals. The last sessions for retrieval of avoidance strategy A1-5 and A2-5 and the discrimination training sessions D1 through D3 on the same day are covered. Top: Both strongly and weakly relearning animals retrieved the avoidance strategy in sessions A1-5 and A2-5. After change from GO- to NO-GO-meaning associated to tone a2 in discrimination training the performance in session D-1 dropped to about chance level. No differences between the two groups were found. The discrimination performance in strongly relearning individuals significantly increased in sessions D-2 and D-3 in comparison to weekly relearning individuals. Bottom: Relative prefrontal dopamine content in dialysate samples of strongly and weakly relearning animals across the avoidance training sessions A1-5 and A2-5 and the discrimination training sessions D-1, D-2, and D-3. In contrast to weakly relearning animals the strongly relearning individuals showed a significant extra dopamine increase during the sessions D-1, D-2, and D-3. Note that the extra dopamine increase was maximally in strongly relearning animals in session D-1 while there were no differences in discrimination behavior between strongly and weakly relearning animals.

Thus, only strongly relearning animals were able to realize with increasing distinctness the context-adequate consequences of tones a1 and a2 in GO- and NO-GO-trials during initial discrimination training.

The recombination of the two tone signals, the footshock, and the shuttle-box compartments as well as the temporal relationships between tone signals and footshock punishment [Barnet et al., 1991; Barnet and Miller, 1996; Meck, 1996] had to be established. The increasing frequency of correct GO- and NO-GO-responses resulted in decreasing punishments as consequence of their own actions in the shuttle-box. This process could mediate in strongly relearning individuals internally a reward percept which signals that the development of the discrimination strategy is well oriented to the goal of conflict solution. This percept could guide the development of the behavioral strategy as internal reinforcement as already mentioned above in context of the establishment of the avoidance strategy.

The different cognitive performances of strongly and weakly relearning animals seemed to be reflected by strong or weak prefrontal dopamine release, respectively. After a moderate dopamine release in sessions A1-5 and A2-5 prefrontal dopamine was strongly elevated in the sessions D-1 through D-3 in strongly relearning animals in contrast to weakly relearning animals. Dopamine became attenuated during sessions D-2 and D-3 (Figure 4 bottom). These results confirmed the hypothesis that the acquisition of a new behavioral strategy causes an extra dopamine release in medial prefrontal cortex indicating the involvement of working memory [Goldman-Rakic, 1992; Goldman-Rakic, 1995; Baddeley, 1998; Durstewitz et al., 1999; Dreher and Burnod, 2002; Deco and Rolls, 2003]. The strong activation of prefrontal dopamine system in session D-1 indicated a type of information processing in strongly relearning animals which resulted in a subsequent rapid development of discrimination behavior in the following sessions D-2 and D-3.

Generally, a learning process stops when the appropriate behavior is acquired, i.e. when the trial outcomes are estimated by the individual as context-adequate in terms of conflict solution. The attenuation of the extra dopamine release in strongly relearning individuals in sessions D-2 and D-3 could indicate a reduction of the demand on the working memory system at an advanced stage of the development of the discrimination strategy. At this stage a partial retrieval of the conditioned response to conditioned tone stimuli is presumably permitted from the by then memorized discrimination strategy. However, the retrieval of the discrimination strategy requires always working memory because the animal has to decide in each trial whether the detected tone signal is associated with a GO- or a NO-GO-meaning, respectively, resulting in a certain strength of prefrontal dopamine release. In comparison, the retrieval of the avoidance response in sessions A1-5 and A2-5 resembled rather a sensory-guided task based only on the detection of the tone signal and was accompanied by an only moderate dopamine increase [Watanabe et al., 1997; Stark et al., 1999; Stark et al., 2000].

The relearning experiment confirmed (1) the coincidence of the formation of important associations and of transient extra prefrontal dopamine release at the beginning of relearning, i.e. the development of a new behavioral strategy indicating working memory functions. Obviously, the perception of an internal reward can guide the individual towards the goal of learning. The results obtained so far led us inescapably to the assumption that (2) the dopamine systems are learning stage-dependent tuned for fast and goal-directed adaptation of an individual to the requirements of environment.

Division of the Avoidance Strategy Formation into Discrete Learning Dependent Stages by Characteristic Changes of Cortical Theta Activity

From the aversive motivated learning experiments – avoidance as well as discrimination conditioning in the shuttle-box - we conclude that (1) the learning process is initiated by the unconditioned footshock punishment evoking a conflict in the individual. (2) The activity of cortical and prefrontal dopamine systems seems to increase during maturation of the avoidance or discrimination strategy, respectively, by associating the conditioned tone stimulus with the unconditioned footshock to build up a reliable behavioral strategy. Presumably in this stage, working memory with attributes like error processing, planning, decision making, and feedback processing is highly involved. The question arises whether there exist learning stage dependent signals governing the development of an adequate behavioral strategy for conflict solving as the goal of learning. Therefore, we used recording of electroencephalograms during avoidance conditioning with following theta analysis to warrant a sufficient temporal resolution for a close correlation between behavioral and learning relevant physiological data, a prerequisite for detection of such strategy-ruling signals.

Theta activity defined by the frequency range from 4 to 8 Hz in accordance with other studies in the gerbil [Bonner and Martinez, 1975], the rat [Krügel et al., 2003], or the mouse [Seidenbecher et al., 2003] appears to be a correlate for the intensity of information processing specifically during associative learning [Balleine and Curthoys, 1991; Asada et al., 1999; Ishii et al., 1999]. Accordingly, if the acquisition of the avoidance strategy consists of stages defined by behavioral and physiological observables, the stepwise learning could be reflected by fast changes of theta activation. The basic hypothesis of the experiment was that the strength of theta activity may characterize the course of intensity of information processing from the start of learning up to the retrieval of the matured behavioral strategy.

Generally, theta activity seems to be involved in brain states of arousal and consciousness specifically appearing during associative learning [Asada et al., 1999; Ishii et al., 1999]. Physiological studies in rat and human have also indicated that mental tasks involving working memory are accompanied by synchronized neuronal activity in the theta-frequency range [Givens, 1996; Sarnthein et al., 1998]. Oscillations of brain potentials between 4 and 8 Hz are generated in subjects during decision making [Jacobs et al., 2006]. Hippocampal theta activity involved in communication between prefrontal cortex and hippocampus plays a crucial role in encoding of information in working memory which is later retrieved for use in problem solving [Givens, 1996; Sarnthein et al., 1998; Jensen, 2005; Jones and Wilson, 2005]. The maintenance of hippocampal theta activity is essential in initial learning in rats [McNaughton et al., 2006]. Theta rhythms generated in hippocampus and cortex may nevertheless link hippocampal and cortical neuron ensembles that participate in representing different aspects of the training situation in discriminative avoidance conditioning [Talk et al., 2004]. Theta synchronization in humans coordinates the central executive circuits, including medial prefrontal cortex [Ishii et al., 1999; Mizuhara and Yamaguchi, 2007]. Together, such results suggest that theta activity as correlate for the intensity of information processing may also reflect learning during the formation of behavioral strategies that require a continuous updating of information.

We found an overall negative correlation of theta activity in the intertrial interval after compartment change with individual learning progress [Stark et al., 2007]. Beyond this general trend, a detailed comparison of actual theta activity with behavioral events in a trial by trial analysis could disclose markers for the formation of relevant associations and for the separation of stages of the learning process [Stark et al., 2008]. For a detailed analysis the theta activity in the intertrial epochs after compartment change until the start of a new trial was chosen. In these trial epochs an animal can update the previous cumulative behavioral feedback experience with the actual outcome of the preceding trial. The result of this processing may be used behaviorally for planning in the next trials. We assumed that during this epoch, the intensity of information processing in the course of learning is reflected most prominently.

As a fundamental result, the process of avoidance strategy formation was divided into four cognitive stages by unique marker trials (Figure 5). After an initial theta activity maximum the sharpest decline in theta power between any two trials (two big open circles on the left in Figure 5) was defined as the transition from stage 1 "signal detection" to stage 2 "escape learning" which started at the marker trial with lower theta activation. Subsequently, the theta power decreased gradually over a number of trials accompanied by a decrease of latency of the unconditioned responses after footshock. Across the trials with unconditioned responses during "escape learning" animals already showed reaction times shorter than 5 s, i.e. with reactions before the onset of the footshock, in some interspersed trials. While these singular events initially remained without consequences in the theta power there was always found one trial in each animal where such an avoidance of the footshock was followed by a sudden marked increase of theta power as referred to theta power in the preceding trials with reaction times shorter than 5 s. This trial was used as marker for the first conditioned response (big filled circle inside left in Figure 5). Subsequently, the number of conditioned responses to the tones increased and their response latencies steeply shortened even though there were still intermingled unconditioned responses. After the marker trial with a conspicuous increase of theta power the previous trend of decrease of theta power was reversed to an increase in trials with an unconditioned response. We consider this reversal at the marker trial as the boundary between stage 2 "escape learning" and stage 3 "avoidance learning". The reliability of this division was confirmed by behavioral data. The number of trials with a reaction time shorter than 5 s was lower than the number of trials with unconditioned responses before the marker trial and, vice versa, after the marker trial. During stage 3 "avoidance learning" mistakes in terms of unconditioned responses with footshocks were still made but with decreasing tendency concomitant with an increase of theta power after these mistakes. The stages "escape learning" and "avoidance learning" as result of theta activity analysis replaced the non-differentiated stage "signal evaluation" determined earlier using prefrontal dopamine values [Stark et al., 2000]. At some maximum of theta power (second maximum; big open circle in the center in Figure 5) this trend reversed in stage 4 "retrieval of avoidance response" to a slow decrease of theta activity after the remaining occasional mistakes. Assumingly, the conjunction of a mistake with a subsequent maximum of theta power represented the crucial event separating stage 3 from stage 4. The post hoc determination of stages in avoidance conditioning was performed by combining of theta power analysis with behavioral analysis. The four stages appear to be clearly distinguishable using the obtained behavioral events.

The close correlation between behavioral data and theta activations determined with high temporal precision during avoidance learning allows us to interpret our finding with respect to the already described cognitive learning stages. At the start of avoidance training in the stage of "signal detection" the tone stimuli are still meaningless for the animals, and they just try to flee from the sudden footshock punishment in an apparently uncoordinated and confused fashion. Analysis of video recordings revealed the strong excitement of the animals caused by the high degree of uncertainty. The theta power within these initial trials reaches the first and highest maximum indicating strong information processing by the animals. Assumingly, stress is involved in these first trials due to unpredictability of the context and drives the animal to search the contralateral shuttle-box compartment to escape the footshock punishment.

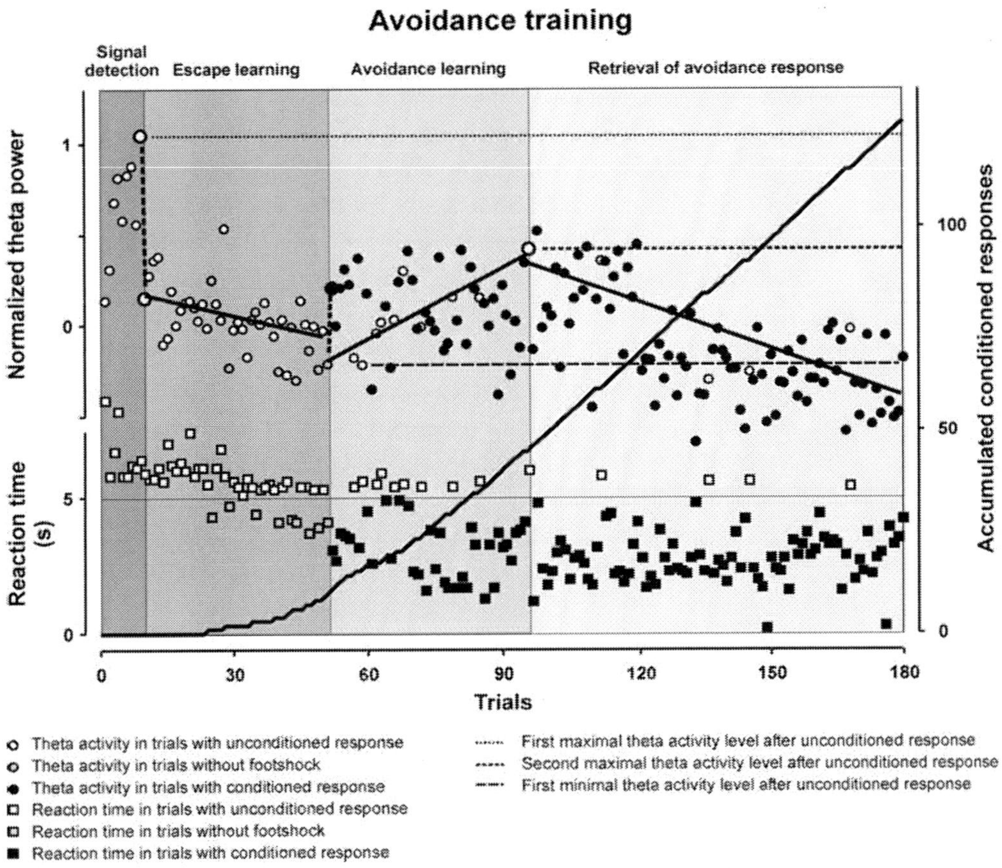

Figure 5. Stage-dependent theta activity in the trial periods after compartment change and corresponding reaction times after tone onset in a gerbil during avoidance conditioning in the shuttle-box. Upper part shows the normalized theta power in the period after compartment change in 180 successive trials with unconditioned responses (open circles) and conditioned responses (filled circles) plotted over the stages 1 "signal detection", 2 "escape learning", 3 "avoidance learning", and 4 "retrieval of avoidance response". After an initial theta power maximum (upper thin dotted line) the sharpest decline of theta power between trial 9 and trial 10 (big open circles connected by fat dotted line, falling) is defined as the event that separates the stages 1 and 2. The regression line of gradually falling theta power in stage 2 "escape learning" is computed from values in trials with unconditioned responses (fat line, falling). The beginning of stage 3 "avoidance learning", by our definition, is marked by the trial 52 with a reaction time lower than 5 s that entails a conspicuous increase of theta power; assumingly the first conditioned response (big filled circle, fat dotted, rising line indicating marked theta power increase). Note that previous trials with reaction time lower than 5 s do not show a substantial increase of theta power. In the neighborhood there is always a trial that shows the absolute theta power minimum of all unconditioned responses (lower thin dotted line connecting to the open circle). The regression line of gradually increasing theta power in stage 3 "avoidance learning" is

computed from values in trials with unconditioned responses (fat solid line, rising). The line stops at the trial 96 with an unconditioned response that forms the second theta power maximum between stages 3 "avoidance learning" and 4 "retrieval of avoidance response" (big open circle; middle thin dotted line), defined as the end of stage 3. Lower part shows reaction times in trials with unconditioned responses (open squares) and conditioned responses (filled squares). The horizontal 5-s line (footshock onset) separates unconditioned and conditioned responses.

Nevertheless, after several hurdle crossings animals can make the sudden experience, that the contralateral compartment is safe. As can be observed in the video recordings, this immediately leads to a coordinated escape behavior, i.e. after compartment change animals turn already during the intertrial interval towards the hurdle awaiting the next footshock punishment. The sharp decrease of theta power from one trial to the next may indicate that the demand of information processing is strongly reduced because the tone stimulus just became a conditioned signal announcing the footshock. By this, the initial stress as possible source of theta activation is largely reduced [Coover et al., 1973; Knardahl and Murison, 1989; Shors et al., 1997; van der Borght et al., 2005]. The association of the tone stimulus with the following footshock enhances strongly the predictability of the punishment. We assume that the sharp decline of theta power indicates the transition from completed stage 1 "signal detection" to the following stage 2 "escape learning". Paired tone and footshock stimuli in further trials optimize the instrumental response in animals, speeding up the reaction times. The perfection of the escape strategy is accompanied by a gradual drop in theta power in these trials with unconditioned responses. During "escape learning" animals occasionally change the compartment already before footshock onset without salient change of theta power compared with theta power in preceding trials with unconditioned responses. Presumably, the animals do not notice yet the contingency between the early reaction time and drop-out of footshock. Several such compartment changes before footshock seem to be required until the animals perceive the contingency between tone onset and the possibility of footshock avoidance. It is assumingly the trial in which the theta power markedly increases, in which the first conditioned response is performed by the animal. At the same time the theta power in trials with unconditioned responses adjacent to the first conditioned response reaches a first minimum. The first conditioned response to tone onset with elevated theta power marks probably the beginning of stage 3 "avoidance learning". After the first conditioned response the animals react more and more to tone onset and no longer to footshock onset, and thus receive the reward by "success" of footshock avoidance more and more frequent. From the video recordings it can be seen, that immediately after tone onset, animals are positioned in front of the hurdle. Often they move the head back and forth as external sign for internal indecision to jump or to stay. At the beginning of this stage, the poorly defined contingency between tone and footshock onset is subjected to an intensive error processing, decision making, and planning indicated by a renewed increase of theta activation immediately after remaining unconditioned responses up to a second maximum of theta activity, i.e. remaining mistakes become the main focus of attention and processing activity interpreted as learning from mistakes [Frank et al., 2004]. In this error processing the footshock punishment as a consequence of exceeding the 5-s latency after tone onset is compared to the consequence of the growing experience to change the shuttle-box compartment with respect to the time schedule followed by footshock avoidance. Feedback processing using short term memory could serve to compare the plan [Tanji and Hoshi, 2001; Tanji et al., 2007] - change the compartment or stay - with the outcome of action – footshock avoidance or punishment. In this respect the individual learns stepwise by unconditioned responses that the compartment change pursued to the reaction time proves the plan and that the conditioned response is the goal of learning. In this way the individual may perform the goal-directed and memory-guided learning process [Goldman-Rakic, 1992; Goldman-Rakic, 1995].

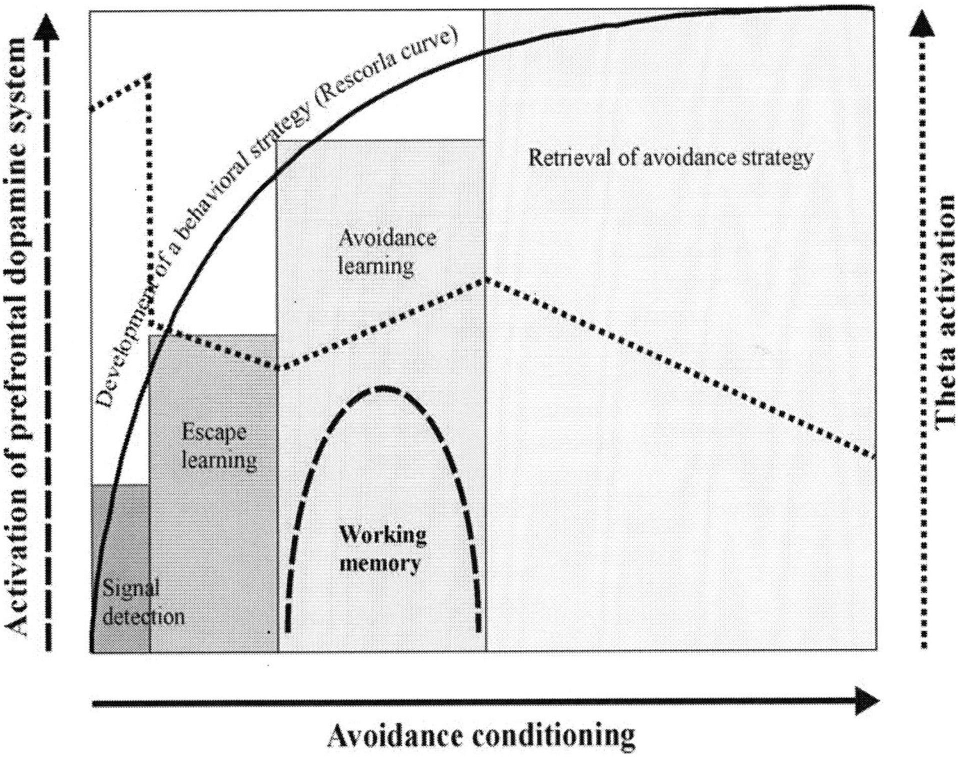

Figure 6. Dynamics of activation of prefrontal dopamine system and changes in cortical theta activity in the course of aversively motivated associative conditioning. The transient increase of prefrontal dopamine was found in the stage of avoidance learning during formation of relevant associations underlying a goal-directed, i.e. problem-solving behavioral strategy. During this stage presumably processes of internal reinforcement are involved to rule the behavioral strategy reducing stepwise the at the beginning of learning evoked conflict. Theta power presumably reflecting the current demand of information processing decreases differently in the stages "signal detection" and "escape learning" in trials with unconditioned responses. Theta activity increases up to a second theta activity maximum in the stage of "avoidance learning" presumably demanding working memory. In the following stage of "retrieval of avoidance strategy" theta activity steadily decreases. The correlation of dopamine and theta activity data with recorded behavioral events during associative learning allows the division of the development of the tested avoidance strategy into discrete learning dependent stages.

In that trial in which the animal experiences the congruity between the plan to reduce sufficiently the conflict and the goal of learning to avoid the footshock theta activity conspicuously increases at the first conditioned response. Possibly, we characterized the physiological substrate of suddenly increasing theta activation as indicator for internal reinforcement. However, in which way this crucial signal is produced is an open question requiring further investigations. Assumingly, dopamine systems of cortical and limbic brain areas are involved [Dayan and Balleine, 2002; Salamone and Correa, 2002; Bouret and Sara, 2004; Dalley et al., 2004; Nieuwenhuis et al., 2004; Kim et al., 2006; Izhikevich, 2007; Doya, 2008; Rushworth and Behrens, 2008]. The renewed increase of theta activity in trials with unconditioned responses during "avoidance learning" up to the second theta maximum presumably reflects an increasing demand on decision making, planning and feedback processing as attributes of working memory. The stage of "avoidance learning" is accompanied by further shortening of reaction times. We assume that the trial with unconditioned response showing the second maximum of theta activity marks the end of "avoidance learning", i.e. the temporal contingencies of the successful avoidance strategy have been acquired.

In the following stage 4 "retrieval of avoidance strategy" the theta power in further sporadic trials with unconditioned responses as a consequence of a "sloppy response" is steadily decreased obviously indicating a decreasing demand of information processing. Alternatively, sporadic trials with unconditioned responses which are normal even in highly trained animals may be interpreted as a check of still valid behavioral contingencies. The omission of footshocks would induce an extinction as a relearning process. The described markers used for division of the avoidance learning into different stages are found in all animals. However, the duration of the stages is individually different [Stark et al., 2008].

The hierarchy of stages and the processes within these stages during avoidance conditioning show the accumulation of partial experiences from trial to trial to a context-adequate memory-guided mature avoidance strategy [Rescorla, 1988; Goldman-Rakic, 1992]. However, very different aspects of the structure of the shuttle-box paradigm are learned before the avoidance response is fully consolidated. The demand of information processing as presumably reflected by theta activity shows several rising and falling phases with singularities in between. Our detailed trial by trial analysis suggests that experiences from two or few successive trials at a given stage of learning determine the further course of information processing under different aspects. This is the case for tone-shock association, for escape optimization, for the initial conditioned response, i.e. the first success, and for the subsequent clarification of remaining mistakes. As previously suggested [Sternberg, 1969; Goldman-Rakic, 1992; Stark et al., 2000; Luu et al., 2004; Krigolson and Holroyd, 2006] the demand of information processing is particularly strong during error analysis. But as judged from the theta activity being highest during initial tone-shock association in the stage of "signal detection", we assume that theta activation reflects the load of information processing in a rather comprehensive way including the state of arousal. In comparison the prefrontal dopamine system seems to be exclusively activated during learning the importance of associated tone signal and footshock stimulus responsible for the successful behavioral strategy.

Conclusion

Simultaneous recording of behavioral data and physiological data like dopamine release and theta activations from the beginning of a learning process up to the retrieval of memorized acquired facts and procedures allowed the investigation of the formation of behavioral strategies and revealed a cascade of discrete learning-dependent stages (Figure 6).

The activation of prefrontal dopamine system seems to reflect information processing related to the stage of formation of relevant associations for a successful behavioral strategy in which the animal realizes problem solving as the consequence of its own successful action. Working memory principles seem to be involved with attributes like error processing, decision making, planning, and feedback processing. Associative learning always demands working memory. Also, during the retrieval of behavioral strategies requiring decision making, working memory is activated. However, the retrieval of a memorized procedure requires obviously no activation of working memory. Cortical theta activity presumably indicates more general demand of information processing, inclusively, the state of arousal to certain moments during stage-dependent learning. The dynamics of dopamine and theta activity data related to behavioral events converge in the assumption that the formation of a behavioral strategy may be divided into discrete learning-dependent stages.

The learning process is initiated by a conflict. Seemingly, in the stage of association of key stimuli activating working memory, a stepwise conflict reduction, which is critical for finding the sufficient and context-adequate problem solution as goal of learning, is performed. We assume that the reflection of successful punishment reduction by the animal acts as an "emotional ruler" to determine the direction of successful development of the behavioral strategy, i.e., animals learn from mistakes. Possibly, the trial-specific theta activation at the first conditioned response indicates a relevant reinforcing signal. Nevertheless, up to now many reports from literature about internal reinforcement may not explain comprehensively the source, the formation and the moment of triggering of the learning stage-dependent signal for internal reinforcement.

The increase in activity of the prefrontal dopamine system during the formation of relevant associations by working memory functions as prerequisite for the presumable perception of an internal reward to guide the individual to the goal of learning indicates that dopamine systems are involved in goal-directed learning-dependent reinforcement.

Acknowledgments

I thank Thomas Rothe and Matthias Deliano for critical reading of the manuscript.

References

Abercrombie, E. D., Keefe, K. A., DiFrischia, D. S., and Zigmond, M. J. (1989). Differential effect of stress on in vivo dopamine release in striatum, nucleus accumbens, and medial frontal cortex. *J. Neurochem.*, 52, 1655-1658.

Arnsten, A. F. T., Cai, J. X., Murphy, B. L., and Goldman-Rakic, P. S. (1994). Dopamine D1 receptor mechanisms in the cognitive performance of young adult and aged monkeys. *Psychopharmacology* (Berl), 116, 143-151.

Asada, H., Fukuda, Y., Tsunoda, S., Yamaguchi, M., and Tonoike, M. (1999). Frontal midline theta rhythms reflect alternative activation of prefrontal cortex and anterior cingulate cortex in humans. *Neurosci. Lett.*, 274, 29-32.

Atkinson, R. C. and Shiffrin, R. M. (1968). Human memory: a proposed system and its control processes. In K. W. Spence and J. T. Spence (Eds.), *The Psychology of Learning and Motivation,* Vol.2 (pp. 89-195). London: Academic Press.

Baddeley, A. (1998). Recent developments in working memory. *Curr. Opin. Neurobiol.*, 8, 234-238.

Balleine, B. W. and Curthoys, I. S. (1991). Differential effects of escapable and inescapable footshock on hippocampal theta activity. *Behav. Neurosci.*, 105, 202-209.

Barnet, R. C., Arnold, H. M., and Miller, R. R. (1991). Simultaneous conditioning demonstrated in second order conditioning: evidence for similar associative structure in forward and simultaneous conditioning. *Learn. Motiv.*, 22, 253-268.

Barnet, R. C. and Miller, R. R. (1996). Temporal encoding as a determinant of inhibitory control. *Learn. Motiv.*, 27, 73-91.

Bischof, A., Stark, H., Wagner, T., and Scheich, H. (2000). The inhibitory influence of an acquired escape strategy on subsequent avoidance learning in gerbils. *Neurosci. Lett.*, 281, 175-178.

Bonner, S. J. and Martinez, J. L. (1975). The early development of the EEG in the gerbil. *Behav. Biol.,* 14, 367-372.

Bouret, S. and Sara, S. J. (2004). Reward expectation, orientation of attention and locus coeruleus-medial frontal cortex interplay during learning. *Eur. J. Neurosci.,* 20, 791-802.

Broersen, L. M., Heinsbroek, R. P. W., de Bruin, J. P. C., Uylings, H. B. M., and Olivier, B. (1995). The role of the medial prefrontal cortex of rats in short-term memory functioning: further support for involvement of cholinergic, rather than dopaminergic mechanisms. *Brain Res.,* 674, 221-229.

Brozoski, T. J., Brown, R. M., Rosvold, H. E., and Goldman, P. S. (1979). Cognitive deficit caused by regional depletion of dopamine in prefrontal cortex of rhesus monkey. *Science,* 205, 929-932.

Coover, G. D., Ursin, H., and Levine, S. (1973). Plasma-corticosterone levels during active-avoidance learning in rats. *J. Comp. Physiol. Psychol.*, 82, 170-174.

Dalley, J. W., Cardinal, R. N., and Robbins, T. W. (2004). Prefrontal executive and cognitive functions in rodents: neural and neurochemical substrates. *Neurosci. Biobehav. Rev.*, 28, 771-784.

Dayan, P. and Balleine, B. W. (2002). Reward, motivation, and reinforcement learning. *Neuron*, 36, 285-298.

Deakin, J. F. W. and Graeff, F. G. (1991). 5-HT and mechanisms of defence. *J. Psychopharmacol.*, 5, 305-315.

Deco, G. and Rolls, E. T. (2003). Attention and working memory: a dynamical model of neuronal activity in the prefrontal cortex. *Eur. J. Neurosci.*, 18, 2374-2390.

Doya, K. (2008). Modulators of decision making. *Nat. Neurosci.*, 11, 410-416.

Dreher, J. C. and Burnod, Y. (2002). An integrative theory of the phasic and tonic modes of dopamine modulation in the prefrontal cortex. *Neural. Netw.*, 15, 583-602.

Durstewitz, D., Kelc, M., and Güntürkün, O. (1999). A neurocomputational theory of the dopaminergic modulation of working memory functions. *J. Neurosci.*, 19, 2807-2822.

Eichenbaum, H. (2008). *Learning and memory*. New York, NY: Norton and Company.

Eysenck, M. W., Ellis, A., Hunt, E., and Johnson-Laird, P. (1994). *The Blackwell Dictionary of Cognitive Psychology* (pp. 333-335). Oxford: Blackwell.

Feenstra, M. G. P. and Botterblom, M. H. A. (1996). Rapid sampling of extracellular dopamine in the rat prefrontal cortex during food consumption, handling and exposure to novelty. *Brain Res.*, 742, 17-24.

Feenstra, M. G. P. (2000). Dopamine and noradrenaline release in the prefrontal cortex in relation to unconditioned and conditioned stress and reward. *Prog. Brain Res.*, 126, 133-163.

Fibiger, H. C. and Phillips, A. G. (1986). Reward, motivation, cognition: psychobiology of mesotelencephalic dopamine systems. In F. E. Bloom (Ed.), *Handbook of Physiology. The Nervous System.* Intrinsic Regulatory Systems of the Brain (pp. 647-675). Bethesda, MD: Am. Physiol. Soc.

Fiorillo, C. D., Tobler, P. N., and Schultz, W. (2003). Discrete coding of reward probability and uncertainty by dopamine neurons. *Science*, 299, 1898-1902.

Frank, M. J., Seeberger, L. C., and O'Reilly, R. C. (2004). By carrot or by stick: cognitive reinforcement learning in parkinsonism. *Science*, 306, 1940-1943.

Fuster, J. M. (1989). *The Prefrontal Cortex: Anatomy, Physiology, and Neuropsychology of the Frontal Lobe* (2 ed., pp. 179-187). New York, NY: Raven Press.

Givens, B. (1996). Stimulus-evoked resetting of the dentate theta rhythm: relation to working memory. *Neuroreport,* 8, 159-163.

Glass, J. D., Hauser, U. E., Randolph, W. W., Rea, M. A., and De Vries, M. J. (1993). In vivo microdialysis of 5-hydroxyindoleacetic acid and glutamic acid in the hamster suprachiasmatic nuclei. *Amer. Zool.*, 33, 212-218.

Goldman-Rakic, P. S. (1992). Dopamine-mediated mechanisms of the prefrontal cortex. *Semin. Neurosci.,* 4, 149-159.

Goldman-Rakic, P. S. (1995). Cellular basis of working memory. *Neuron*, 14, 477-485.

Graeff, F. G. (1993). Role of 5-HT in defensive behavior and anxiety. *Rev. Neurosci.*, 4, 181-211.

Granon, S., Passetti, F., Thomas, K. L., Dalley, J. W., Everitt, B. J., and Robbins, T. W. (2000). Enhanced and impaired attentional performance after infusion of D1 dopaminergic receptor agents into rat prefrontal cortex. *J. Neurosci.*, 20, 1208-1215.

Herman, J. P., Guillonneau, D., Dantzer, R., Scatton, B., Semerdjian-Rouquier, L., and Le Moal, M. (1982). Differential effects of inescapable footshocks and of stimuli previously paired with inescapable footshocks on dopamine turnover in cortical and limbic areas of the rat. *Life Sci.*, 30, 2207-2214.

Hernandez, L. and Hoebel, B. G. (1990). Feeding can enhance dopamine turnover in the prefrontal cortex. *Brain Res. Bull.*, 25, 975-979.

Imperato, A., Puglisi-Allegra, S., Scrocco, M. G., Casolini, P., Bacchi, S., and Angelucci, L. (1992). Cortical and limbic dopamine and acetylcholine release as neurochemical correlates of emotional arousal in both aversive and non-aversive environmental changes. *Neurochem. Int.,* 20 Suppl, 265S-270S.

Ishii, R., Shinosaki, K., Ukai, S., Inouye, T., Ishihara, T., Yoshimine, T., Hirabuki, N., Asada, H., Kihara, T., Robinson, S. E., and Takeda, M. (1999). Medial prefrontal cortex generates frontal midline theta rhythm. *Neuroreport,* 10, 675-679.

Izaki, Y., Hori, K., and Nomura, M. (1998). Dopamine and acetylcholine elevation on lever-press acquisition in rat prefrontal cortex. *Neurosci. Lett*., 258, 33-36.

Izhikevich, E. M. (2007). Solving the distal reward problem through linkage of STDP and dopamine signaling. *Cereb. Cortex*, 17, 2443-2452.

Jacobs, J., Hwang, G., Curran, T., and Kahana, M. J. (2006). EEG oscillations and recognition memory: Theta correlates of memory retrieval and decision making. *Neuroimage,* 32, 978-987.

Jensen, O. (2005). Reading the hippocampal code by theta phase-locking. *Trends Cogn. Sci,* 9, 551-553.

Jones, M. W. and Wilson, M. A. (2005). Theta rhythms coordinate hippocampal-prefrontal interactions in a spatial memory task. *PLoS Biol.,* 3, e402.

Kim, H., Shimojo, S., and O'Doherty, J. P. (2006). Is Avoiding an Aversive Outcome Rewarding? Neural Substrates of Avoidance Learning in the Human Brain. *PLoS Biol.,* 4, e233.

Knardahl, S. and Murison, R. (1989). Plasma corticosterone and renin activity during two-way active avoidance learning in spontaneously hypertensive and Wistar-Kyoto rats. *Behav. Neural. Biol.,* 51, 389-400.

Koob, G. F. (1992). Dopamine, addiction and reward. *Semin. Neurosci.,* 4, 139-158.

Krigolson, O. E. and Holroyd, C. B. (2006). Evidence for hierarchical error processing in the human brain. *Neuroscience,* 137, 13-17.

Krügel, U., Kittner, H., Franke, H., and Illes, P. (2003). Purinergic modulation of neuronal activity in the mesolimbic dopaminergic system in vivo. *Synapse*, 47, 134-142.

Luu, P., Tucker, D. M., and Makeig, S. (2004). Frontal midline theta and the error-related negativity: neurophysiological mechanisms of action regulation. *Clin. Neurophysiol*., 115, 1821-1835.

McNaughton, N., Ruan, M., and Woodnorth, M. A. (2006). Restoring theta-like rhythmicity in rats restores initial learning in the Morris water maze. *Hippocampus*, 16, 1102-1110.

Meck, W. H. (1996). Neuropharmacology of timing and time perception. *Cogn. Brain Res*., 3, 227-242.

Mizuhara, H. and Yamaguchi, Y. (2007). Human cortical circuits for central executive function emerge by theta phase synchronization. *Neuroimage*, 36, 232-244.

Nieuwenhuis, S., Holroyd, C. B., Mol, N., and Coles, M. G. H. (2004). Reinforcement-related brain potentials from medial frontal cortex: origins and functional significance. *Neurosci. Biobehav. Rev*., 28, 441-448.

Ohl, F. W. and Scheich, H. (1996). Differential frequency conditioning enhances spectral contrast sensitivity of units in auditory cortex (field Al) of the alert Mongolian gerbil. *Eur. J. Neurosci*., 8, 1001-1017.

Rescorla, R. A. (1988). Pavlovian conditioning. It's not what you think it is. *Am. Psychol.*, 43, 151-160.

Riess, D. (1972). Vicarious conditioned acceleration: successful observational learning of an aversive Pavlovian stimulus contingency. *J. Exp. Anal. Behav.,* 18, 181-186.

Rushworth, M. F. and Behrens, T. E. (2008). Choice, uncertainty and value in prefrontal and cingulate cortex. *Nat. Neurosci.*, 11, 389-397.

Salamone, J. D. (1994). The involvement of nucleus accumbens dopamine in appetitive and aversive motivation. *Behav. Brain Res.*, 61, 117-133.

Salamone, J. D. and Correa, M. (2002). Motivational views of reinforcement: implications for understanding the behavioral functions of nucleus accumbens dopamine. *Behav. Brain Res.,* 137, 3-25.

Sarnthein, J., Petsche, H., Rappelsberger, P., Shaw, G. L., and von Stein, A. (1998). Synchronization between prefrontal and posterior association cortex during human working memory. *Proc. Natl. Acad. Sci. USA*, 95, 7092-7096.

Sawaguchi, T., Matsumura, M., and Kubota, K. (1990). Effects of dopamine antagonists on neuronal activity related to a delayed response task in monkey prefrontal cortex. *J. Neurophysiol.,* 63, 1401-1412.

Sawaguchi, T. and Goldman-Rakic, P. S. (1991). D1 dopamine receptors in prefrontal cortex: involvement in working memory. *Science*, 251, 947-950.

Sawaguchi, T. and Goldman-Rakic, P. S. (1994). The role of D1-dopamine receptor in working memory: local injections of dopamine antagonists into the prefrontal cortex of rhesus monkeys performing an oculomotor delayed-response task. *J. Neurophysiol.*, 71, 515-528.

Scheich, H. and Zuschratter, W. (1995). Mapping stimulus features and meaning in gerbil auditory cortex with 2-deoxyglucose, and c-Fos antibodies. *Behav. Brain Res.*, 66, 195-205.

Schultz, W. (1992). Activity of dopamine neurons in the behaving primate. *Semin. Neurosci.*, 4, 129-139.

Schultz, W., Apicella, P., and Ljungberg, T. (1993). Responses of monkey dopamine neurons to reward and conditioned stimuli during successive steps of learning a delayed response task. *J. Neurosci.,* 13, 900-913.

Schultz, W., Dayan, P., and Montague, P. R. (1997). A neural substrate of prediction and reward. *Science*, 275, 1593-1599.

Schultz, W. (2002). Getting formal with dopamine and reward. *Neuron*, 36, 241-263.

Seamans, J. K., Floresco, S. B., and Phillips, A. G. (1998). D1 receptor modulation of hippocampal-prefrontal cortical circuits integrating spatial memory with executive functions in the rat. *J. Neurosci.,* 18, 1613-1621.

Seidenbecher, T., Laxmi, T. R., Stork, O., and Pape, H. C. (2003). Amygdalar and hippocampal theta rhythm synchronization during fear memory retrieval. *Science*, 301, 846-850.

Shors, T. J., Gallegos, R. A., and Breindl, A. (1997). Transient and persistent consequences of acute stress on long-term potentiation (LTP), synaptic efficacy, theta rhythms and bursts in area CA1 of the hippocampus. *Synapse*, 26, 209-217.

Sokolowski, J. D., McCullough, L. D., and Salamone, J. D. (1994). Effects of dopamine depletions in the medial prefrontal cortex on active avoidance and escape in the rat. *Brain Res.,* 651, 293-299.

Spanagel, R. and Weiss, F. (1999). The dopamine hypothesis of reward: past and current status. *Trends Neurosci.,* 22, 521-527.

Stark, H. and Scheich, H. (1997). Dopaminergic and serotonergic neurotransmission systems are differentially involved in auditory cortex learning: a long-term microdialysis study of metabolites. *J. Neurochem*., 68, 691-697.

Stark, H., Bischof, A., and Scheich, H. (1999). Increase of extracellular dopamine in prefrontal cortex of gerbils during acquisition of the avoidance strategy in the shuttle-box. *Neurosci. Lett.,* 264, 77-80.

Stark, H., Bischof, A., Wagner, T., and Scheich, H. (2000). Stages of avoidance strategy formation in gerbils are correlated with dopaminergic transmission activity. *Eur. J. Pharmacol.,* 405, 263-275.

Stark, H., Rothe, T., Wagner, T., and Scheich, H. (2004). Learning a new behavioral strategy in the shuttle-box increases prefrontal dopamine. *Neuroscience*, 126, 21-29.

Stark, H., Rothe, T., Deliano, M., and Scheich, H. (2007). Theta activity attenuation correlates with avoidance learning progress in gerbils. *Neuroreport*, 18, 549-552.

Stark, H., Rothe, T., Deliano, M., and Scheich, H. (2008). Dynamics of cortical theta activity correlates with stages of auditory avoidance strategy formation in a shuttle-box. *Neuroscience,* 151, 467-475.

Sternberg, S. (1969). The discovery of processing stages: extensions of Donder's method. *Acta Psychol*., 30, 276-315.

Talk, A., Kang, E., and Gabriel, M. (2004). Independent generation of theta rhythm in the hippocampus and posterior cingulate cortex. *Brain Res.,* 1015, 15-24.

Tanji, J. and Hoshi, E. (2001). Behavioral planning in the prefrontal cortex. *Curr. Opin. Neurobiol., 11,* 164-170.

Tanji, J., Shima, K., and Mushiake, H. (2007). Concept-based behavioral planning and the lateral prefrontal cortex. *Trends Cogn. Sci., 11,* 528-534.

Van der Borght, K., Meerlo, P., Luiten, P. G. M., Eggen, B. J. L., and Van der Zee, E. A. (2005). Effects of active shock avoidance learning on hippocampal neurogenesis and plasma levels of corticosterone. *Behav. Brain Res*., 157, 23-30.

Wasserman, E. A. and Miller, R. R. (1997). What's elementary about associative learning? *Annu. Rev. Psychol.,* 48, 573-607.

Watanabe, M., Kodama, T., and Hikosaka, K. (1997). Increase of extracellular dopamine in primate prefrontal cortex during a working memory task. *J. Neurophysiol*., 78, 2795-2798.

Wetzel, W., Wagner, T., Ohl, F. W.,Scheich, H. (1998). Categorical discrimination direction in frequency-modulated tones by Mongolian gerbils. *Behav. Brain Res*., 91, 29-39.

Wightman, R. M. and Robinson, D. L. (2002). Transient changes in mesolimbic dopamine and their association with 'reward'. *J. Neurochem*., 82, 721-735.

Yamamuro, Y., Hori, K., Iwano, H., and Nomura, M. (1994). The relationship between learning performance and dopamine in the prefrontal cortex of the rat. *Neurosci. Lett*., 177, 83-86.

Young, A. M. J. (1993). Intracerebral microdialysis in the study of physiology and behaviour. *Rev. Neurosci.,* 4, 373-395.

Zuschratter, W., Gass, P., Herdegen, T., and Scheich, H. (1995). Comparison of frequency-specific c-Fos expression and fluoro-2-deoxyglucose uptake in auditory cortex of gerbils (Meriones unguiculatus). *Eur. J. Neurosci.*, 7, 1614-1626.

In: Prefrontal Cortex: Roles, Interventions and Traumas ISBN 978-1-60692-415-0
Editors: Lorenzo LoGrasso and Giovanni Morretti

Chapter 5

The Orbitofrontal Cortex and Emotional Decision-Making: The Neglected Role of Anxiety

Sabine Windmann **and** ***Martina Kirsch***
Goethe University, Department of General Psychology II
Institute of Psychology and Sports Sciences
Mertonstr.17, 60054 Frankfurt/Main, Germany

Abstract

The orbital part of the prefrontal cortex is known to be crucially involved in emotional decision-making. Its function seems to be, first, to associate affective value with behavioral bias (i.e., approach or withdrawal) in complex choice situations, and secondly, to flexibly control and transiently inhibit affective and behavioral impulses. Dysfunction of this region due to damage or immaturity of OFC cells leads to impulsiveness, behavioral perseveration, and reduced sensitivity for risk, as observed in children as well as various patients groups. We review the evidence with a focus on the much less investigated question of whether and how *hyper*activation (or hyperfunctioning of modules and processes) involving OFC leads to the opposite behavioral tendencies, namely risk-aversion, enhanced inhibition, undecidedness and higher risk sensitivity including heightened anxiety. We identify two perspectives with opposing views onto this issue, and report some unpublished studies of populations with children and patients with anxiety disorders using the Iowa gambling task, a task that is presumed to be sensitive to OFC function. We find that, if anything, anxiety has the same beneficial effects onto performance as cortical maturation. Although effects of anxiety are much weaker and less conclusive than those of age during childhood, it seems that there are situations in which enhanced anxiety can support advantageous decision-making. Our results highlight the important role of orbitofrontal cortex in integrating approach- and withdrawal-tendencies mediated by mesolimbic and mesostriatal structures on the one hand and higher cognitive centres on the other, with the latter ones

* Phone: +44 69/798-22905; Fax: +44 69/798-23457; Email: Sabine.Windmann@psych.uni-frankfurt.de

recruiting more dorsal parts of the prefrontal cortex and allowing for conscious thinking, reasoning, and problem-solving. Behavioral interventions as in education, cognitive training, and psychotherapy are most effective when they take into account the motivational and evaluative function of this region.

The ventral surface of the frontal lobe is known as the orbitofrontal cortex (OFC) as it is located above the eyeballs and their muscles. It comprises Brodman areas14 medially and 13/25 caudally as well as areas 11 and 12 around the ventral convexity. As part of the prefrontal cortex, these regions are among the last to mature during ontogenesis, to be completed usually only during early adulthood (e.g., Diamond, 2002; Fuster, 2008; Schore, 1999).

Functions of the OFC have been linked to higher emotion control in the broadest sense. Animal and neuroimaging work has shown that on the input side, the OFC responds to primary as well as secondary rewards and punishments of various sensory modalities and mediates anticipation of such events (Breiter, Aharon, Kahneman, Dale, and Shizgal, 2001; Elliott, Dolan, and Frith, 2000; Gottfried, O'Doherty, and Dolan, 2003; Kirsch, Schienle, Stark, Sammer, Blecker, Walter, Ott, Burkart, and Vaitl, 2003; Knutson, Fong, Adams, Varner, and Hommer, 2001; O'Doherty, 2004; Rogers, Owen, Middleton, Williams, Pickard, Sahakian, and Robbins,1999; Rolls, 1996, 2002; Rolls, Kringelbach, and de Araujo, 2003; Rolls, O'Doherty, Kringelbach, Francis, Bowtell, and McGlone, 2003; Small, Zatorre, Dagher, Evans, and Jones-Gotman, 2001). On the output side, the OFC is involved in controlling the flexible adjustment of behavior according to expected and changing outcomes (Baxter, Parker, Lindner, Izquierdo, and Murray, 2000; Bechara, 2004; Damasio, 1996; Fellows, 2007; O'Doherty, 2007; O'Doherty, Critchley, Deichmann, and Dolan, 2003; Pickens, Saddoris, Gallagher, and Holland, 2005). Thus, the region is thought to be involved in the dynamical linking of higher affective evaluation with behavior control.

Response control in accordance with higher affective evaluation often involves inhibition of primary, conditioned, or otherwise automatic affective responses, particularly fear. It is mostly relevant in situations that were previously dangerous or risky, or otherwise resulted in negative outcome, but have changed and are now useful, attractive response options. For instance, a food source that had been contaminated before may have been cleared and now provide good quality food. An elevator that got stuck a couple of days ago can have been repaired and might be functioning properly again, to be preferred to the stairs. A person who was upset and angry when we met them the first time may be more relaxed when we meet them again and actually turn out to become a very good friend. In all these situations, what needs to be inhibited is feelings of fear, risk, or anxiety (and the accompanying withdrawal behaviors) that are no longer adaptive motives as the circumstances have changed.

The orbitofrontal cortex with its bilateral connections to the amygdala on the one hand and goal-related thinking centres like dorsolateral prefrontal cortex on the other is best suited to mediate these functions. In fact, animal electrophysiology as well as human imaging studies have often demonstrated the crucial role of OFC subregions in extinguishing conditioned fear, recovering extinguished fear, regulating anticipatory emotions in general, and inhibiting previously established responses (Milad and Quirk, 2002; Schoenbaum, Setlow, Saddoris, and Gallagher, 2003). Accordingly, damage to the OFC leads to ignorance towards danger and threat, and to inflexible behavior that is not dynamically adjusted to changing outcome contingencies in the environment. Neuropsychology has demonstrated many times how patients with damage to regions of the OFC fail to control affect, to inhibit impulsive behavior, and to choose the behavioral option that is in the best of their long-term interests in complex decision-making tasks as well as everyday life situations. The famous case of Phineas Gage, alongside more systematic patient studies, illustrates this point (Bechara, Damasio, Tranel, and Damasio, 1997; Bechara, Tranel, and Damasio, 2000; Damasio, 1994).

The same tendency can be found in children and adolescents whose OFC neurons and connections are still underdeveloped; these show increased impulsiveness (Chambers and Potenza, 2003), reduced inhibition (Bunge, Dudukovic, Thomason, Vaidya, and Gabrieli, 2002), and a choice pattern in complex decision-making tasks like the Iowa gambling task (see below) that is similar to that of patients with OFC lesions (Crone, Bunge, Latenstein, and van der Molen, 2005; Hooper, Luciana, Conklin, and Yarger, 2004; Letho and Elorinne, 2003). Like patients with OFC dysfunction, the children tend to choose risky behavioral options without much worry or care, alongside reduced anticipatory physiological reactions (like skin conductance response) that normally accompany such decisions. The behaviour resembles that found in individuals with antisocial tendencies such as substance abuse, pathological gambling, and psychopathy, conditions which therefore have also been linked to orbitofrontal dysfunction (Forbush, Shaw, Graeber, Hovick, Meyer, Moser, Bayless, Watson, and Black, 2008; van Honk, Hermans, Putman, Montagne, and Schutter, 2002). More generally, failure to experience a healthy amount of fear and to appropriately process risk and punishment signals are considered part of psychopathy (Blair, 2008; Sommer, Hajak, Dohnel, Schwerdtner, Meinhardt, and Muller, 2006; van Honck and Schutter, 2006).

How then does the intact orbitofrontal cortex "know" what amount of fear is healthy and appropriate? Normally, this information should be deduced from behavioral outcomes and is mediated by interaction of various brain regions, including amygdale and striatum. Successful behavior, that is, decisions whose rewarding outcomes exceed expectations, should reinforce existing stimulus-response associations, while lack of success or unexpected misfortune (punishment) should weaken these connections and bias withdrawal behavior. This is the central assumption of temporal difference error reinforcement learning theories (McClure, Daw, and Montague, 2003; Schultz, Dayan, and Montague, 1997). However, in a damaged, immature (as in children), or otherwise malfunctioning OFC that is less flexible and plastic than normal, the system may get stuck in a state where behavioral options with the strongest associations are repeatedly activated, regardless of outcome, while alternative behaviors are never tried, and their outcomes never experienced. To some degree, this conflict between exploitation (continuing to choose one particular behavioral option) and exploration (choosing alternative behaviors to see whether these lead to better outcomes) is present in all individuals. However, in cases with diminished functionality of OFC circuits, the right balance between these two tendencies could be shifted towards exploitation, regardless of long-term costs. As a matter of fact, patients with damage to the OFC show perseveration, a reduced capability to switch from a previously reinforced behavior to novel behaviors (Fellows and Farah, 2003, 2005).

From a purely psychofunctional point of view, if malfunctioning of OFC regions leads to perseveration, impulsivity, and reduced sensitivity towards fear and risk, then "hyperfunctioning" of those same modules should lead to enhanced inconsistency, higher avoidance of risk, heightened concern about long-term outcomes, and a generally heightened level of fear or worries. This notion is reminiscent of what many decades ago the German psychiatrist Lungwitz (1955, Becker, 1993) described as a manifestation of 'hypertrophy of anxiety feeling cells'. In his conception, termed the "Theory of Psychobiology", there are five types of feeling cells, all of which are seen in connection with their afferent and efferent connections including peripheral autonomic nerves and effector systems (as part of what is called a "reflex system"). The type of feeling cells that are concerned with anxiety mediate the feeling of "being cornered, beset, of compulsion, of inhibition, of astonishment, of defiance, of withdrawal, shame, shyness, carefulness, care, etc." (Becker, 1993, p. 41). 'Hypertrophy' of those cells is described as the psychobiological basis of anxiety neuroses. The condition lets the patients' cognitive styles and attitudes towards the world regress towards a more self-absorbed and less sophisticated way of thinking that Lungwitz described as 'infantilistic' and based on immature (or underdeveloped) reflex systems. This theory would predict that due to their "immature" feeling cells (perhaps situated in OFC), patients with anxiety neurosis think and behave similarly to children (whose OFC neurons are not mature yet). Clearly, Lungwitz did not have any knowledge of modern neuroscience and of the precise role and function of neurons (he seems to identify these with a muscle rather than with an information processing device), but at a very functional-descriptive level, his conception fits with existing evidence of the role of dysfunctional OFC sensitivity for risk and inhibition of impulsiveness in both children and patients with anxiety disorders (c.f., Kalin, Shelton, and Davidson, 2007).

What happens according to the Theory of Psychobiology when children are neurotic themselves? Lungwitz proposed that neuroses of childhood do not differ in principle from neuroses of adults: Neurotic children with high anxiety show a yet more "infantilistic" and evolutionarily "primitive" thinking style than do their healthy peers because of underdeveloped anxiety reflex systems (see Becker, 1993, page 107). Thus, not only do the effects of neurotic anxiety and young age lie on the same dimension (as they both rely on immature "reflex systems"), they are also presumed to have additive effects. When applied to a decision making task that tests OFC function, the theory would predict that highly anxious children perform worst, followed by healthy children and adult patients with anxiety disorders, who both perform worse than do healthy adults.

The theory also knows of intermediate forms of anxiety that lie in between healthy and "neurotic" states, suggesting that Lungwitz held a dimensional perspective onto mental illnesses rather than a categorical one with discrete boundaries between healthy and ill, in line with modern psychological theories of anxiety (e.g., Endler and Kocovski, 2002; Hansell and Damour, 2008). These intermediate conditions are referred to as nervousness: "'Nervousness' is commonly used as a description of mild forms of neurosis; namely, degrees of excitability of the reflex system approaching the normal, but already of pathological grade. Less frequently, it is used to describe still normal degrees of excitability of the reflex systems that approach the abnormal, especially in the anxiety and pain reflex systems" (Becker, 1993, p. 9). Consequently we would expect to find not only individuals with pathological anxiety, but also with heightened levels of normal anxiety who are on the borderline between healthy and ill to behave more like children, albeit not as much as patients with anxiety disorders.

Modern theories of anxiety disorders describe the patients as overly sensitive to risk and threat (Clark, 1986; Ehlers, Margraf, Davies, and Roth, 1988; McNally, 1994, 1995, 1997; Williams, Watts, MacLeod, and Mathews, 1997). The idea is that the patients hold an abnormal attentional bias, higher sensitivity, and higher anticipatory fear towards threat signals that can be either internal (body) or external (world). It has been speculated many times that imbalanced interaction between limbic centres, including the amygdala, and prefrontal regions, particularly orbitofrontal cortex, could be involved in the underlying neural pathology (Davidson, 2002; Gorman, Kent, Sullivan, and Coplan, 2000; LeDoux and Müller, 1997; Milad and Rauch, 2007; Windmann, 1998; Windmann, Sakhavat, and Kutas, 2002). These descriptions have been made independently of Damasios (1994, 1996) and Becharas (2004) work on the role of somatic markers in risk anticipation.

Recent neuroimaging studies have begun to confirm the speculations on the role of OFC in anxiety disorders (Domschke, Ohrmann, Braun, Suslow, Bauer, Hohoff, Kersting, Engelien, Arolt, Heindel, Deckert, and Kugel, 2008; Monk, Nelson, McClure, Mogg, Bradley, Leibenluft, Blair, Chen, Charney, Ernst, and Pine, 2006; Monk, Telzer, Mogg, Bradley, Mai, Louro, Chen, McClure-Tone, Ernst, and Pine, 2008). The patients tend towards higher activation or higher involvement of OFC regions, contrary to patients with OFC lesions or psycho-/sociopathy. Healthy individuals under induction of "worry" show the same tendency (Hoehn-Saric, Lee, McLeod, and Wong, 2005) as do individuals who are high at risk for anxiety and depression when reading negative emotional words (Wolfensberger, Veltman, Hoogendijk, De Ruiter, Boomsma, and de Geus, in press). This further adds to the notion that there is a continuum between normal (state) and pathological (trait) forms of anxiety.

If patients with damage to OFC and patients are more prone to risky and impulsive behavior that is not in the best of their long-term interest, and patients with anxiety disorder do the opposite due to increased activation/recruitment of OFC circuits, then this difference between the two groups should manifest in decision-making tasks designed to test OFC function. One of those tasks is the Iowa gambling tasks established by Bechara, Damasio, Damasio, and Anderson (1994). This refers to a card playing game where the subject is asked to collect points by drawing cards from four decks, two of which return 100 points whereas the other two return only 50 points with each card, which the subjects quickly learns. However, what takes longer to appreciate is that some of the cards with the higher returns are associated with severe losses, up to 1250 points, or very frequent losses, such that the expectancy value is negative (-25 points per card). It is therefore not advantageous in the long run to draw cards from those decks (the "bad" decks). The cards from the other two decks are associated with occasional losses too, but frequency and/or amounts of the losses are fewer so that the expectancy value is still positive (+25 points per card, "good" decks). Players who want to maximize their profit on the task should therefore draw from the cards that at first appear to be associated with only small wins, and avoid the risky bad decks even though their immediate return value appears high.

Healthy individuals do indeed learn these associations and gradually increase their payoff across blocks of trials (Bechara et al., 1997). However, patients with damage to OFC are unable to do that; they keep drawing from the bad decks even though many of themunderstand at some point that these are risky choices. They also fail to develop skin conductance responses when drawing from the bad decks indicating that their emotional system does not signal to them the presence of imminent risk. Children, due to immature prefrontal circuits, show similarly impulsive choice behavior on this task (Crone and van der Molen, 2004, 2007).

How do patients with anxiety disorders behave in the Iowa gambling task? Lungwitz (1955) would have predicted that their performance is reduced, like the ones of the children, due to their "infantilistic" thinking styles. On the other hand, modern cognitive theories on anxiety disorders as well as neuroscience evidence pointing to a tendency towards "hyperactivation" of OFC regions in these individuals would probably predict the opposite, namely, that they learn the task better than do healthy adults due to their enhanced sensitivity to risk (see also Must, Szabó, Bódi, Szász, Janka, and Kéri, 2006; Smoski, Lynch, Rosenthal, Cheavens, Chapman, and Krishnan, 2008, for a similar logic in depressed individuals).

In a series of experiments, we failed to find any consistent differences between patients with highly somatic anxiety disorders (i.e., panic disorder) and healthy control subjects in the original and an inverted version (see Bechara et al., 2000) of the Iowa gambling task (Guse, 2006; Wischniewski, 2007), although we did confirm in a study with healthy subjects that both these tasks activate medial and lateral orbitofrontal cortex (Windmann, Kirsch, Mier, Stark, Walter, Güntürkün, and Vaitl, 2006). This failure to find any differences between the groups could at least in part be due to the chosen payoff values used in the card game which followed very literally the procedures described in Bechara et al. (2000, Figure 1). It was only later during personal communication with Antoine Bechara (the latest on 15/10/2007) that we learnt that he had used different payoff amounts in his studies that were dynamically adapted to subject's decisions, as in the commercial version of the Iowa gambling task. We are now working with these probabilistic payoffs in present and future studies.

Another possibility is that panic disorder and generalized anxiety disorder are not based on the same mechanisms, and that only generalized anxiety disorder is related to the hypothesized effects of OFC 'hyperactivation'. We are currently exploring this possibility in ongoing studies with a computerized version of the Iowa gambling task. However, one thing we did find is that children with high anxiety showed higher performance in the Iowa gambling task than their healthy peers (Kirsch, Kirsch, Mier, and Windmann, 2007). Although the effect is relatively weak, it seems to conform to some other reports in the literature (Garon, Moore, and Waschbusch, 2006; Schmitt, Brinkley, and Newman, 1999). Surprisingly though, another study reported in the literature found the contrary effects of anxiety on performance in the Iowa gambling task in healthy adults (Miu, Heilman, and Houser, 2008). The crucial factor explaining the inconsistency could be the question of whether enhanced anxiety and risk sensitivity can be directed to or linked with the task at hand, or, alternatively, comes from other sources and distracts participants during task performance, as some authors have speculated (Lösel and Schmucker, 2004; Preston, Buchanan, Stansfield, and Bechara, 2007). Clearly, more research is needed on that side of the spectrum of abnormal OFC function.

Depending on the outcome of this research it would be recommendable to reconsider in education, psychotherapy, and other interventions that in some populations, OFC dysfunction may be causal to the underlying problem. If this is the case, then the intervention program would be most successful if it contained measures to help, first, accurate and clear affective evaluation of situations and choice options, and second, self-controlled adjustments in behavior. For instance, for children and individuals with deficits in OFC function like ADHD, impulsive personality disorder, and addiction, it could be helpful to make incentives and long-term benefits of the desired behavior more transparent to increase consistency in decision-making. An example would be attaching a picture of a wanted camera on the wallet or the piggybank to foster the long-term motivation to save the required money, or engaging in imagination of the beneficial effects of a proper meal at home before opening the bag of potato chips in the car. An example of an intervention measure helping to self-control behavior would be the employment of a reinforcement scheme according to which reinforcers accumulate in a nonlinear fashion over time: The longer the individual inhibits impulsive responses, the more reinforcement (e.g., money) they will gain until they have reached their long-term goal.

For patients with negative affect like anxiety and depression, where OFC mediated functions may be overly sensitive, the problem seems to be not so much the inhibition of behavior but, on the contrary, motivating and initiating behavior. These patients are known to often overgeneralize their negative evaluation of stimuli and response options and as a result become quite passive and socially isolated. The reason is that they do not find the available behavioral options attractive and/or safe enough to promote activity. The patients should therefore be taught how to better differentiate between actually harmful and actually harmless stimuli/situations (Windmann, 1998; Windmann et al., 2002), as proposed by cognitive therapy (Beck, 1970, 1976; Beck, Emery, and Greenberg, 2005). Learning how to relax probably needs to be part of this program, if it is true that the patients' abnormally high risk perception is further supported by increased sensitivity to bodily fear signals (Clark, 1986; Ehlers et al., 1988). In addition, these patients could be motivated to act on the basis of revised affective evaluations by helping them focus on (and keep record of) expected and experienced positive outcomes, such as, keeping a diary of the events and activities that they did not want to take part in at first, but in the end were glad having joined. Some of these measures are part of the classical behavioral intervention program designed by Lewinsohn, Clarke, Hops, and Andrews (1990). A combination of both cognitive and behavioral elements would probably be most successful paired with psychoactive medication in select cases.

Acknowledgment

Work described in this article was supported by a research grant from the Lungwitz foundation, Berlin (Germany).

References

Baxter, M. G., Parker, A., Lindner, C. C., Izquierdo, A. D., and Murray, E. A. (2000). Control of response selection by reinforcer value requires interaction of amygdala and orbital prefrontal cortex. *J. Neurosci., 20*(11), 4311-4319.

Bechara, A. (2004). The role of emotion in decision-making: evidence from neurological patients with orbitofrontal damage. *Brain Cogn., 55*(1), 30-40.

Bechara, A., Damasio, A. R., Damasio, H., and Anderson, S. W. (1994). Insensitivity to future consequences following damage to human prefrontal cortex. *Cognition, 50*(1-3), 7-15.

Bechara, A., Damasio, H., Tranel, D., and Damasio, A. R. (1997). Deciding advantageously before knowing the advantageous strategy. *Science, 275*(5304), 1293-1295.

Bechara, A., Tranel, D., and Damasio, H. (2000). Characterization of the decision-making deficit of patients with ventromedial prefrontal cortex lesions. *Brain, 123 (Pt 11)*, 2189-2202.

Beck, A. T. (1970). Cognitive therapy: Nature and relation to behavior therapy. *Behav. Ther.* (1), 184-200.

Beck, A. T. (1976). *Cognitive Therapy and the Emotional Disorders*. New York: International Universities Press.

Beck, A. T., Emery, G., and Greenberg, R. L. (2005). *Anxiety Disorders and Phobias: A Cognitive Perspective*. New York: Basic Books.

Becker, R. (Ed.). (1993). *Hans Lungwitz: Psychobiology and Cognitive Therapy of the Neuroses*. Basel: Birkhäuser Verlag.

Blair, R. J. (2008). Review. The amygdala and ventromedial prefrontal cortex: functional contributions and dysfunction in psychopathy. *Philos. Trans R Soc. Lond B Biol. Sci.*

Breiter, H. C., Aharon, I., Kahneman, D., Dale, A., and Shizgal, P. (2001). Functional imaging of neural responses to expectancy and experience of monetary gains and losses. *Neuron, 30*(2), 619-639.

Bunge, S. A., Dudukovic, N. M., Thomason, M. E., Vaidya, C. J., and Gabrieli, J. D. (2002). Immature frontal lobe contributions to cognitive control in children: evidence from fMRI. *Neuron, 33*(2), 301-311.

Chambers, R. A., and Potenza, M. N. (2003). Neurodevelopment, impulsivity, and adolescent gambling. *J. Gambl. Stud, 19*(1), 53-84.

Clark, D. M. (1986). A cognitive approach to panic. *Behav. Res. Ther., 24*(4), 461-470.

Crone, E. A., Bunge, S. A., Latenstein, H., and van der Molen, M. W. (2005). Characterization of children's decision making: sensitivity to punishment frequency, not task complexity. *Child Neuropsychol, 11*(3), 245-263.

Crone, E. A., and van der Molen, M. W. (2004). Developmental changes in real life decision making: performance on a gambling task previously shown to depend on the ventromedial prefrontal cortex. *Dev. Neuropsychol., 25*(3), 251-279.

Crone, E. A., and van der Molen, M. W. (2007). Development of decision making in school-aged children and adolescents: evidence from heart rate and skin conductance analysis. *Child Dev., 78*(4), 1288-1301.

Damasio, A. R. (1994). *Descartes' Error: Emotion, Reason, and the Human Brain*. New York: Putnam Pub Group.

Damasio, A. R. (1996). The somatic marker hypothesis and the possible functions of the prefrontal cortex. *Philos Trans R Soc Lond B Biol Sci, 351*(1346), 1413-1420.

Davidson, R. J. (2002). Anxiety and affective style: role of prefrontal cortex and amygdala. *Biol. Psychiatry, 51*(1), 68-80.

Diamond, A. (2002). Normal Development of Prefrontal Cortex, from Birth to Young Adulthood: Cognitive Functions, Anatomy and Biochemistry. In D. T. Stuss and R. T. Knight (Eds.), *Principles of Frontal Lobe Function*. Oxford: Oxford University Press.

Domschke, K., Ohrmann, P., Braun, M., Suslow, T., Bauer, J., Hohoff, C., Kersting, A., Engelien, A., Arolt, V., Heindel, W., Deckert, J., and Kugel, H. (2008). Influence of the catechol-O-methyltransferase val158met genotype on amygdala and prefrontal cortex emotional processing in panic disorder. *Psychiatry Res., 163*(1), 13-20.

Ehlers, A., Margraf, J., Davies, S., and Roth, W. T. (1988). Selective Processing of Threat Cues in Subjects with Panic Attacks. *Cognition and Emotion, 2*, 201 – 219.

Elliott, R., Dolan, R. J., and Frith, C. D. (2000). Dissociable functions in the medial and lateral orbitofrontal cortex: evidence from human neuroimaging studies. *Cereb. Cortex, 10*(3), 308-317.

Endler, N. S., and Kocovski, N. L. (2002). Personality disorders at the crossroads. *J. Personal. Disord., 16*(6), 487-502.

Fellows, L. K. (2007). The role of orbitofrontal cortex in decision making: a component process account. *Ann. N Y Acad. Sci., 1121*, 421-430.

Fellows, L. K., and Farah, M. J. (2003). Ventromedial frontal cortex mediates affective shifting in humans: evidence from a reversal learning paradigm. *Brain, 126*(Pt 8), 1830-1837.

Fellows, L. K., and Farah, M. J. (2005). Different underlying impairments in decision-making following ventromedial and dorsolateral frontal lobe damage in humans. *Cereb. Cortex, 15*(1), 58-63.

Fuster, J. (2008). *The Prefrontal Cortex*. London: Academic Press.

Garon, N., Moore, C., and Waschbusch, D. A. (2006). Decision making in children with ADHD only, ADHD-anxious/depressed, and control children using a child version of the Iowa Gambling Task. *J Atten Disord, 9*(4), 607-619.

Gorman, J. M., Kent, J. M., Sullivan, G. M., and Coplan, J. D. (2000). Neuroanatomical hypothesis of panic disorder, revised. *Am. J. Psychiatry, 157*(4), 493-505.

Gottfried, J. A., O'Doherty, J., and Dolan, R. J. (2003). Encoding predictive reward value in human amygdala and orbitofrontal cortex. *Science, 301*(5636), 1104-1107.

Guse, B. (2006). *Entscheidungsverhalten bei Personen mit klinisch relevanter Angst.* Unpublished Internal Report [Diploma Thesis], University of Bochum, Germany.

Forbush, K.T., Shaw, M., Graeber, M.A., Hovick, L., Meyer, V.J., Moser, D.J., Bayless, J., Watson, D., and Black, D.W. (2008). Neuropsychological characteristics and personality traits in pathological gambling. *CNS Spectr, 13(4),* 306-315.

Hansell, J. H., and Damour, L. (2008). *Abnormal Psychology*. New York: Wiley.

Hoehn-Saric, R., Lee, J. S., McLeod, D. R., and Wong, D. F. (2005). Effect of worry on regional cerebral blood flow in nonanxious subjects. *Psychiatry Res., 140*(3), 259-269.

Hooper, C.J., Luciana, M., Conklin, H.M., Yarger, R.S. (2004). Adolescents' performance on the Iowa Gambling Task: implications for the development of decision making and ventromedial prefrontal cortex. *Dev. Psychol., 40 (6),* 1148-1158.

Kalin, N. H., Shelton, S. E., and Davidson, R. J. (2007). Role of the primate orbitofrontal cortex in mediating anxious temperament. *Biol. Psychiatry, 62*(10), 1134-1139.

Kirsch, M., Kirsch, P., Mier, D., and Windmann, S. (2007). Entscheidungsverhalten von Kindern in der IOWA-Gambling-Task: Der Einfluss von Alter und Ängstlichkeit. *Zeitschrift für Neuropsychologie, 18*, 126.

Kirsch, P., Schienle, A., Stark, R., Sammer, G., Blecker, C., Walter, B., Ott, U., Burkart, J., and Vaitl, D. (2003). Anticipation of reward in a nonaversive differential conditioning paradigm and the brain reward system: an event-related fMRI study. *Neuroimage, 20*(2), 1086-1095.

Knutson, B., Fong, G. W., Adams, C. M., Varner, J. L., and Hommer, D. (2001). Dissociation of reward anticipation and outcome with event-related fMRI. *Neuroreport, 12*(17), 3683-3687.

Ledoux, J. E., and Muller, J. (1997). Emotional memory and psychopathology. *Philos. Trans R Soc Lond B Biol. Sci., 352*(1362), 1719-1726.

Lehto, J.E. and Elorinne, E. (2003). Gambling as an executive function task. *Appl. Neuropsychol.* 10(4), 234-238.

Lewinsohn, P. M., Clarke, G. N., Hops, H., and Andrews, J. (1990). Cognitive-behavioral treatment for depressed adolescents. *Behav. Ther., 21*, 385-401.

Losel, F., and Schmucker, M. (2004). Psychopathy, risk taking, and attention: a differentiated test of the somatic marker hypothesis. *J. Abnorm. Psychol., 113*(4), 522-529.

Lungwitz, H. (1955). *Die Neurosenlehre – Die Erkenntnistherapie [2 Bände]*. Berlin: de Gruyter.

McClure, S. M., Daw, N. D., and Montague, P. R. (2003). A computational substrate for incentive salience. *Trends Neurosci., 26*(8), 423-428.

McNally, R. J. (1994). *Panic Disorder: A Critical Analysis*. New York: Guildford Press.

McNally, R. J. (1995). Automaticity and the anxiety disorders. *Behav. Res. Ther., 33*(7), 747-754.

McNally, R. J. (1997). Memory and anxiety disorders. *Philos. Trans R Soc. Lond B Biol. Sci., 352*(1362), 1755-1759.

Milad, M. R., and Quirk, G. J. (2002). Neurons in medial prefrontal cortex signal memory for fear extinction. *Nature, 420*(6911), 70-74.

Milad, M. R., and Rauch, S. L. (2007). The role of the orbitofrontal cortex in anxiety disorders. *Ann. N Y Acad. Sci., 1121*, 546-561.

Miu, A. C., Heilman, R. M., and Houser, D. (2008). Anxiety impairs decision-making: psychophysiological evidence from an Iowa Gambling Task. *Biol. Psychol., 77*(3), 353-358.

Monk, C. S., Nelson, E. E., McClure, E. B., Mogg, K., Bradley, B. P., Leibenluft, E., Blair, R. J., Chen, G., Charney, D. S., Ernst, M., and Pine, D. S. (2006). Ventrolateral prefrontal cortex activation and attentional bias in response to angry faces in adolescents with generalized anxiety disorder. *Am. J. Psychiatry, 163*(6), 1091-1097.

Monk, C. S., Telzer, E. H., Mogg, K., Bradley, B. P., Mai, X., Louro, H. M., Chen, G., McClure-Tone, E. B., Ernst, M., and Pine, D. S.(2008). Amygdala and ventrolateral prefrontal cortex activation to masked angry faces in children and adolescents with generalized anxiety disorder. *Arch. Gen. Psychiatry, 65*(5), 568-576.

Must, A., Szabo, Z., Bodi, N., Szasz, A., Janka, Z., and Keri, S. (2006). Sensitivity to reward and punishment and the prefrontal cortex in major depression. *J. Affect Disord., 90*(2-3), 209-215.

O'Doherty, J., Critchley, H., Deichmann, R., and Dolan, R. J. (2003). Dissociating valence of outcome from behavioral control in human orbital and ventral prefrontal cortices. *J. Neurosci., 23*(21), 7931-7939.

O'Doherty, J. P. (2004). Reward representations and reward-related learning in the human brain: insights from neuroimaging. *Curr. Opin. Neurobiol., 14*(6), 769-776.

O'Doherty, J. P. (2007). Lights, camembert, action! The role of human orbitofrontal cortex in encoding stimuli, rewards, and choices. *Ann. N Y Acad. Sci., 1121*, 254-272.

O'Doherty, J. P., Dayan, P., Friston, K., Critchley, H., and Dolan, R. J. (2003). Temporal difference models and reward-related learning in the human brain. *Neuron, 38*(2), 329-337.

Pickens, C. L., Saddoris, M. P., Gallagher, M., and Holland, P. C. (2005). Orbitofrontal lesions impair use of cue-outcome associations in a devaluation task. *Behav. Neurosci., 119*(1), 317-322.

Preston, S. D., Buchanan, T. W., Stansfield, R. B., and Bechara, A. (2007). Effects of anticipatory stress on decision making in a gambling task. *Behav. Neurosci., 121*(2), 257-263.

Quirk, G. J., Russo, G. K., Barron, J. L., and Lebron, K. (2000). The role of ventromedial prefrontal cortex in the recovery of extinguished fear. *J. Neurosci., 20*(16), 6225-6231.

Rogers, R. D., Owen, A. M., Middleton, H. C., Williams, E. J., Pickard, J. D., Sahakian, B. J., and Robbins, T. W. (1999). Choosing between small, likely rewards and large, unlikely rewards activates inferior and orbital prefrontal cortex. *J. Neurosci., 19*(20), 9029-9038.

Rolls, E. T. (1996). The orbitofrontal cortex. *Philos. Trans R Soc. Lond B Biol. Sci., 351*(1346), 1433-1443; discussion 1443-1434.

Rolls, E. T. (2002). The functions of the orbitofrontal cortex. In D. T. Stuss, and Knight, R.T. (Ed.), *Principles of frontal lobe function*. Oxford, UK: Oxford University Press.

Rolls, E. T., Kringelbach, M. L., and de Araujo, I. E. (2003). Different representations of pleasant and unpleasant odours in the human brain. *Eur. J. Neurosci., 18*(3), 695-703.

Rolls, E. T., O'Doherty, J., Kringelbach, M. L., Francis, S., Bowtell, R., and McGlone, F. (2003). Representations of pleasant and painful touch in the human orbitofrontal and cingulate cortices. *Cereb. Cortex, 13*(3), 308-317.

Schmitt, W. A., Brinkley, C. A., and Newman, J. P. (1999). Testing Damasio's somatic marker hypothesis with psychopathic individuals: risk takers or risk averse? *J. Abnorm. Psychol., 108*(3), 538-543.

Schoenbaum, G., Setlow, B., Saddoris, M. P., and Gallagher, M. (2003). Encoding predicted outcome and acquired value in orbitofrontal cortex during cue sampling depends upon input from basolateral amygdala. *Neuron, 39*(5), 855-867.

Schore, A. N. (1999). *Affect Regulation and the Origin of the Self: The Neurobiology of Emotional Development*. Philadelphia: Lawrence Erlbaum Associates Inc.

Schultz, W., Dayan, P., and Montague, P. R. (1997). A neural substrate of prediction and reward. *Science, 275*(5306), 1593-1599.

Small, D. M., Zatorre, R. J., Dagher, A., Evans, A. C., and Jones-Gotman, M. (2001). Changes in brain activity related to eating chocolate: from pleasure to aversion. *Brain, 124*(Pt 9), 1720-1733.

Smoski, M. J., Lynch, T. R., Rosenthal, M. Z., Cheavens, J. S., Chapman, A. L., and Krishnan, R. R. (2008). Decision-making and risk aversion among depressive adults. *J. Behav. Ther. Exp. Psychiatry.*

Sommer, M., Hajak, G., Dohnel, K., Schwerdtner, J., Meinhardt, J., and Muller, J. L. (2006). Integration of emotion and cognition in patients with psychopathy. *Prog. Brain Res., 156*, 457-466.

van Honk, J., Hermans, E.J., Putman, P., Montagne, B., and Schutter, D.J. (2002). Defective somatic markers in sub-clinical psychopathy. *Neuroreport, 13(8),* 1025-1027.

van Honk, J., and Schutter, D. J. (2006). Unmasking feigned sanity: a neurobiological model of emotion processing in primary psychopathy. *Cognit Neuropsychiatry, 11*(3), 285-306.

Williams, J. M. G., F. N. Watts, C. MacLeod and A. Mathews. (1997). *Cognitive Psychology and Emotional Disorders*. Chichester: Wiley.

Windmann, S. (1998). Panic disorder from a monistic perspective: integrating neurobiological and psychological approaches. *J. Anxiety Disord, 12*(5), 485-507.

Windmann, S., Kirsch, P., Mier, D., Stark, R., Walter, B., Güntürkün, O., and Vaitl, D. (2006). On framing effects in decision making: linking lateral versus medial orbitofrontal cortex activation to choice outcome processing. *J. Cogn. Neurosci., 18*(7), 1198-1211.

Windmann, S., Sakhavat, Z., and Kutas, M. (2002). Electrophysiological evidence reveals affective evaluation deficits early in stimulus processing in patients with panic disorder. *J. Abnorm. Psychol., 111*(2), 357-369.

Wischniewski, J. (2006). *Treffen Panikpatienten Entscheidungen anders? Eine Untersuchung mit der Iowa Gambling Task.* Unpublished Internal Report [Diploma Thesis], University of Bochum, Germany.

Wolfensberger, S. P., Veltman, D. J., Hoogendijk, W. J., De Ruiter, M. B., Boomsma, D. I., and de Geus, E. J. (in press). The neural correlates of verbal encoding and retrieval in monozygotic twins at low or high risk for depression and anxiety. *Biol. Psychol.*

In: Prefrontal Cortex: Roles, Interventions and Traumas
Editors: Lorenzo LoGrasso and Giovanni Morretti
ISBN 978-1-60692-415-0

Chapter 6

PEEF: Premotor Ear-Eye Field. A New Vista of Area 8B

Bon Leopoldo, Marco Lanzilotto and Cristina Lucchetti
Department of Biomedical Sciences,
University of Modena and Reggio Emilia,
Via Campi 287, 41100 Modena, Italy

Abstract

In macaque monkeys, area 8B may be considered cytoarchitectonically as a transitional area between the granular area 9, rostrally, and the rostral part of the dorsal agranular area 6 (FC or F7), caudally. This area is anatomically connected with auditory cortical areas, cerebellum and superior colliculus. Microstimulation of area 8B evokes ear movements or eye movements in some sites; in other sites, it evokes both ear and eye movements by varying the intensity of electric stimulation. Unit activity recording shows that neurons in area 8B have a role in encoding different auditory environmental stimuli and movements of the ear and eye. In addition, fixation of a visual stimulus, when attention is engaged, modulates the discharge of auditory environmental neurons, and sensory-motor neurons.

Current functional and anatomical evidences strongly support the proposal that area 8B is a specific Premotor Ear-Eye Field (PEEF) involved in the recognition of auditory stimuli and in orienting processes. Moreover, activation by specific environmental auditory stimuli, suggests that PEEF is an important node in the hierarchical organisation of the auditory network. The inhibitory effects on neural discharge of auditory and auditory-motor cells might be a consequence of the engagement of attention during visual fixation. This phenomenon may be the expression of a combination of a covert orienting of attention relative to eye effectors, and an overt orienting of attention relative to ear effectors. It seems that attention may affect more than one channel at the same time during a conditioned task or during natural behaviour. Then the PEEF, based on its connections and functional characteristics may be involved in three circuits: 1) an auditory circuit, 2) an oculomotor circuit, 3) and a fronto-cerebellar circuit.

I. Introduction

The prefrontal cortex is the rostral part of the frontal cortex. It is subdivided in many cytoarchitectonic areas with different functions. The prefrontal cortex is more developed in non-human and human primates than in other animals. The anatomical interconnections and physiological data suggest that the prefrontal cortex is involved in high-order brain functions and in the organization of motor behaviour (Tanji and Hoshi 2008).

In this review we will talk about area 8B, which has remained relatively an unexplored part of the prefrontal cortex. Area 8B, together with area 6 and 8A, based on cytoarchitecture, anatomical connections and electrophysiological data, may be considered as part of the premotor cortex (Pandya and Yeterian 1985, Mann et al. 1988, Passingham 1993, Bon and Lucchetti 1994, Lucchetti et al. 1998, Moschovakis et al. 2004) and area 8B may be considered a "premotor ear-eye field" (PEEF) (Lucchetti et al. 2008).

II. Anatomical Background

Cytoarchitecture

In macaque monkeys area 8B may be considered cytoarchitectonically as a transitional area between the granular area 9, rostrally, and the rostral part of the dorsal agranular area 6 (FC or F7), caudally (Von Bonin and Bailey 1947). The first scientist to identify this area was Walker (1940), and successively Von Bonin and Bailey (1947) and Matelli et al. (1991) confirmed this statement. Some neuroanatomists considered area 8B as the dorso-mesial caudal part of area 9 (Barbas and Pandya 1989, Pandya and Yeterian 1990, Barbas et al. 1999). Petrides and Pandya (1999) re-examined, in a comparative cytoarchitectonic analysis the dorsolateral prefrontal cortex of the human and the macaque brain. They identified an area interposed between area 9 and the dorsal part of area 6 and following Walker (1940) they defined this area as 8B. In the original paper they described this area as follows:

> "Its posteroventral part is located in the rostralmost section of the superior limb of the arcuate sulcus. Dorsally, it extends up to the midline, and it continues medially as far as the border of the cingulate sulcus. In this area, layer II is well defined and blends gently with layer III. Layer III is sparse and contains small- to medium-sized pyramidal neurons; only a few neurons in this layer are as large as those encountered in 8A. Layer IV is poorly developed and layer V almost blends with layer VI. A few darkly stained cells can be distinguished in layer Va."

Neuroanatomy

Anatomical investigations showed the complex connections of area 8B with cortical and subcortical structures. The study by Barbas and Pandya (1989) showed that dorsal prefrontal areas (9, 8, 46) are strongly interconnected and area 9 sends a robust projection toward dorsal area 6. Recent anatomical investigations showed that area 8B sends robust projections to SEF (Luppino et al. 2003, Wang et al. 2005).

Barbas and Mesulam (1981) showed prominent projections from auditory association cortices: in particular from the superior temporal gyrus and part of the dorsal bank of the superior temporal sulcus, to the rostral part of area 8A and contiguous area 8B. Subsequent investigations pointed out the reciprocal connections between auditory association area AA1 and area 8A, and between area AA2 and dorsal prefrontal cortex areas 9 and 10 (Pandya and Yeterian 1990, Barbas et al. 1999). Quantitative investigations have addressed the anatomical interactions between prefrontal areas 9 and 10 and inhibitory neurons in superior temporal cortices involved in auditory perception (Barbas et al. 2005).

It has been suggested that the prefrontal cortex is devoted to the integration of "what" and "where" in non human-primates for the visual cortical system: neurons that are object-tuned, location-tuned or are have both what and where tuning were found in the dorsolateral and ventrolateral prefrontal cortex (Rao et al. 1997). Using anatomical and electrophysiological recordings methods, Romanski et al. (1999) also identified two different auditory streams in non-human primates, which originate from the caudal and rostral auditory belt cortex and project to different areas of the frontal lobe. The rostral belt is reciprocally connected to the frontal pole (area 10), rostral principal sulcus (area 46) and ventral prefrontal region (areas 12 and 45), whereas the caudal belt is mainly connected with caudal principal sulcus (area 46), frontal eye fields (area 8A) and with area 8B. They suggested that two streams originate from caudal and rostral auditory cortices and target areas associated with spatial "where" and non spatial "what" processes in the prefrontal cortex. Moreover, investigations using fMRI and ERPs (event related potentials) methods have shown both streams for sound identity and sound spatial location in humans, suggesting that ventral and dorsal prefrontal areas are involved in representing the "what" and "where" respectively (Alain et al. 2001)

In addition, the prefrontal cortex is highly connected with the parietal lobe. In particular the medial surface of parietal lobe area PGm sends projections to the rostral part of dorsal area 6, area 8, dorsal areas 46 and 9, while area 9 sends back projections to area PGm (Pandya and Yeterian 1990). Electrical stimulation of area PGm evokes eye and ear movements in non human-primates (Thier and Andersen 1998). Kelly and Strick (2003) showed anatomical cerebro-cerebellum connections through the basilar pons and thalamus. The strongest projections to the basilar pons derive from the dorsolateral prefrontal convexity, including rostral area 8A, area 9 and dorsal area 46. Area 8B sends projections to the paramedian nucleus, peripeduncular nucleus and nucleus reticularis tegmentum ponti (NRTP) (Schmahmann and Pandya 1997). Middleton and Strick (2001) showed that area 9 and area 46 receive a consistent input from the cerebellum through thalamic regions, and proposed distinct cerebellum output channels to the prefrontal and motor cortices.

Auditory neurons were described in different part of cerebellum: in the middle part of the vermis (Snider and Stowell 1944; Fadiga and Pupilli 1964), in the nuclei interpositi and dentate nucleus (Mortimer 1975). The dentate nucleus, as shown by Lynch et al. (1994), projects to area 8B. Moreover, areas 8A, 8B and 9 project to the deep layers of the superior colliculus and pretectum (Fries 1984, Tanila et al. 1993). The deep layers of the superior colliculus project to the reticular formation and to the cervical spinal cord where the neck is represented (Raybourn and Keller 1977, Kuypers 1981). Electrophysiological evidence shows a clear relationship between superior colliculus stimulation and head movements in the monkey (Corneil et al. 2002). The projections from the cerebellum (vermis), the superior and the inferior colliculus and auditory cortex onto the pontine nulei, suggest a role of the dorsolateral pontine nulei in the integration of visual and auditory information. It appears that this complex system of multiple loops of cerebellar connections with the presence of auditory neurons represent a substantial sensory input for the cerebellar motor control.

The dorsomedial frontal cortex (areas 9,8B, 6 and 4) receives dopaminergic projections from cells of type A9 located dorsally to the substantia nigra pars compacta and to the retro rubral area, from cells of type A10 in the parabrachial pigmented nucleus and linear nuclei. This suggests that area 8B is part of the mesofrontal dopamine system implicated in psychiatric disorders (schizophrenia, psychotic status) (Williams and Goldman-Rakic 1998). Finally, the injection of rabies virus into lateral rectus muscle of the macaque monkey showed the presence of labelled neurons in area 8B and 9, as well as in area 8A (FEF), area F7 (SEF) and F6 (Moschovakis et al 2004) (Fig. 1).

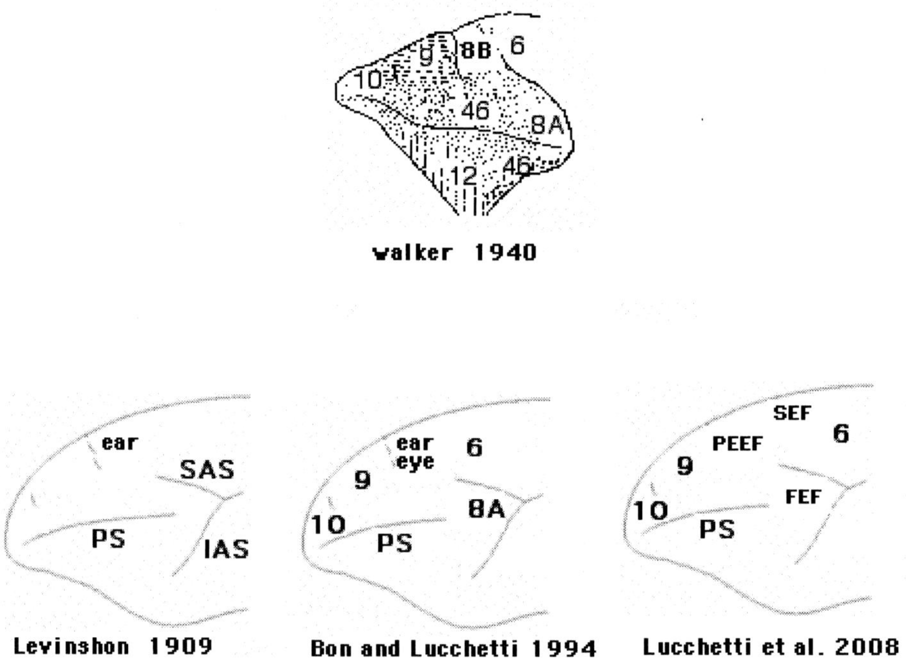

Figure 1. Cytoarchitectonic map of Walker (1940). Stimulation studies of Levinshon (1909). Representation of the stimulation and recording study of Bon and Lucchetti 1994. The actual vision of frontal fields by Lucchetti et al. (2008).

III. Lesions Studies

Many studies of clinical human disorders following natural lesions, and experimental prefrontal lesions in monkeys showed the involvement of prefrontal cortex in personality, motor behaviour, working memory and in temporal encoding to execute a motor act (Harlow 1848, Fuster 1997).

Specific lesion studies showed that animals with prefrontal cortex damage exhibited a deficit in auditory discrimination tasks (Rosenkilde 1979) and that this deficit was manifested when the lesion included areas 8A and 8B (Wegener 1973). Localised lesions in area 8A (FEF) gave rise to a transitory deficit in attention, eye movements and eye-head orienting toward a visual stimulus (Rizzolatti et al. 1983, van der Steen et al. 1986, Schiller et al 1987).

One case with lesion in the monkey, extending from area 8B throughout dorsal area 6, showed initially tilting neck movements. In the days following the lesion, the animal performed saccades and fixation tasks correctly in all directions, while contralateral arm reaching movements were severely impaired. Pleasant stimuli, presented in the ipsilateral or contralateral hemifield, readily drew the attention of the animal. If the same stimuli were presented simultaneously in both hemifields, the monkey oriented itself only toward the ipsilateral one. Aversive stimuli evoked an aggressive reaction only when the stimulus was localized in the ipsilateral hemifield. The animal clearly neglected the aversive stimulus presented in the contralateral hemifield. The animal recovered completely in 30 days. The postmortem examination revealed a lesion in the dorsomedial frontal cortex. The combined attentional and motor deficits suggest that area 6 and 8B, called dorsomedial frontal cortex (DMFC) may be involved in the preparation and execution of movements triggered by the affective meaning of the stimulus (Lucchetti et al. 1998).

On the other hand, combined lesions of dorsal area 46 and 9 produced different deficits in memory tasks. The dorsal prefrontal region receives visuospatial information from areas 8A, 6 and 46. The ventrolateral prefrontal cortex receives non-spatial visual information. Consequently, a lesion of the dorsal part of prefrontal cortex affects visuospatial input and does not affect nonspatial visual object information. Lesions limited to area 9 produced a mild impairment in memory task performance (Petrides 2000).

IV. Neurophysiology

Electrophysiological investigation of area 8B started with the experiments of Ferrier in 1875. In those experiments the author electrically stimulated a large frontal region: areas 9, 8B, 8A, 46 and dorsal area 6 and evoked eye movements. Later Levinsohn (1909) used electric stimulation to evoke eye movements in dorsal area 6 and ear movements in area 8B.

Many years later an explosion of investigations pointed out relevant neuronal characteristics of area 8A (FEF), and the rostral part of dorsal area 6 (SEF). For a detailed vision about FEF and SEF see Tehovnik et al. (2000), and about the cortical and subcortical networks see Lynch and Tian (2006).

Area 8B had been neglected until 1994 when experiments of microstimulation and unit activity recording in macaque monkey pointed out the role of this area in ear and eye motor control in spontaneous behaviours (Bon and Lucchetti 1994). Microstimulation in some sites evoked only ear movements or only eye movements; in other locations it evoked both ear and eye movements by varying the intensity of electrical stimulation. The electrically evoked ear movements were forward, or backward or oblique (upward-forward; upward-backward). The evoked eye movements were mostly fixed vector saccades, contralateral and with an upward orientation of about 45 degrees. If we consider only the sites where the threshold was equal to or lower than 50 μA, mostly of the evoked ear movements were position dependent (Fig. 2).

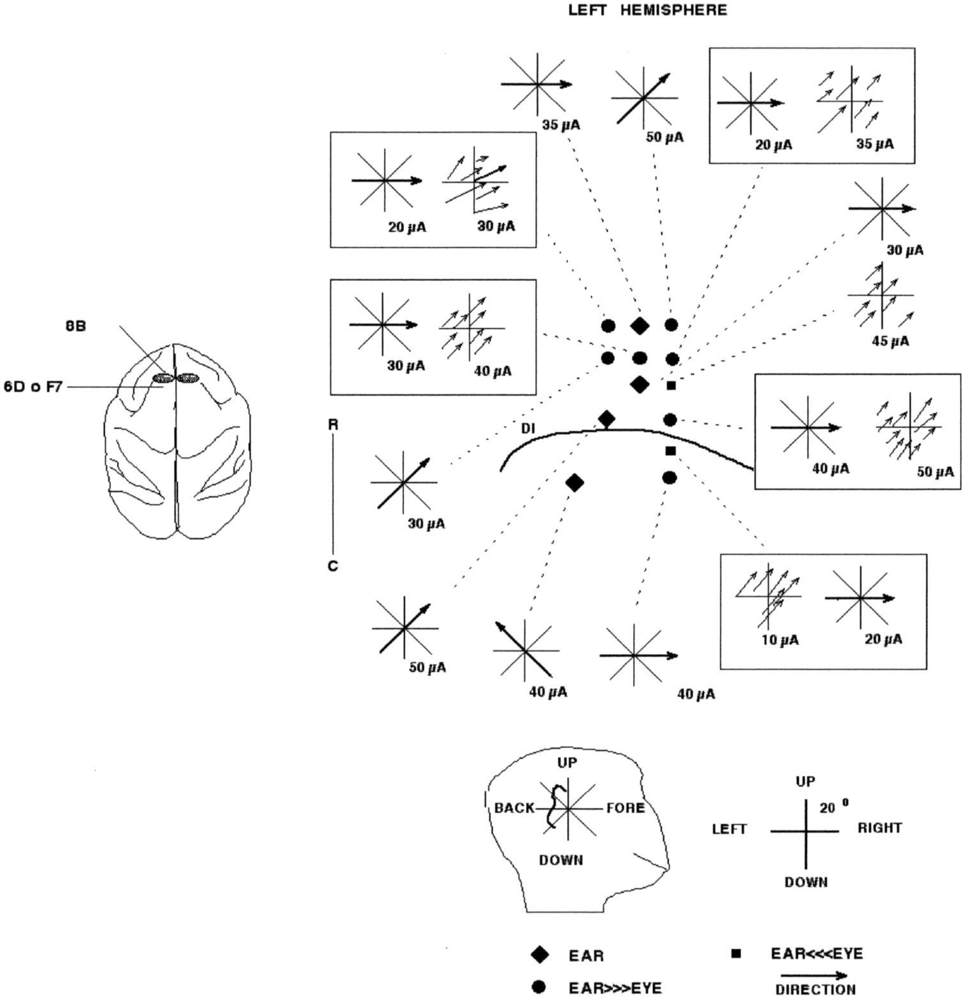

Figure 2. Microstimulation map of area 8B. Representation of ear, eye, and both ear and eye movements evoked with a current threshold equal or lower than 50 μA. DI: dimple. (R rostral, C caudal). Arrows represent the mean direction of ear and eye movements in each site. (Exp Brain Res, 102, 1994, 259-71, "Ear and eye representation in the frontal cortex, area 8b, of the macaque monkey: an elettrophysiological study", Bon L and Lucchetti C, Figure 2-Figure 5, With kind permission of Springer Science+ Business Media).

In addition, neurons discharged before ear movements, and before ear and eye movements, or only before eye movements. The majority of ear and ear-eye cells had a preferred direction for ear movements. Eighty-five percent of cells did not have a preferred direction for visual guided saccades and were active when the monkey made saccades toward the unlit targets (checking saccades). This type of saccades were found and defined previously in SEF (Bon and Lucchetti, 1992).

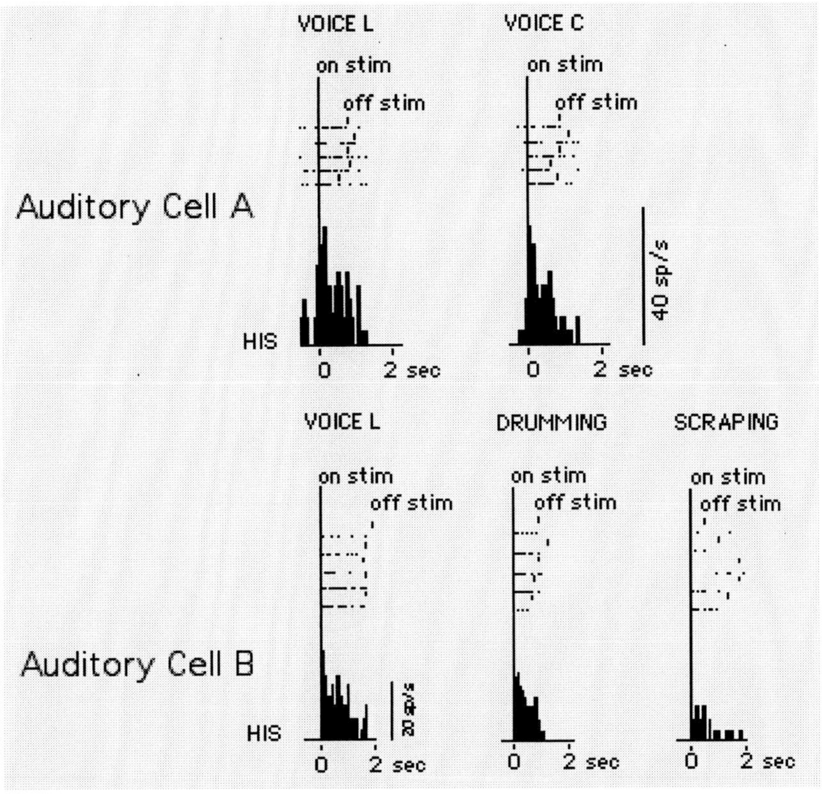

Figure 3. Example of auditory cell. A: auditory cell active for experimenters' voices. B: Auditory cell active for experimenter's voice and environmental stimuli. Raster: each dot is one spike. HIS: unit activity histogram. Bin width: 50 ms. (Exp Brain Res, 168, 2006, 441-9, "Auditory environmental cells and visual fixation effect in area 8B of macaque monkey", Bon L and Lucchetti C, Figure 2, With kind permission of Springer Science+ Business Media).

Further investigations showed new and interesting aspects for auditory, motor and attentional characteristics of neurons of area 8B (Bon and Lucchetti 2006; Lucchetti et al. 2008). Auditory neurons, were active only for environmental auditory stimuli: experimenter's voices, opening and closing of the lab doors, scraping of feet. However, the best stimuli were represented by the experimenters' voices (Fig.3).

In addition, some auditory cells showed activity directionally tuned with the stimulus. The stimulus in these cases was represented by the experimenters' footsteps. In other words, the cell activity increased or decreased when the experimenter moved toward the Faraday cage and viceversa when he/she moved away. Cells that showed activity synchronized with the onset of auditory stimuli and with the onset of an orienting saccade and/or an orienting ear movement were defined as "auditory-motor". For the sensory aspects of neural activity, the unit's discharge rates could be modulated in relation to one or more types of environmental stimuli. With some stimuli, this activity could be very weak and show rapid adaptation.

One part of auditory-motor cells presented a discharge synchronized with the onset of orienting movements of both the eye and ear (Fig. 4). Few of these neurons showed activity that correlated only with the onset of orienting eye movements, other neurons had activity that correlated only with the onset of orienting ear movements (Fig. 5).

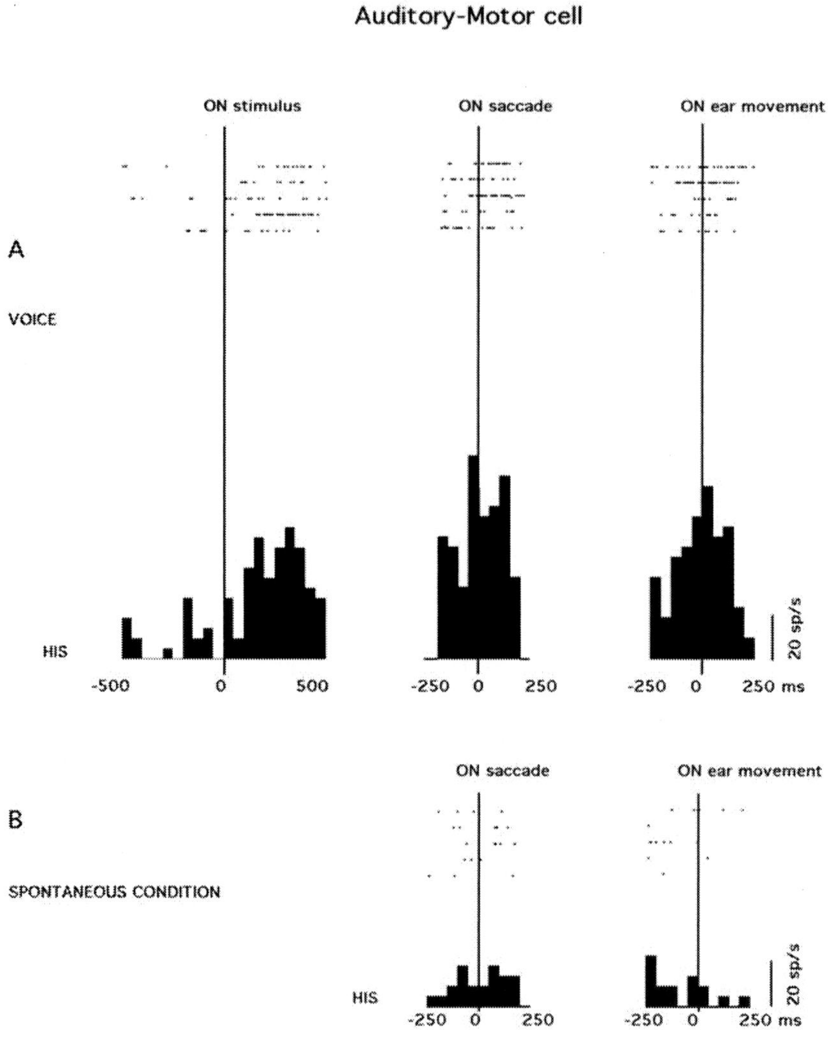

Figure 4. Example of auditory motor cell. A: This cell is active for auditory environmental stimuli, for orienting saccades, and orienting ear movements. B: In spontaneous condition the discharge is not synchronized with saccades or with ear movements. Raster: each dot is one spike. HIS: unit activity histogram. Bin width: 50 ms. (Exp Brain Res, 186, 2008, 131-41, "Auditory-motor and cognitive aspects in area 8B of macaque monkey's frontal cortex: a premotor ear–eye Weld (PEEF)", Lucchetti C et al. , Figure 3, With kind permission of Springer Science+ Business Media).

Those cells that did not show activity synchronized with the onset of auditory stimuli, but only with orienting ear movements, were defined as motor. The motor cells showed phasic, tonic, and phasic-tonic activity. An example of phasic-tonic activity is presented in Figure 6, where we can see a phasic discharge related to orienting ear movements and a tonic discharge in relation to ear position. These cells sometimes showed directional selectivity, forward and backward, and only a few cells discharged for oblique, upward and downward movements of the ear.

In addition different types of cells were found: "complex behaviour" cells showed inhibition of discharge by an auditory stimulus only when the ear was in a posterior position. "Novel visual stimuli" cells discharged at the presentation of different objects (mirror, cans, tools). Finally, cells showed neural activity for the experimenter's body or for a white coat presented on a stick. Similar cells were described by Tanila et al. (1992) in the prefrontal cortex.

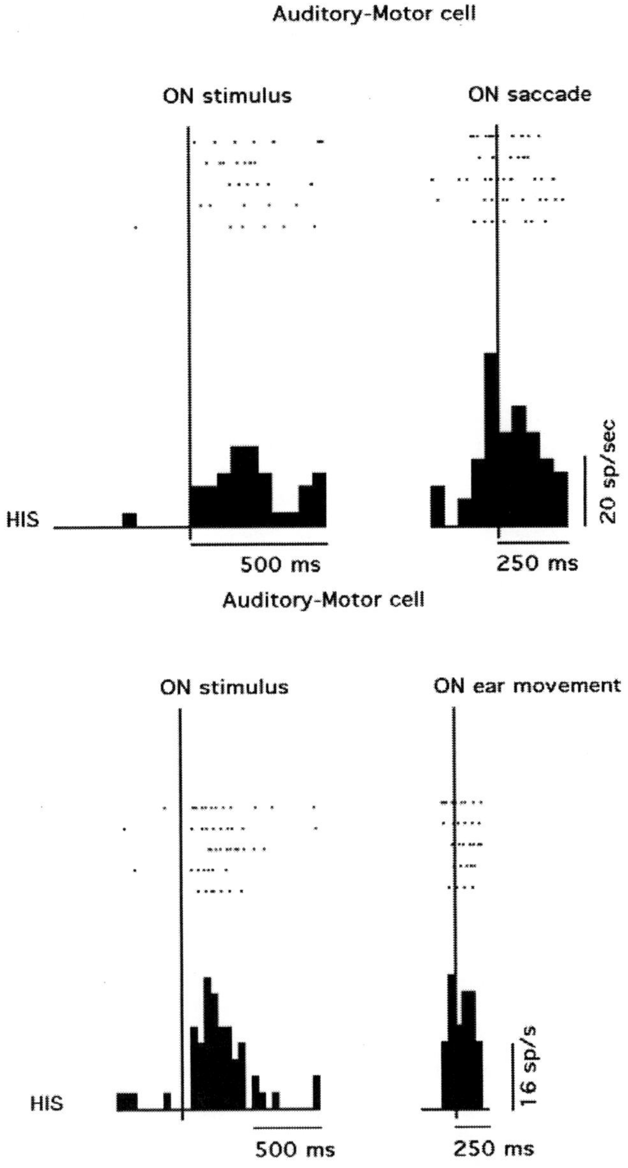

Figure 5. Auditory motor cells. Top: auditory-eye cell. Bottom: auditory-ear cell. Raster: each dot is one spike. HIS: unit activity histogram. Bin width: 50 ms. (Exp Brain Res, 186, 2008, 131-41, "Auditory-motor and cognitive aspects in area 8B of macaque monkey's frontal cortex: a premotor ear–eye Weld (PEEF)", Lucchetti C et al. , Figure 4-Figure 5, With kind permission of Springer Science+ Business Media).

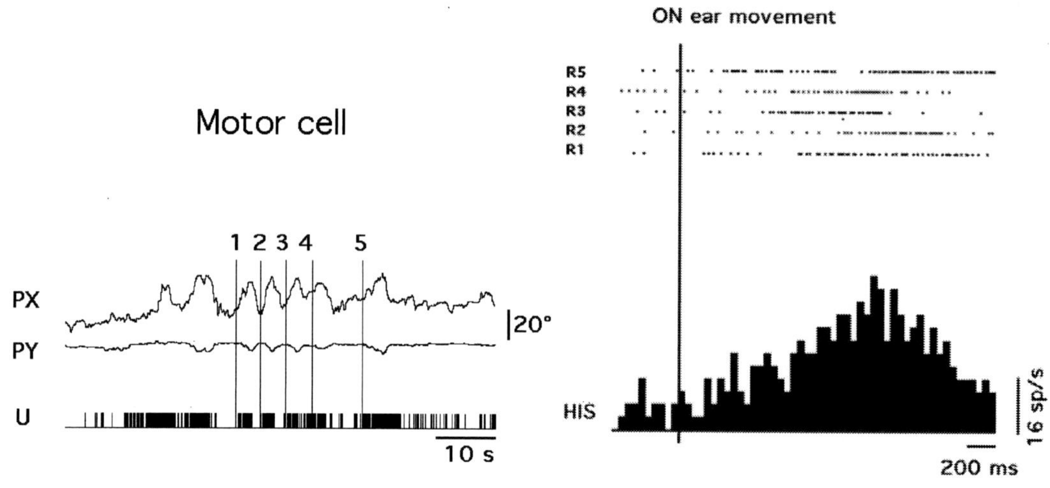

Figure 6. Example of motor cell. In this example, we can see a relationship to ear movement and a different tonic discharge in relation to ear position. PX: horizontal ear component, PY: vertical ear component. U: unit activity, each bar is one spike. Raster: each dot is one spike. HIS: unit activity histogram. Bin width: 50 ms. (Exp Brain Res, 186, 2008, 131-41, "Auditory-motor and cognitive aspects in area 8B of macaque monkey's frontal cortex: a premotor ear–eye Weld (PEEF)", Lucchetti C et al. , Figure 6, With kind permission of Springer Science+ Business Media).

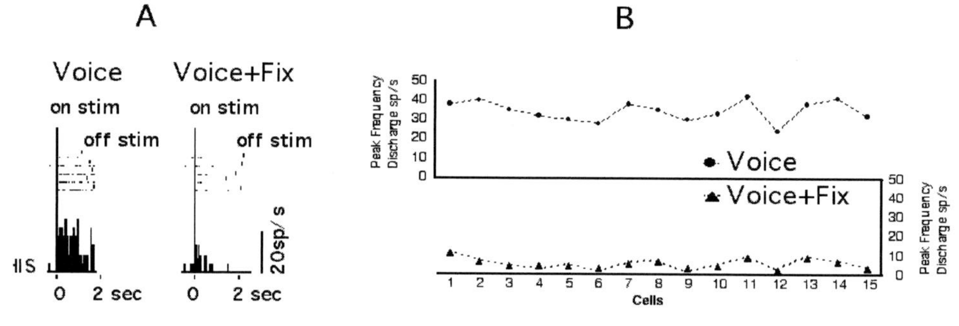

Figure 7. Inhibitory effect of visual fixation on auditory cells. Left: example of auditory cell (VOICE) and an inhibitory effect during visual fixation (FIX-VOICE). Each dot in the raster represents one spike. HIS: unit activity histogram. Bin width: 50 ms. Right: population analysis of 15 auditory cells influenced by fixation, Bi-Polar Chart Plot (Exp Brain Res, 168, 2006, 441-9, "Auditory environmental cells and visual fixation effect in area 8B of macaque monkey", Bon L and Lucchetti C, Figure 5-Figure 6, With kind permission of Springer Science+ Business Media).

Moreover, the auditory cells and the auditory-motor cells were tested when the animal performed a visual fixation in primary position in which the attention was engaged. Fifty percent of auditory cells showed a significantly lower activity when auditory stimuli were generated during the execution of visual fixation task, instead of when the same stimuli were generated in spontaneous conditions (Fig. 7). The same effect was present also in about fifty percent of the auditory-motor cells, related only to the orienting ear movement. These neurons showed a significantly lower activity level, in both their auditory and motor components, when auditory stimuli were presented during the execution of visual fixation task, as opposed to when the same stimuli were presented out of the task (Fig. 8).

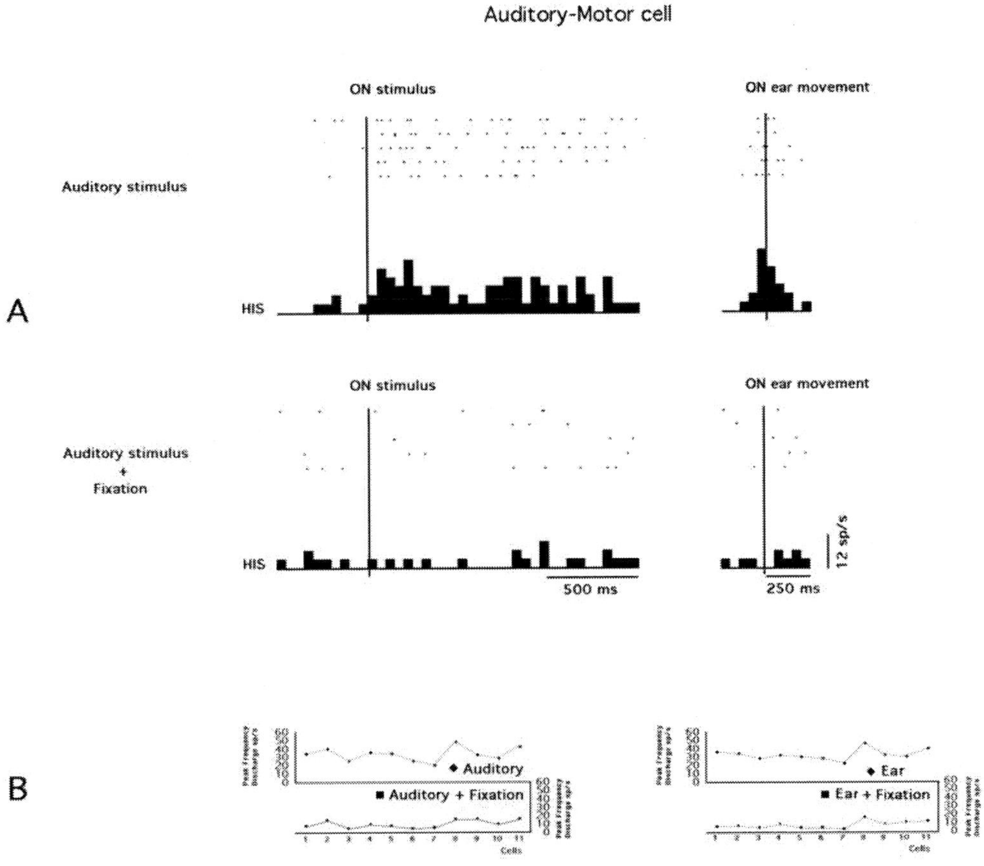

Figure 8. Inhibitory effect of visual fixation on auditory-motor cells. A: Example of auditory–motor cell in spontaneous condition and during visual fixation. In spontaneous condition, the activity is brisk for both auditory stimulus and ear movement, while during a visual fixation task the discharge is weak for both auditory stimulus and ear movement. Each dot in the raster represents one spike. HIS: unit activity histogram. Bin width: 50 ms. B: population analysis of 11 auditory-motor cells influenced by visual fixation. Left: auditory component, right: motor component (Exp Brain Res, 186, 2008, 131-41, "Auditory-motor and cognitive aspects in area 8B of macaque monkey's frontal cortex: a premotor ear–eye Weld (PEEF)", Lucchetti C et al. , Figure 8-Figure 9, With kind permission of Springer Science+ Business Media).

Conclusion

Considerations

If we observe the natural behaviour of an animal pointing to an another animal that may be a prey (cat and rat) and at the same time an auditory stimulus is produced, we may note two different reactions: the animal maintains its gaze towards the prey and orients its ears towards the auditory stimulus, or the animal orients both gaze and ears towards the auditory stimulus. A similar behaviour may be seen in humans, for example when we are reading a book and an external sound is produced, for example a message on a cellular phone, we may continue to read the book or we may orient the head toward the phone.

The electrophysiological investigations show that area 8B is involved in ear-eye motor control and in the auditory perception of environmental auditory stimuli. Other studies, carried out in the lateral belt area and in the core of the auditory cortex, connected to area 8B and other prefrontal cortices, showed neurons with discharge related to complex stimuli, vocalizations, and to faces and conspecific vocalizations (Rauschecker et al. 1995, Recanzone 2000, Ghanzanfar et al. 2005).

Three issues are relevant at this moment about area 8B (Bon and Lucchetti 1994, 2006, Lucchetti et al. 2008): a) the presence of auditory environmental neurons, b) the presence of auditory-motor neurons; c) the involvement of attentional processes.

A) Auditory Environmental Neurons

That environmental or naturalistic stimuli are more efficient has already been suggested by experimental evidence in the midbrain and inferior colliculus, and it has been proposed that this aspect is related to the intrinsic properties of the signal (Attias and Schreiner 1997, Escabì et al. 2003). More recent studies indicate that neurons of the lateral belt area, discharge better for complex stimuli and vocalisation, which may suggest, as argued by the authors, that this field is processing "what" information (Rauschecker et al. 1995, Recanzone 2000). Fuster et al. (2000) showed that neurons in area 8B, but also in area 9 and 6 were active when the animal performed correctly an association task between tone and colour.

The activity related to environmental auditory stimuli, found in area 8B, suggests a natural behavioural meaning in a cross-modal association between stimulus-subject (voice-experimenter) and between stimulus-motor act (footstep-walking). Even if largely speculative, this natural cross-modal association may represent an abstraction of auditory stimuli or alternatively may be an expression of auditory recognition based on emotion.

B) Auditory-Motor Neurons

Auditory-motor neurons, sensory and motor in nature, were tested without any behavioural constraints imposed by operant conditioning. These neurons were specific for environmental auditory stimuli and also showed properties of motor integration with two effectors: ear and/or eye. The animals oriented their gaze, in natural behaviour, turning their ears towards a stimulus presented in front of them or behind them. Accordingly, the neural activity could reflect a general aspect of orienting that involves the spatial localization of an acoustic stimulus.

The above evidences suggest that area 8B may be involved not only in the recognition of auditory stimuli but also in orienting processes (Romanski et al. 1999, Rao et al. 1997, Alain et al. 2001). In addition, activation for specific environmental auditory stimuli and the presence of auditory-motor and complex cells suggest that area 8B has an important place in the hierarchical organisation of the auditory system (Kaas and Hackett 2000, Wessinger et al. 2001). According to the model proposed by Kaas and Hackett (2000), area 8B may be considered together with areas 8A, 46, 12 and 10 at the fourth level of this hierarchical organisation of auditory system in primates.

C) Attentional Processes

Some considerations are necessary to explain the inhibitory effects that visual fixation tasks have on auditory and auditory-motor neurons. Similar results were found in the superior colliculus of the cat, when two visual stimuli were presented at the same time (Rizzolatti et al. 1974) and when visual fixation inhibited the auditory response (Populin and Yin 2002). Moreover, a similar effect has been found in the superior colliculus and in the posterior parietal cortex of the macaque monkey for visual and auditory peripheral stimuli (Bell et al. 2003, Gifford and Cohen 2004, Cohen et al. 2005). In the experiments of Rizzolatti et al. (1974), carried out with curare, both stimuli were visual. The authors explained the inhibitory effect as a consequence of orienting attention. Our experimental approach was similar to that of Bell et al. (2003), since one stimulus was visual and the other one is auditory. The inhibitory effect on neural discharge of both auditory and auditory-motor cells might be a consequence of the engagement of attention during visual fixation (Bon and Lucchetti 1997). This issue may be the expression of a combination of covert orienting of attention relative to eye position (i.e., nonfoveal locations), similar to the classic finding of Cherry (1953), and an overt orienting of attention relative to orientation of the ear. Accordingly, it seems that attention may affect more than one channel at the same time during a conditioned task or during natural behaviour (Turatto et al. 2004). Moreover, the inhibitory effect of auditory and auditory-motor neuron activity suggests that attention may filter or attenuate the auditory signals while a subject is orienting attention toward a visual stimulus (Treisman 1960). If we accept the attention as a link between sensory input and motor output, the involvement of attention in the gaze and ear motor control is also in agreement with the premotor theory of attention (Rizzolatti and Craighero 1998). All together, based on its functional characteristics and anatomical connections, area 8B may be part of the inhibitory network for gaze shift and ear orienting (Schiller and Tehovnik 2005).

Why "PEEF"?

There is a debate about whether area 8 (area 8A plus 8B) should be treated as a premotor or a prefrontal area. In macaque monkeys area 8B may be considered cytoachitectonically a transitional area between the granular area 9, rostrally, and the rostral part of the dorsal agranular area 6 caudally (Walker, 1940, Von Bonin a Bailey 1947, Matelli et al. 1991). Pandya and Yeterian (1985) used the term "premotor" to include both areas 8 and 6. Subsequently, other authors also treated area 6 and 8 as premotor cortex (Mann et al., 1988, Passingham, 1993, Bon and Lucchetti, 1994, Lucchetti et al. 1998, Lucchetti et al. 2008). In addition, the cytoarchitecture of area 8B differs from the granular area 8A (FEF), located latero-caudally to it in the prearcuate region (Barbas and Mesulam, 1981, Petrides and Pandya, 1994, Petrides and Pandya 1999). Transneuronal transfer of rabies virus and a functional imaging study clearly show that area 8B is involved with SEF in eye motor control (Moschovakis et al. 2004).

Area 8B is reciprocally connected with the auditory cortex (Barbas and Mesulam 1981), receives projections from the dentate nucleus of cerebellum via the thalamus, much like FEF

(Lynch et al 1994), and projects to the superior colliculus, also like FEF (Fries 1984). Recent anatomical studies show that area 8B sends robust projections to (SEF) (Luppino et al. 2003, Wang et al. 2005).

The neural activity of area 8B is prevalently related to ear or to ear-eye movement and to auditory environmental stimuli (Bon and Lucchetti 1994, 2006). In contrast, neural activity in SEF is related to eye movement, eye fixation, ear and neck movement (Schlag and Schlag-Rey 1987, Bon and Lucchetti 1990, 1991,1992, Tehovnik and Lee 1993, Tehovnik and Sommer 1997, Chen and Walton 2005), auditory stimuli (Schall 1991) and attentional processes (Bon and Lucchetti 1997). Neural activity in the FEF is related to eye movement, neck movement, auditory and visual stimuli and attentional processes (Schall 1997).

Microstimulation of area 8B predominantly evoked small fixed-vector saccades and ear movement, as well as ear-eye movement (Levinshon 1909, Bon and Lucchetti 1994). Microstimulation of SEF predominantly evoked goal directed saccades and, in a few penetrations, also ear movements (Schlag and Schlag-Rey 1987, Bon and Lucchetti 1992, Tehovnik et al. 2000). In contrast, microstimulation of FEF evoked small fixed-vector saccades in the inferior part, and large fixed-vector saccades in the superior part (Bruce et al. 1985).

Taking these results together, the principal difference between area 8B and SEF/FEF is that the neurons in area 8B are rarely related to saccades and visual fixation, and they are more related to ear movement. Moreover, microstimulation of area 8B predominantly evokes activation of ear muscles or a coactivation of ear and eye muscles.

In the first report by Bon and Lucchetti (1994) about area 8B, they said that this area "may be considered a rostral extension of supplementary eye field (SEF) or a different region". Considering, the functional differences between area 8B and both the SEF and FEF (area 8A), as well as the differences in cytoarchitecture and anatomical projections, we can now consider area 8B as a separate field, a Premotor Ear-Eye Field (PEEF).

Acknowledgments We wish to thank Dr, Helen Barbas for helpful suggestions in revising this review.

References

Alain, C; Arnott, SR; Hevenor, S; Graham, S; Grady, CL. "What" and "Where" in the human auditory system. *Proc. Natl. Acad. Sci. USA,* 2001 98, 12301-12306.

Attias, H; Schreiner, C. Temporal low-order statistics of natural sounds. In: Mozer MC, Jordan MI, Petsche T, editor. *Advances in neural information processes systems.* Cambridge MA: MIT Press; 1997; 27-33.

Barbas, H; Mesulam, MM. Organization of afferent input to subdivisions of area 8 in the rhesus monkey. *J. Comp. Neurol.*, 1981 200, 407-431.

Barbas, H; Ghashghaei, H; Dombrowski, SM; Rempel-Clower, NL. Medial prefrontal cortices are unified by common connections with superior temporal cortices and distinguished by input from memory-related areas in the rhesus monkey. *J. Comp. Neurol.,* 1999 410, 343-67.

Barbas, H; Medalla, M; Alade, O; Suski, J; Zikopoulos, B; Lera, P. Relationship of prefrontal connections to inhibitory systems in superior temporal areas in the rhesus monkey. *Cerebral Cortex,* 2005 15, 1356-1370.

Barbas, H; Pandya, DN. Architecture and intrinsic connections of the prefrontal cortex in the rhesus monkey. *J. Comp. Neurol,* 1989 286, 353-375.

Bell, AH; Corneil, BD; Munoz, DP; Meredith, MA. Engagement of visual fixation suppresses sensory responsiveness and multisensory integration in the primate superior colliculus. *Eur J. Neurosci.*, 2003 18, 2867-2873.

Bon, L; Lucchetti, C. Neurons signalling the maintenance of attentive fixation in frontal area 6aß of macaque monkey. *Exp. Brain Res.,* 1990 82, 231-233.

Bon, L; Lucchetti, C. Behavioral and motor mechanisms of dorsomedial frontal cortex in Macaca monkey. *Intern J. Neuroscience*, 1991 60, 187-193.

Bon, L; Lucchetti, C. The dorsomedial frontal cortex of the macaca monkey: fixation and saccade-related activity. *Exp. Brain Res.*, 1992 89, 571-580.

Bon, L; Lucchetti, C. Ear and eye representation in the frontal cortex, area 8b, of the macaque monkey: an electrophysiological study. *Exp. Brain Res.*, 1994 102, 259-271.

Bon, L; Lucchetti, C. Attentional-related neurons in the supplementary eye field of the macaque monkey. *Exp. Brain Res.*, 1997 113, 180–185.

Bon, L; Lucchetti, C. Auditory environmental cells and visual fixation effect in area 8B of macaque monkey. *Exp. Brain Res.,* 2006 168, 441-449.

Bruce, CJ; Goldberg, ME; Bushnell, MC; Stanton, GB. Primate frontal eye fields: II. Physiological and anatomic correlates of electrically evoked eye movements. *J. Neurophysiol,* 1985 54, 714-734.

Chen, LL; Walton, MMG. Head movement evoked by electric stimulation in the supplementary eye field of the rhesus monkey. *J. Neurophysiol.,* 2005 94, 4502-4519.

Cherry, EC. Some experiments on the recognition of speech with one and with two ears. *J. Acustical Soc of America,* 1953 25, 975-979.

Cohen, YE; Russ, BE; Gifford III, GW. Auditory processing in the posterior parietal cortex. *Behavioural and Cognitive Neuroscience Reviews*, 2005 4, 218-231.

Corneil, BD; Olivier, E; Munoz, DP. Neck muscle responses to stimulation of monkey superior colliculus. I. Topography and manipulation of stimulation parameters. *J. Neurophysiol.*, 2002 88, 1980-1999.

Escabì, MA; Miller, LM; Read, HL; Schreiner, CE. Naturalistic auditory contrast improves spectrotemporal coding in the cat inferior colliculus. *J. Neurosci.,* 2003 23, 11489-11504.

Fadiga, E; Pupilli, GC. Teleceptive components of the cerebellar functions. *Physiol Rev,* 1964 44, 432-486.

Ferrier, D. Experiments on the brains of monkeys. *Philos. Trans R Soc Lond B Biol. Sci.,* 1875 165, 433-488.

Fries, W. Cortical projections to the superior colliculus in the macaque monkey: a retrograde study using horseradish peroxidase. *J. Comp. Neurol.,* 1984 230, 55-76.

Fuster, JM. *The prefrontal cortex.* 3rd Edition. Philadelphia-New York: Lippincot-Raven publishers; 1997.

Fuster, JM; Bodner, M; Kroger, JK. Cross-modal and cross-temporal association in neurons of frontal cortex. *Nature,* 2000 405, 347-351.

Ghazanfar, AA; Maier, JX; Hoffman, KL; Logothetis, NK. Multisensory integration of dynamic faces and voices in rhesus monkey auditory cortex. *J. of Neuroscience,* 2005 18, 5004-5012.

Gifford III, GW; Cohen, YE. The effect of a central fixation light on auditory spatial responses in area LIP. *J. of Neurophysiol.,* 2004 91, 2929-2933.

Harlow, JM. Passage of an iron rod through the head. *Boston med surg J.,* 1848 39, 389-393.

Kaas, JH; Hackett, TA. Subdivision of auditory cortex and processing streams in primates. *Proc. Natl. Acad. Sci. USA,* 2000 97, 11793-11799.

Kelly, RM; Strick, PL. Cerebellar loops with motor cortex and prefrontal cortex of a nonhuman primate. *J. Neurosci.,* 2003 23, 8432-8444.

Kuypers, HGJM. Anatomy of the descending pathways. In: Brooks V, editor. *Handbook of Physiology, Vol 2.* Bethesda, MA: Am Physiol Soc; 1981; 63-86.

Levinsohn, G. Uber die beziehungen der grosshirnrinde beim affen zu den bewegungen des auges. *Graefes Archive for Clinical and Experimental Ophthalmology,* 1909 71, 313-378.

Lynch, JC; Hoover, JE; Strick, PL. Input to the primate frontal eye field from the substantia nigra, superior colliculus, and dentate nucleus demonstrated by transneuronal transport. *Exp. Brain Res.,* 1994 100, 181-186.

Lynch, JC; Tian, JR. Cortico-cortical networks and cortico-subcortical loops for the higher control of eye movements. *Progress in Brain research,* 2006 151, 461-501.

Lucchetti, C; Lanzilotto, M; Bon, L. Auditory-motor and cognitive aspects in area 8B of macaque monkey's frontal cortex: a premotor ear-eye field (PEEF). *Exp. Brain Res.,* 2008 186, 131-141.

Lucchetti, C; Lui, F; Bon, L. Neglect syndrome for aversive stimuli in a macaque monkey with dorsomedial frontal cortex lesion. *Neuropsychologia,* 1998 36, 251-257.

Luppino, G; Rozzi, S; Calzavara, R; Matelli, M. Prefrontal and agranular cingulate projections to the dorsal premotor areas F2 and F7 in the macaque monkey. *Eur. J. Neurosci.,* 2003 17, 559-578.

Mann, SE; Thau, R; Schiller, PH. Conditional task-related responses in monkey dorsomedial frontal cortex. *Exp. Brain Res.,* 1988 69, 460-468.

Matelli, M; Luppino, G; Rizzolatti, G. Architecture of superior and mesial area 6 and adiacent cingulate cortex in the macaque monkey. *J. Comp. Neurol.,* 1991 311, 445-462.

Middleton, FA; Strick, PL. Cerebellar projections to the prefrontal cortex of the primate. *J. Neuroscience,* 2001 21, 700-712.

Mortimer, JA. Cerebellar responses to teleceptive stimuli in alert monkeys. *Brain Research,* 1975 83, 369-390.

Moschovakis, AK; Gregoriou, GG; Ugolini, G; Doldan, M; Graf, W; Guldin, W; Hadjidimitrakis, K; Savaki, HE. Oculomotor areas of the primate frontal lobes: a transneuronal transfer of rabies virus and [^{14} C]-2-deoxyglucose functional imaging study. *J. Neurosci.,* 2004 24, 5726-5740.

Pandya, DN; Yeterian, EH. Architecture and connections of cortical association areas. In: Peters A, Jones EG, editor. *Association and auditory cortices*. New York: Plenum; 1985; 3-61.

Pandya, DN; Yeterian, EH. Prefrontal cortex in relation to other cortical areas in rhesus monkey: architecture and connections. *Progr. Brain Res.,* 1990 85, 63-94.

Passingham, R. *The frontal lobes and voluntary action*. Oxford: Oxford University Press; 1993.

Petrides, M; Pandya, DN. Comparative architectonic analysis of the human and the macaque frontal cortex. In: Boller F, Grafman J, editors. *Handbook of Neuropsychology, vol 9.*, Amsterdam: Elsevier; 1994; 17-57.

Petrides, M; Pandya, DN. Dorsolateral prefrontal cortex: comparative cytoarchitectonic analysis in the human and the macaque brain and corticocortical connections patterns. *European Journal of Neurosciences,* 1999 11, 1011-1036.

Petrides, M. The role of the mid-dorsolateral prefrontal cortex in working memory. *Exp. Brain Res.,* 2000 133, 44-54.

Populin, LC; Yin, TCT. Bimodal interactions in the superior colliculus of the behaving cat. *J Neuroscience,* 2002 22, 2826-2834.

Rao, SC; Rainer, G; Miller, EK. Integration of what and where in the primate prefrontal cortex. *Science,* 1997 276, 821-824.

Rauschecker, JP; Tian, B; Hauser, M. Processing of complex sounds in the macaque non primary auditory cortex. *Science*, 1995 268, 111-114.

Raybourn, MS; Keller, EL. Colliculoreticular organization in primate oculomotor system. *J. Neurophysiol.*, 1977 40, 861-878.

Recanzone, GH. Spatial processing in the auditory cortex of the macaque monkey. *Proc. Natl. Acad Sci USA,* 2000 97, 11829-11835.

Rizzolatti, G; Camarda, R; Grupp, LA; Pisa, M. Inhibitory effect of remote visual stimuli on visual responses of cat superior colliculus: spatial and temporal factors. *J. Neurophysiol.,* 1974 37, 1262-1275.

Rizzolatti, G; Matelli, M; Pavesi, G. Deficits in attention and movement following the removal of postarcuate (area 6) and prearcuate (area 8) cortex in macaque monkeys. *Brain,* 1983 106, 655-673.

Rizzolatti, G; Craighero, L. Spatial attention: mechanisms and theories. In: Sabourin M, Craik F, Robert M, editors. *Advances in psychological science vol. 2: biological and cognitive aspects.* Psychological Press; 1998; 171-198.

Romanski, LM; Bates, JF; Goldman-Rakic, PS. Auditory belt and parabelt projections to the prefrontal cortex in the rhesus monkey. *J. Comp. Neurol.,* 1999 403, 141-157.

Rosenkilde, CE. Functional eterogeneity of the prefrontal cortex in the monkey: a review. *Behav. Neural. Biol.,* 1979 25, 301-345.

Schall, JD. neural activity related to visual saccadic eye movements in the supplementary motor area of rhesus monkey. *J. Neurophysiology,* 1991 66, 530-558.

Schall, JD. Visuomotor areas of the frontal lobe in Cerebral Cortex Vol.12. In: Rockland KS, Kaas JH, PetersA, editors. *Extrastriate cortex in primates*. New York and London: Plenum Press; 1997; 527-616.

Schiller, PH; Sandell, JH; Maunsell, JHK. The effect of frontal eye field and superior colliculus lesions on saccadic latencies in the rhesus monkey. *J Neurophysiol,* 1987 57, 1033-1049.

Schiller, PH; Tehovnik, EJ. Neural mechanisms underlying target selection with saccadic eye movements. *Progress in Brain Research,* 2005 149, 157-171.

Schlag, J; Schlag-Rey, M. Evidence for a supplementary eye field. *J. Neurophysiol.,* 1987 57, 179-200.

Schmahmann, JD; Pandya, DN. Anatomic organization of the basilar pontine projections from prefrontal cortices in rhesus monkey. *J. Neurosci.,* 1997 17, 438-458.

Snider, RS; Stowell, A. The receiving areas of the tactile, auditory and visual systems in the cerebellum. *J. Neurophysiol.,* 1944 7, 331-357.

van der Steen, J; Russell, IS; James, GO. Effects of unilateral frontal eye-field lesions on eye-head coordination in monkey. *J. Neurophysiol.,* 1986 55, 696-713.

Tanila, H; Carlson, S; Linnankoski, I; Lindros, F; Kahila, H. Functional properties of dorsolateral prefrontal cortical neurons in awake monkey. *Behav. Brain Res.,* 1992 47, 169-180.

Tanila, H; Carlson, S; Linnankoski, I; Kahila, H. Regional distribution of functions in dorsolateral prefrontal cortex of the monkey. *Behav. Brain Res.,* 1993 53, 63-71.

Tanji, J; Hoshi, E. Role of the lateral prefrontal cortex in executive behavioral control. *Physiol. Rev.*, 2008 88, 37-57.

Tehovnik, EJ; Lee, KM. The dorsomedial frontal cortex of the rhesus monkey. Topographic representation of saccades evoked by electric stimulation. *Exp. Brain Res.,* 1993 96, 430-442.

Tehovnik, EJ; Sommer, MS. Electrically evoked saccades from the dorsomedial frontal cortex and frontal eye field: a parametric evaluation reveals differences between areas. *Exp. Brain Res.,* 1997 117, 369-378.

Tehovnik, EJ; Sommer, MA; Chou, IH; Slocum, WM; Schiller, PH. Eye fields in the frontal lobes of primates. *Brain Res. Rev.,* 2000 32, 413-448.

Thier, P; Andersen, RA. Eletrical microstimulation distinguishes distinct saccade-related areas in the posterior parietal cortex. *J. Neurophysiol.,* 1998 80, 1713-1735.

Treisman, AM. Contextual cues in selective listening. *Quarterly Journal of Experimental Psycholology: Human Perception and Performance,* 1960 12, 242-248.

Turatto, M; Galfano, G; Bridgeman, B; Umiltà, C. Space-independent modality-driven attentional capture in auditory, tactile and visual systems. *Exp Brain Res,* 2004 155, 301-310.

Von Bonin, G; Bailey, P. *The neocortex of macaca mulatta.* Urbana: University of Illinois: Press; 1947.

Walker, AE. A cytoarchitectural study of frontal area of the Macaque monkey. *J. Comp Neurol.*, 1940 73, 59-86.

Wang, YW; Isoda, M; Matsuzaka, Y; Shima, K; Tanji, J. Prefrontal cortical cells projecting to the supplementary eye field and presupplementary motor area in the monkey. *Neuroscience Research,* 2005 53, 1-7.

Wegener, JG. The sound localizing behavior of normal and brain damaged monkeys. *J. Auditory Res.*, 1973 13, 191-219.

Wessinger, CM; Van Meter, J; Tian, B; Van Lare, J; Pekar, J; Rauschecker, JP. Hierarchical organization of the human auditory cortex revealed by functional magnetic resonance imaging. *J. Cognitive Neurosci.,* 2001 13, 1-7.

Williams, SM; Goldman–Rakic, P. Widespread origin of the primate mesofrontal dopamine system. *Cerebral Cortex*, 1998 8, 321-345.

In: Prefrontal Cortex: Roles, Interventions and Traumas ISBN 978-1-60692-415-0
Editors: Lorenzo LoGrasso and Giovanni Morretti

Expert Commentary A

Prefrontal Cortex: Its Roles in Cognitive Impairment in Parkinson's Disease Revealed by PET

***Qing Wang*[ab*]*, Kelly A. Newell*[a]*, Peter T. H. Wong*[d] *and Ying Lu*[c]

[a]Neurobiology Research Centre, School of Health Sciences,
University of Wollongong, NSW 2522, Australia
[b]Department of Neurology, the Third Hospital of Sun Yat-Sen University,
600 Tianhe Road, Guangzhou, Guangdong 510630, P.R.China
[c]Department of Radiology and Biostatistics, University of California,
San Francisco, CA 94143, USA
[d]Departments of Pharmacology, Yong Loo Lin School of Medicine,
National University of Singapore 117597, Singapore

Parkinson's disease (PD) is a neurodegenerative disorder, classically characterized by the chronic loss of dopaminergic neurons primarily in substantia nigra pars compacta, which leads to a reduction of dopamine levels in the striatum. The motor symptoms do not become obvious until at least an 80% reduction in striatal dopamine levels. Recent works have demonstrated that cognitive impairment occurs even in the early course of PD which is correlated with dopaminergic dysfunctions in the prefrontal cortex (Brück, 2005b; Chudasama and Robbins, 2006) and not necessarily related to motor disorders. This commentary will discuss the current knowledge of the prefrontal cortex and its association with cognitive deficits in PD.

Increasing evidence show that profound dopamine depletion not only occurs in the striatum but also in the prefrontal cortex (Scatton, 1982), and this may be associated with the cognitive deficits in PD (Roberts, 1994; Goldman-Rakic, 1998; Kulisevsky, 2000). L-dopa is widely used for the treatment of PD and shows beneficial effects on the cognitive

* Corresponding author: Dr. Qing Wang, Neurobiology Research Centre, School of Health Sciences, University of Wollongong, NSW 2522, Australia. Phone: +61 2 4221 3199; Fax: +61 2 4221 4096; Email: denniswq@yahoo.com or dwang@uow.edu.au

dysfunctions among PD patients. One study by Shohamy, based on electrophysiological and computational examination, demonstrated that the loss of dopamine in PD led to specific learning impairment, and that enhancing dopamine levels with L-dopa treatment alleviated the impairment of feedback-based sequence learning (Shohamy, 2005). Mollion also showed that in two conditional associative learning tasks, the increase in response time and the decrease in errors found in L-dopa medicated PD patients compared to non-L-dopa medicated patients reflected enhancement of working memory, suggesting the L-dopa treatment improve the cognitive impairment in PD patients (Mollion, 2003). More evidence indicated that mesocortical regions, especially prefrontal cortex, may be the key locus for cognitive functional improvement following dopaminergic enhancement (Arnsten, 1998; Mattay, 2000; Mehta, 2000). Interestingly, L-dopa was also found to exert detrimental effects on cognition related functions like extinction learning (Czernecki, 2002) and probabilistic reversal learning (Cools, 2001). For these contrasting effects, Cools proposed that increases of dopamine transmission in prefrontal cortex and its reductions in striatum contribute to the cognitive stability; however, cognitive flexibility benefited from potentiated phasic striatal dopamine transmission and its reduction in the prefrontal cortex (Cools, 2006).

Literature shows that disruption of the prefrontal cortex in PD leads to considerable cognitive dysfunction, which is likely related to metabolic and cerebral blood flow changes in prefrontal cortex and associated with the striatal dysfunction in PD patients. Early in 1985, Globus examined regionally reduced cerebral blood flow using a 133Xenon inhalation technique, and evaluated cognitive dysfunction in PD patients (Globus, 1985). However, with technological advancement, positron emission tomography (PET) has become a very useful tool in investigating, among other things, the dopaminergic system. PET is an imaging method used to track the regional distribution and kinetics of chemical compounds in the living body by labelling them with short-lived positron-emitting isotopes. It was the first and most precise technology to directly measure components of the dopamine system like dopamine uptake and release, dopamine transport, dopamine receptors, and cerebral blood flow in the living human brain (Volkow, 1996).

In the MPTP-induced Parkinson's disease monkey model, a significant decrease of blood flow and dopamine transporters was observed by PET in mesolimbicortical regions like putamen, caudate, and primary motor cortex (Brownell, 2003). Playford firstly used PET to examine regional cerebral blood flow in PD patients and found the obvious reduction in the prefrontal cortical cerebral blood flow when compared to control subjects (Playford, 1992). An obvious decrease of cerebral blood flow in bilateral prefrontal cortex of PD patients during central sensory processing was determined through PET (Boecker, 1999); whilst the dopamine agonist apomorphine profoundly induced decreases of regional cerebral blood flow in the primary motor cortex, the medial and dorsolateral prefrontal cortex as evidenced by PET (Hosey, 2005). Similarly, recent work using PET showed a significant correlation between L-dopa-induced blood flow decreases in the dorsolateral prefrontal cortex and cognitive functional changes in performance on the planning task and spatial working memory in PD patients (Cools, 2002). The work suggested that high-level cognitive impairment in PD patients could be ameliorated by L-dopa through inducing relative blood flow changes in the dorsolateral prefrontal cortex (Cools, 2002).

Consistent with Cools work (Cools, 2002)., with the help of fMRI, Mattay and colleagues (Mattay, 2002) demonstrated that prefrontal cortex, subserving working memory, displayed higher activation during the hypodopaminergic state, and increased activation in prefrontal cortex during the working memory task in the hypodopaminergic state was positively associated with errors in task performance. These results suggest that prefrontal cortex exert important roles in modulating cognitive function like working memory via mesocortical dopaminergic system, and hypodopaminergic state is likely related to the decreased efficiency of prefrontal cortical information processing.

In a study by Owen (Owen, 1998), a Tower of London planning task was performed to present abnormal spatial working memory in PD patients, which was associated with a regional decrease of cerebral blood flow as a metabolic marker in the basal ganglia. This study is similar to Dagher's work, showing abnormal blood flow in the basal ganglia of PD patients with `frontal' cognitive deficits (Dagher, 2001). Besides the L-dopa mediated cerebral blood flow changes in PD patients, PET study also showed an obvious atrophy associated with cognitive impairment which was observed in the right and the left prefrontal cortex in early stage PD patients (Brück, 2004).

With the help of PET, a profound reduction of Fluorodopa uptake in frontal cortex of PD patients was observed, and this reduction was positively correlated with cognitive deficits including verbal fluency, working memory, and attentional functioning reflecting frontal lobe function (Rinne, 2000). In contrast, using 6-[^{18}F]fluoro-l-dopa (Fdopa) as the tracer in PET, Brück observed an *upregulation* of cortical Fdopa uptake in early non-medicated PD patients, and indicated that the increase in dorsolateral prefrontal cortical Fdopa uptake was associated with cognitive deficits in early PD (Brück, 2005a). This increase of Fdopa uptake in prefrontal cortex might result from the compensatory process in the cortical-subcortical dopamine loops among PD patients (Cropley, 2006).

In addition to the dopamine transmission, various receptors in the cortical regions also contribute to cognitive deficits in PD. It is interesting to find that in animal studies dopamine D1 and D2 receptors, muscarinic receptors and serotonin receptors in prefrontal cortex were involved in regulating cognitive activity in various PD animal models (Tzavara, 2004; Wang, 2005; Cao, 2007). Clinical studies showed that dopamine D2/3 receptors in the dorsolateral prefrontal cortex of advanced PD patients were significantly decreased, and slightly declined in early stage of PD (Kaasinen, 2000). Meoni found that NMDA NR1 expression was decreased in the prefrontal cortex of PD patients, and indicated that this downregulation may result from the degeneration of the dopaminergic input to the prefrontal cortex in PD (Meoni, 1999). Also, it was shown that nicotinic ACh receptors were reduced in cortical regions of PD patients (Perry, 1993).

Prefrontal cortex is increasingly recognized to be the important brain region in mediating cognitive dysfunctions among different stages in the progression of PD. However, more work needs to explore how cognitive dysfunctions are affected through prefrontal cortex modulating interventions in PD. Future work should address the functional correlations of mesocortical and nigrostriatal regions in mediating cognitive impairment in PD. Moreover, experimental and preclinical data should be converted to clinical practice and provide novel strategies in slowing down the progression of cognitive deficits in PD patients.

References

Arnsten AFT (1998) Catecholamine modulation of prefrontal cortical cognitive function. *Trends Cogn. Sci.* 2:436-447.

Boecker H, Ceballos-Baumann, A., Bartenstein, P., Weindl, A., Siebner, H.R., Fassbender, T., Munz, F., Schwaiger, M., Conrad, B. (1999) Sensory processing in Parkinson's and Huntington's disease: investigations with 3D H(2)(15)O-PET. *Brain* 122 (Pt 9):1651-1665.

Brownell AL, Canales, K., Chen, Y.I., Jenkins, B.G., Owen, C., Livni, E., Yu, M., Cicchetti, F., Sanchez-Pernaute, R., Isacson, O. (2003) Mapping of brain function after MPTP-induced neurotoxicity in a primate Parkinson's disease model. *Neuroimage* 20(2):1064-1075.

Brück A, Aalto, S., Nurmi, E., Bergman, J., Rinne, J.O. (2005a) Cortical 6-[18F]fluoro-L-dopa uptake and frontal cognitive functions in early Parkinson's disease. *Neurobiol. Aging* 26(6):891-898.

Brück A, Aalto, S., Nurmi, E., Bergman, J., Rinne, J.O. (2005b) Cortical 6-[18F]fluoro-L-dopa uptake and frontal cognitive functions in early Parkinson's disease. *Neurobiol. Aging* 26(6):891-898.

Brück A, Kurki, T., Kaasinen, V., Vahlberg, T., Rinne, J.O. (2004) Hippocampal and prefrontal atrophy in patients with early non-demented Parkinson's disease is related to cognitive impairment. *J. Neurol. Neurosurg. Psychiatry* 75(10):1467-1469.

Cao J, Liu, J., Zhang, Q.J., Wang, T., Wang, S., Han, L.N., Li, Q. (2007) The selective 5-HT1A receptor antagonist WAY-100635 inhibits neuronal activity of the ventromedial prefrontal cortex in a rodent model of Parkinson's disease. *Neurosci. Bull.* 23(6):315-322.

Chudasama Y, Robbins TW (2006) Functions of frontostriatal systems in cognition: comparative neuropsychopharmacological studies in rats, monkeys and humans. *Biol. Psychol.* 73(1):19-38.

Cools R (2006) Dopaminergic modulation of cognitive function-implications for L-DOPA treatment in Parkinson's disease. *Neurosci. Biobehav. Rev.* 30(1):1-23 Review.

Cools R, Barker, R.A., Sahakian, B.J., Robbins, T.W. (2001) Enhanced or impaired cognitive function in Parkinson's disease as a function of dopaminergic medication and task demands. *Cereb. Cortex* 11(12):1136-1143.

Cools R, Stefanova, E., Barker, R.A., Robbins, T.W., Owen, A.M. (2002) Dopaminergic modulation of high-level cognition in Parkinson's disease: the role of the prefrontal cortex revealed by PET. *Brain* 125(Pt 3):584-594.

Cropley VL, Fujita, M., Innis, R.B., Nathan, P.J. (2006) Molecular imaging of the dopaminergic system and its association with human cognitive function. *Biol. Psychiatry* 59(10):898-907.

Czernecki V, Pillon, B., Houeto, J.L., Pochon, J.B., Levy, R., Dubois, B. (2002) Motivation, reward, and Parkinson's disease: influence of dopatherapy. *Neuropsychologia* 40(13):2257-2267.

Dagher A, Owen, A.M., Boecker, H., Brooks, D.J. (2001) The role of the striatum and hippocampus in planning: a PET activation study in Parkinson's disease. *Brain* 124(Pt 5):1020-1032.

Globus M, Mildworf, B., Melamed, E. (1985) Cerebral blood flow and cognitive impairment in Parkinson's disease. *Neurology* 35(8):1135-1139.

Goldman-Rakic PS (1998) The cortical dopamine system: role in memory and cognition. *Adv. Pharmacol.* 42:707-711.

Hosey LA, Thompson, J.L., Metman, L.V., van den Munckhof, P., Braun, A.R. (2005) Temporal dynamics of cortical and subcortical responses to apomorphine in Parkinson disease: an H2(15)O PET study. *Clin. Neuropharmacol.* 28(1):18-27.

Kaasinen V, Någren, K., Hietala, J., Oikonen, V., Vilkman, H., Farde, L., Halldin, C., Rinne, J.O. (2000) Extrastriatal dopamine D2 and D3 receptors in early and advanced Parkinson's disease. *Neurology* 54(7):1482-1487.

Kulisevsky J (2000) Role of dopamine in learning and memory: implications for the treatment of cognitive dysfunction in patients with Parkinson's disease. *Drugs Aging* 16(5):365-379.

Mattay VS, Callicott, J.H., Bertolino, A., Heaton, I., Frank, J.A., Coppola, R., Berman, K.F., Goldberg, T.E., Weinberger, D.R. (2000) Effects of dextroamphetamine on cognitive performance and cortical activation. *Neuroimage* 12(3):268-275.

Mehta M, Owen, A.M., Sahakian, B.J., Mavaddat, N., Pickard, J.D., Robbins, T.W. (2000) Ritalin and working memory modulation in humans: ritalin enhances working memory by modulating discrete frontal and parietal lobe regions in the human brain. *J. Neurosci.* 20:RC1-6.

Meoni P, Bunnemann, B.H., Kingsbury, A.E., Trist, D.G., Bowery, N.G. (1999) NMDA NR1 subunit mRNA and glutamate NMDA-sensitive binding are differentially affected in the striatum and pre-frontal cortex of Parkinson's disease patients. *Neuropharmacology* 38(5):625-633.

Mollion H, Ventre-Dominey, J., Dominey, P.F., Broussolle, E. (2003) Dissociable effects of dopaminergic therapy on spatial versus non-spatial working memory in Parkinson's disease. *Neuropsychologia* 41(11):1442-1451.

Owen AM, Doyon, J., Dagher, A., Sadikot, A., Evans, A.C. (1998) Abnormal basal ganglia outflow in Parkinson's disease identified with PET. Implications for higher cortical functions. *Brain* 121 (Pt 5):949-965.

Perry EK, Irving, D., Kerwin, J.M., McKeith, I.G., Thompson, P., Collerton, D., Fairbairn, A.F., Ince, P.G., Morris, C.M., Cheng, A.V., et al (1993) Cholinergic transmitter and neurotrophic activities in Lewy body dementia: similarity to Parkinson's and distinction from Alzheimer disease. *Alzheimer Dis. Assoc. Disord.* 7:69-79.

Playford ED, Jenkins, I.H., Passingham, R.E., Nutt, J., Frackowiak, R.S., Brooks, D.J. (1992) Impaired mesial frontal and putamen activation in Parkinson's disease: a positron emission tomography study. *Ann. Neurol.* 32(2):151-161.

Rinne JO, Portin, R., Ruottinen, H., Nurmi, E., Bergman, J., Haaparanta, M., Solin, O. (2000) Cognitive impairment and the brain dopaminergic system in Parkinson disease: [18F]fluorodopa positron emission tomographic study. *Arch. Neurol.* 57(4):470-475.

Roberts AC, De Salvia, M.A., Wilkinson, L.S., Collins, P., Muir, J.L., Everitt, B.J., Robbins, T.W. (1994) 6-Hydroxydopamine lesions of the prefrontal cortex in monkeys enhance performance on an analog of the Wisconsin Card Sort Test: possible interactions with subcortical dopamine. *J. Neurosci.* 14(5 Pt 1):2531-2544.

Scatton B, Rouquier, L., Javoy-Agid, F., Agid, Y. (1982) Dopamine deficiency in the cerebral cortex in Parkinson disease. *Neurology* 32(9):1039-1040.

Shohamy D, Myers, C.E., Grossman, S., Sage, J., Gluck, M.A. (2005) The role of dopamine in cognitive sequence learning: evidence from Parkinson's disease. *Behav. Brain Res.* 156(2):191-199.

Tzavara ET, Bymaster, F.P., Davis, R.J., Wade, M.R., Perry, K.W., Wess, J., McKinzie, D.L., Felder, C., Nomikos, G.G. (2004) M4 muscarinic receptors regulate the dynamics of cholinergic and dopaminergic neurotransmission: relevance to the pathophysiology and treatment of related CNS pathologies. *FASEB J.* 18(12):1410-1412.

Volkow ND, Fowler, J.S., Gatley, S.J., Logan, J., Wang, G.J., Ding, Y.S., Dewey, S. (1996) PET evaluation of the dopamine system of the human brain. *J. Nucl. Med.* 37(7):1242-1256.

Wang Q, Wang, P.H., McLachlan, C., Wong, P.T. (2005) Simvastatin reverses the downregulation of dopamine D1 and D2 receptor expression in the prefrontal cortex of 6-hydroxydopamine-induced Parkinsonian rats. *Brain Res.* 1045(1-2):229-233.

Peer-reviewer for this commentary

Dr. Penghua Wang
Department of Internal Medicine
Yale University School of Medicine
Post Box 208022, 300 Cedar Street
New Haven, CT 06510 USA
Tel: 1-203-737-5635, 203-785-4140
FAX: 1-203-785-3864
Email: penghua.wang@yale.edu

In: Prefrontal Cortex: Roles, Interventions and Traumas ISBN 978-1-60692-415-0
Editors: Lorenzo LoGrasso and Giovanni Morretti

Expert Commentary B

Noradrenergic Actions in Prefrontal Cortex: Relevance to AD/HD

Amy F. T. Arnsten*
Yale Medical School, New Haven, Connecticut, USA

Abstract

This chapter reviews the important role of prefrontal cortex (PFC) in the regulation of behavior and attention, and evidence that these processes are weakened in Attention-Deficit/Hyperactivity Disorder (AD/HD). Norepinephrine (NE) has been found to have a critical beneficial effect on PFC function through actions at post-synaptic, α2A-adrenoceptors, while high levels of NE release during stress impair PFC regulation of behavior through actions at α1 adrenoceptors. The PFC regulates its own NE input through projections to NE-containing locus coeruleus (LC) neurons. The LC fires according to arousal state and attentional demands. Most medications effective for the treatment of AD/HD powerfully influence NE transmission, either by blocking reuptake or mimicking its actions at α2A-adrenoceptors. The importance of NE to AD/HD is increasingly appreciated.

Lay Abstract

The symptoms of Attention-Deficit/Hyperactivity Disorder (AD/HD) - impaired regulation of attention and behavior- likely involve weaknesses in higher brain functions. The prefrontal cortex (PFC) is a higher brain region necessary for the appropriate control of behavior, attention and emotion. Imaging studies indicate this brain region is afflicted in AD/HD. The PFC is highly dependent on its neurochemical state, and requires optimal levels of norepinephrine for proper function. Norepinephrine is released in brain according to arousal state and attentional demands. Many AD/HD medications such as

* Correspondence to: Dr. Amy F.T. Arnsten. Department of Neurobiology, Yale Medical School, 333 Cedar St., New Haven, CT 06510; Email: amy.arnsten@yale.edu; Phone: 203-785-4431; Fax: 203-785-5263

methylphenidate (Ritalin), amphetamine (Adderall), atomoxetine (Strattera) and guanfacine, alter norepinephrine actions. It is likely that these medications act, at least in part, by providing a more optimal chemical environment for PFC regulation of behavior and attention.

Keywords: norepinephrine, attention, executive function, hyperactivity, adrenoceptor, guanfacine.

Introduction

Basic science has made great strides in understanding the neurochemical influences needed for optimal prefrontal cortical (PFC) regulation of behavior and attention. Although much research has focused on the important role of dopamine (DA), there is increasing appreciation that norepinephrine (NE) has a vital influence as well. NE plays an essential role in arousal and attention, and may orchestrate the interplay of posterior sensory cortices, subcortical structures mediating primitive responses, and PFC regulation of attention and behavior. The current chapter reviews this literature, and outlines its direct relevance to our understanding and treatment of Attention Deficit Hyperactivity Disorder (AD/HD).

Prefrontal Cortical Cognitive Dysfunction in AD/HD

Neuropsychological and imaging studies have established that PFC executive abilities are weakened in patients with AD/HD (reviewed in Arnsten et al., 1996; Barkley, 1997). The PFC guides behavior and attention using working memory, applying represented information to inhibit inappropriate actions or thoughts. These processes are the basis of the so-called executive functions, including regulation of attention, planning, impulse control, mental flexibility, and the initiation and monitoring of action. Lesions to the PFC produce symptoms such as forgetfulness, distractibility, impulsivity, perseveration, and disorganization.

The PFC is critical for the inhibition of both covert responses, i.e. attention regulation, and overt responses, e.g. impulse control. The role of PFC in attention regulation has been appreciated for many years. While the posterior cortices provide processing resources, allowing us to pay attention as it were, the PFC regulates what we attend to based on represented goals. The PFC inhibits responses to distracting stimuli and suppresses irrelevant thoughts such as proactive interference. Thus, patients with PFC lesions are easily distracted (Woods and Knight, 1986; Godefroy and Rousseaux, 1996), are impaired at gating sensory stimuli (Knight et al., 1989; Yamaguchi and Knight, 1990), have poor concentration and organization, and are more vulnerable to disruption from proactive interference (Thompson-Schill et al., 2002). PFC lesions impair the ability to sustain attention, particularly over long delays (Wilkins et al., 1987). Lesions of the dorsolateral PFC impair the ability to shift attentional set (Manes et al., 2002). PFC lesions also impair divided attention, and these attentional deficits have been associated with lesions in the left, superior PFC (Godefroy and Rousseaux, 1996). Similar results have been seen in animals, where PFC lesions impair attentional regulation in monkeys e.g. (Malmo, 1942; Bartus and Levere, 1977; Dias et al., 1996), and rats (Muir et al., 1996).

The PFC also allows us to regulate overt behaviors including locomotor activity. The right inferior PFC is particularly important for behavioral inhibition (reviewed in (Aron et al., 2004)). Both imaging (Konishi et al., 1999; Rubia et al., 2003) and lesion studies indicate that the right PFC in humans is critical for inhibitory abilities, e.g. performance of the Stop or Go-No Go tasks. The importance of the PFC to inhibitory control has also been shown in monkeys with lesion (Petrides, 1986), electrophysiological (Watanabe, 1986) and imaging studies (Morita et al., 2004). There is also a classic but often forgotten literature demonstrating that PFC lesions cause locomotor hyperactivity in monkeys (Kennard et al., 1941; French, 1959; Gross, 1963; Gross and Weiskrantz, 1964). Monkeys were often observed to circle in their cages following PFC lesions. Thus, some of the locomotor hyperactivity observed in AD/HD may arise from PFC dysfunction.

The Cellular Basis of PFC Cognitive Function

Single unit recording studies in monkeys have shown that PFC neurons are able to hold modality-specific information "on-line" over a delay and use this represented information to guide behavior in the absence of environmental cues (Goldman-Rakic, 1995). PFC neurons can also fire in relationship to an abstract rule that is used to govern action (Wallis et al., 2001). A unique feature of PFC neurons is their ability to maintain information in the presence of interference from distracting stimuli (Miller et al., 1993). Delay-related firing also can serve as the basis for behavioral inhibition, as examined in an anti-saccade task in which monkeys must look away from a remembered visual stimulus (Funahashi et al., 1993). Thus, delay-related activity is observed both when an animal must make a memory-guided action, and when an animal must withhold a prepotent response based on representational knowledge. This cellular marker for working memory has been very useful when examining the neuromodulatory influences of catecholamines on PFC cognitive function (see below).

PFC Dysfunction in AD/HD

Research over the last 20 or more years has established that PFC regulation of behavior is weaker in patients with AD/HD. AD/HD patients are impaired on tasks of behavioral inhibition, reward reversal and working memory that require PFC function e.g. (Itami and Uno, 2002; Bedard et al., 2003; McLean et al., 2004). In contrast, they are not impaired on tasks of covert attentional orienting that depend on posterior parietal association cortex (Swanson et al., 1991).

Conversely, stimulant medication has been found to improve spatial working memory, response inhibition, set-shifting and other PFC cognitive functions in both "normal" college students (Mehta et al., 2000) and in children and adults with AD/HD (Aron et al., 2003;

Bedard et al., 2003; Mehta et al., 2004). Interestingly, in adults with AD/HD, childhood ratings of AD/HD (both self-reported and informant ratings) correlated with response to methylphenidate on the spatial working memory task (Turner et al., 2004). Thus, studies of spatial working memory performance are likely very relevant to the therapeutic effects of AD/HD medications.

Numerous structural imaging studies have shown reduced size of the PFC in AD/HD patients, particularly in the right hemisphere (Castellanos et al., 1996; Casey et al., 1997; Filipek et al., 1997; Giedd et al., 2001; Kates et al., 2002; Hill et al., 2003; Sowell et al., 2003). Imaging studies have also shown evidence of reduced blood flow or metabolism in PFC that correspond with poor PFC cognitive function (Rubia et al., 1999; Yeo et al., 2000). These functional deficits are normalized by stimulant medication (Vaidya et al., 1998). Imaging studies have shown more efficient dorsolateral PFC activity (BOLD) following stimulant treatments that improve spatial working memory, consistent with improved PFC cognitive function (Mehta et al., 2000). Thus, there is an excellent correspondence between AD/HD symptoms, neuropsychological deficits, PFC deficiency with imaging, and normalization with stimulant medication.

There is also suggestive evidence of reduced catecholamine inputs to the PFC in adults with AD/HD based on fluoro-dopa PET imaging (Ernst et al., 1998). These data are especially compelling, given that most medications used to treat AD/HD enhance DA and NE transmission. Although most genetic studies have focused on linkage of AD/HD with genes related to DA (the DA transporter, DA D1 and D4 receptors, and calcyon, a molecule that links D1 receptors to IP3/protein kinase C signaling), NE-related genes have also been associated with AD/HD. Most prominently, the gene for the synthetic enzyme for NE, dopamine β hydroxylase, has been associated with AD/HD (Daly et al., 1999; Roman et al., 2002), and with less consistency, the α2A adrenoceptor (Comings et al., 1999; Xu et al., 2001). It should also be remembered that the D4 receptor has very high affinity for NE (Van Tol et al., 1991) and thus should really be considered a catecholamine receptor. As described below, catecholamines have a critical influence on PFC cognitive function. Thus, it is logical to argue that many AD/HD symptoms may arise from genetic alterations in catecholamine transmission which lead to weakened PFC regulation of attention and behavior. These symptoms would be ameliorated by catecholamine-enhancing medications. An understanding of catecholamine influences on PFC function, including an appreciation for the conditions when NE would normally be released in cortex, can help provide a rational view of AD/HD symptoms and treatment.

NE's Important Roles in Arousal and Attention

The NE-synthesizing cells of the locus coeruleus (LC) project throughout the forebrain, and provide NE to the entire cortical mantle. These neurons are a critical portion of the arousal system, and have been shown to fire according to the sleep/waking state of the animal. LC neurons fire during alert waking,, slow their firing when the animal becomes drowsy and falls into slow wave sleep, and shut off completely during rapid eye movement (REM) sleep (Foote et al., 1980; Aston-Jones et al., 1999).

NE has direct alerting actions on cortical neurons (McCormick et al., 1991), and also has powerful indirect actions, exciting other ascending arousal systems in basal forebrain (Berridge and España, 2000; Berridge and Waterhouse, 2003) and thalamus (McCormick et al., 1991). Both the direct and indirect stimulation of cortical arousal occurs through α1 and β adrenergic receptor stimulation (ibid). In contrast, low levels of NE released in thalamus under drowsy conditions engage α2 receptors, which have higher affinity for NE, and reduce thalamo-cortical stimulation (Buzsaki et al., 1991). The thalamus has a very dense NE innervation, and this input contributes to information transfer through this structure. Thus, under conditions of sufficient NE release to engage α1 and β adrenergic receptors, information is faithfully transmitted from thalamus to cortex, while under conditions of low NE release when α2 receptors are engaged, thalamic neurons are put into a burst mode which prevents information transfer (McCormick et al., 1991). Thus, the varying affinities of NE for α2 vs. α1 or β adrenergic receptors acts as a switch to alter neuronal, and thus behavioral state.

Within the waking state, NE has a key role in modulating attention (reviewed in (Aston-Jones et al., 1999) and contributes to decision-making about relevant vs. irrelevant stimuli (Usher et al., 1999; Rajkowski et al., 2004). Aston-Jones and colleagues have shown that under optimal waking conditions (i.e. alert, unstressed), the LC exhibits modest tonic firing and pronounced phasic firing to relevant stimuli (Rajkowski et al., 1998; Rajkowski et al., 2004). Importantly to AD/HD, the LC also suppresses firing to irrelevant stimuli during these ideal conditions (ibid). In contrast, when animals are stressed or agitated, high levels of tonic activity are recorded from LC, and phasic firing is poorly regulated, including inappropriate responses to distracting stimuli (ibid). Given the extensive projections of NE axons, these response patterns would ramify throughout the neuroaxis, and have widespread effects on cortical processing as described below.

Noradrenergic Modulationof PFC Cognitive Function

NE has powerful, bimodal effects on the higher cognitive functions of the PFC. It has been appreciated for many years that DA has a critical influence on PFC cognitive functions (Brozoski et al., 1979), especially through its actions at the D1 receptor family (Sawaguchi and Goldman-Rakic, 1994). D1 receptor stimulation produces an inverted U dose response, whereby either too much or too little receptor stimulation impairs working memory in mice (Lidow et al., 2002), rats (Zahrt et al., 1997), monkeys (Arnsten and Goldman-Rakic, 1990, 1998), and humans (Kimberg et al., 1997; Egan et al., 2001). However, research indicates that NE has an equally important influence on PFC cognitive function, and this body of work has increasing relevance to AD/HD.

As with DA, NE has dual effects on PFC function depending on the amount of NE release. Moderate levels of NE have important, beneficial effects on PFC function, whereas high concentrations of NE released during stress contribute to impaired PFC function. However, in contrast to DA, the beneficial vs. detrimental actions can be dissociated by actions at different adrenoceptors: moderate levels of NE improve PFC function via α2A adrenoceptors, whereas high levels of NE released during stress impair PFC function by engaging lower affinity α1-adrenoceptors and possibly β1 adrenoceptors (reviewed in Arnsten 2000). This dichotomy is reminiscent of NE dual actions in thalamus. However, the NE innervation of PFC is far more delicate than that in thalamus, and it is likely that higher rates of LC firing (i.e. rates that occur during non-stressed waking) are needed in PFC to release sufficient NE to engage α2A adrenoceptors. Still higher tonic LC firing rates, e.g., during stress, appear to be needed for NE to engage the lower affinity α1 adrenoceptors. Thus, α1 adrenoceptor antagonists have no effect on working memory when infused into the PFC during non-stressful conditions (Li and Mei, 1994; Birnbaum et al., 1999), but protect PFC cognitive function under conditions of uncontrollable stress (Birnbaum et al., 1999). Conversely, infusions of α1 adrenoceptor agonists such as phenylephrine mimic the stress response and impair working memory (Arnsten et al., 1999; Mao et al., 1999). These detrimental actions have been observed at the cellular level as well, where iontophoresis of phenylephrine onto PFC neurons decreased the memory-related cell-firing necessary for working memory function (Birnbaum et al., 2004). These mechanisms are especially relevant to Post-Traumatic Stress Disorder (PTSD), which in children can produce symptoms of distractibility and poor impulse control similar to AD/HD. In this regard, it is noteworthy that the α1 adrenoceptor antagonist, prazosin, is now successfully used to treat PTSD in patients with PTSD (Raskind et al., 2003).

Although AD/HD and stress-induced PFC dysfunction have much in common, a more likely etiology for AD/HD is insufficient catecholamine stimulation in PFC. PFC function is markedly weakened by insufficient NE stimulation of α2A-adrenoceptors in the PFC. Findings reviewed below suggest that moderate levels of NE release during non-stressful conditions normally engage α2A-adrenoceptors and strengthen working memory. Thus, unlike α1 and β blockers which have no effect when infused in PFC under non-stressful conditions, infusion of the α2 antagonist, yohimbine, markedly impairs working memory performance in monkeys (Li and Mei, 1994). Conversely, studies of nonhuman primates have shown that α2A-adrenoceptor agonists such as guanfacine improve working memory (Arnsten et al., 1988; Mao et al., 1999). Remarkably, α2 adrenoceptor agonists have been shown to improve PFC function in mice (Franowicz et al., 2002), rats (Tanila et al., 1996), monkeys (Arnsten et al., 1988; Rama et al., 1996) and humans (Jakala et al., 1999a; Jakala et al., 1999b). The efficacy of these agents to enhance PFC cognitive function can be completely dissociated from the sedating properties of these compounds at higher doses (Arnsten et al., 1988). Much research has focused on elucidating the mechanisms underlying these beneficial actions of PFC cognitive function.

Initial studies demonstrated actions at *post*-synaptic, α2A adrenoceptors. Although original research focused on the role of α2 adrenoceptors at pre-synaptic sites, it is now known that the vast majority of α2 adrenoceptors are localized post-synaptic to NE neurons (MacDonald et al., 1997). In the monkey PFC, α2A adrenoceptors are localized both pre-synaptically on NE terminals, and post-synaptically on the dendritic spines of PFC pyramidal neurons ((Aoki et al., 1998). The post-synaptic α2A adrenoceptors are classically positioned over the post-synaptic density. Pharmacological data indicates that NE acts at these post-synaptic α2 receptors to strengthen PFC cognitive function; i.e. the α2 agonist, clonidine, becomes more potent and more efficacious when the presynaptic NE terminal is destroyed or depleted of NE (Arnsten and Goldman-Rakic, 1985; Cai et al., 1993).

The subtype of α2 receptor underlying the beneficial effects has also been determined. There are 3 subtypes of α2 receptors cloned in humans: the A, B and C subtypes. Both the A and C subtypes can be found in PFC, with the former predominating. Studies in genetically altered mice indicate that the α2A-preferring agonist, guanfacine, loses its enhancing effects when administered to mice with a functional knockout of the α2A-adrenoceptor (Franowicz et al., 2002). Indeed, α2A mutant mice exhibit weaker working memory abilities than wild type mice (ibid). In contrast, mice with a knockout of the α2C receptor show normal cognitive enhancement with α2 agonist treatment (Tanila et al., 1999). Thus, the α2A adrenoceptor subtype mediates the enhancing effects of NE in PFC.

A number of approaches have shown that α2 agonists like guanfacine act directly in the PFC to enhance executive functions. SPECT imaging of monkeys performing a spatial working memory task show that systemic administration of guanfacine increases regional cerebral blood flow in the dorsolateral PFC, the same brain region that is critical for performance of the task (Avery et al., 2000). Furthermore, infusions of guanfacine directly into this same region of the PFC produce a delay-related improvement in working memory performance in young adult monkeys (Mao et al., 1999). Importantly, iontophoresis of the α2 agonist, clonidine, onto PFC neurons in monkeys performing a spatial working memory task increases delay-related firing, the cellular measure of working memory (Li et al., 1999). Systemic administration similarly increases delay-related firing in PFC, and this strengthening of delay-related firing by either systemic or iontophoretic application can be blocked by iontophoresis of the α2 antagonist, yohimbine (ibid). Thus, α2 receptor stimulation in PFC strengthens working memory at the cellular and behavioral levels. Conversely, blockade of α2 receptors with yohimbine infusions directly into PFC dramatically weakens working memory (Li and Mei, 1994) and markedly erodes delay-related activity (Li et al., 1999). As reviewed above, delay-related activity is an important cellular basis for regulating attention, reducing distractibility, and inhibiting prepotent behavioral responses. The finding that α2 receptor stimulation enhances delay-related activity is consistent with findings that agonists such as guanfacine reduce distractibility (Arnsten and Contant, 1992) and enhance behavioral inhibition (Steere and Arnsten, 1997). Most recently, infusion of guanfacine into the ventrolateral PFC in monkeys strengthened associative learning and impulse control (Wang et al., 2004b; Wang et al., 2004a). Thus, α2 receptor stimulation is critical for a variety of PFC cognitive processes at both the behavioral and cellular levels.

Importantly, studies in monkeys indicate that many of the symptoms of AD/HD can be recreated by blocking α2 NE receptors in the PFC (Figure 1). In addition to the weakened working memory and delay-related activity described above, infusions of the α2 antagonist, yohimbine, into PFC increase impulsivity (Ma et al., 2003). Monkeys tested on a go- no go task showed increased errors of commission, but no change in errors of omission, following yohimbine infusion into dorsolateral PFC (Ma et al., 2003). ADHD patients also show errors of commission on the go-no go task, and methylphenidate ameliorates these errors (Trommer et al., 1991).

Most recently, yohimbine infusions into the dorsolateral PFC of rhesus monkeys have been shown to induce locomotor hyperactivity (Ma et al., 2005), reminiscent of the increased activity found with PFC ablations. Infusion of saline was without effect. Many researchers have speculated that striatal DA mechanisms underlie the hyperactivity observed in AD/HD patients.

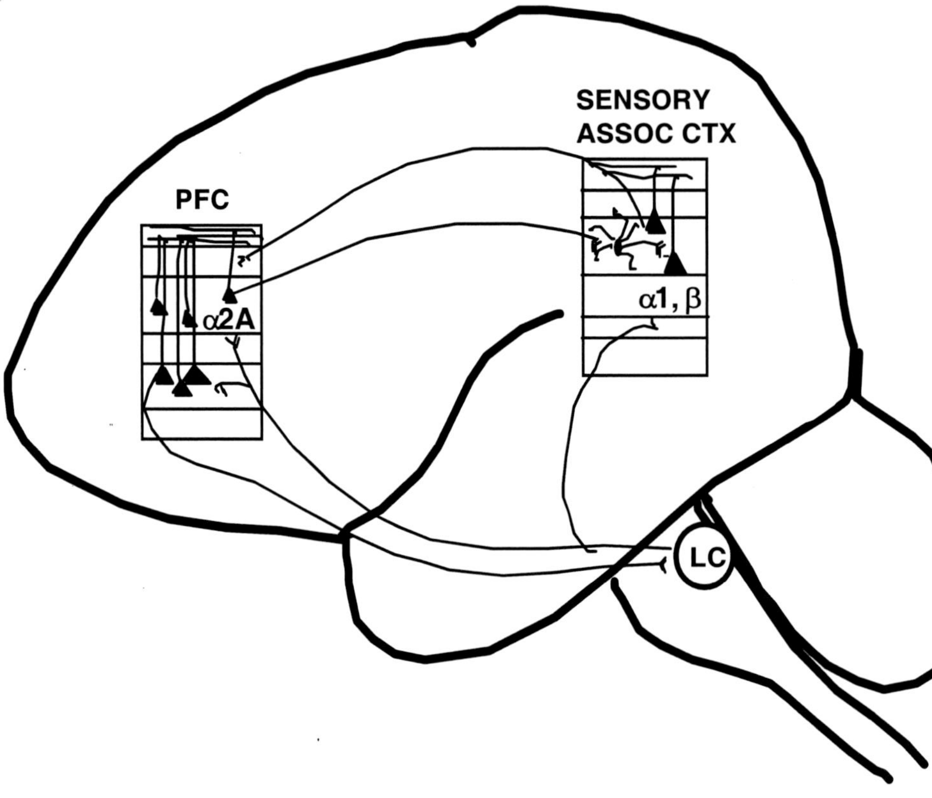

Figure 1. NE cells in the LC project to the PFC, where they improve working memory via α2A receptors, and to the posterior cortices, where they may enhance sensory function via α1 and β receptors. The PFC projects back to the LC and to posterior cortices. Blockade of NE α2A adrenoceptors in the monkey PFC produces behavioral changes similar to AD/HD, including hyperactivity, distractibility, impulsivity and impaired working memory. See text for details.

However, these results in monkeys suggest that PFC dysfunction may contribute to the locomotor hyperactivity, as well as the impulsivity and poor attention regulation/working memory, which form the cardinal symptomatology of AD/HD.

The PFC projects back to posterior sensory cortices (Barbas et al., 2005) and to subcortical structures such as the amygdala (Ghashghaei and Barbas, 2002) in order to gate sensory (Knight et al., 1989; Yamaguchi and Knight, 1990) and affective (Quirk et al., 2003) processing. Thus, NE actions in PFC can indirectly influence posterior and subcortical practices. However, NE also has direct modulatory effects on these brain regions, and these are described below.

NE Influences on Posterior Cortical Functions

NE can influence attention and perception through its actions on sensory and association cortices posterior to the PFC. Thirty years ago, Foote and colleagues first discovered that NE increases the signal/noise properties of neurons in the auditory cortex of monkeys, primarily by suppressing noise (Foote et al., 1975). Since that seminal paper, there have been numerous other examples whereby NE has been shown to enhance signal/noise response, e.g. in hippocampus (Segal and Bloom, 1976), cerebellum (Moises et al., 1981), and in other sensory cortices (Waterhouse et al., 1980, 1981). Waterhouse and colleagues have continued to perform elegant studies of NE actions in somatosensory cortex, demonstrating that NE can enhance inhibitory actions via β adrenergic receptors, while enhancing excitatory actions via α1 adrenergic receptors coupled to protein kinase C signaling (Waterhouse et al., 1980, 1981; Mouradian et al., 1991; Devilbiss and Waterhouse, 2000). For example, subthreshold somatosensory stimulation will come to evoke a response in somatosensory cortical neurons if it is coupled with phasic activation of noradrenergic cells in locus coeruleus the (LC) (Waterhouse et al., 1998). These electrophysiological findings suggest that NE should facilitate sensory perception, although this hypothesis has not been specifically tested at the behavioral level.

In contrast to these in depth studies of NE actions in primary sensory cortex, there has been relatively little research on NE modulation of higher association areas in posterior cortex, perhaps because these studies must be done in primates. For example, the posterior parietal association cortex is essential for paying attention- allocating attentional resources in time and space (Coull and Nobre, 1998). This cortical area receives a dense NE innervation (Morrison and Foote, 1986), but we know little about NE's modulatory actions in this cortical area. Pharmacological and imaging studies in humans and monkeys indicate that α2 adrenoceptor stimulation may impair the attention orienting abilities of posterior parietal cortex (Clark et al., 1987; Witte and Marrocco, 1997; Coull et al., 2001). However, as all these studies involved systemic administration of drug, it is not known if the compounds had actions in parietal cortex, nor whether the drugs acted by decreasing NE release and/or via post-synaptic receptor mechanisms. Even less is known about NE modulation of the ventral stream, e.g. areas V4 and inferior temporal areas which are critically involved in feature extraction and objection perception. These will be important arenas for future research.

NE Influences on Subcortical Functions

NE prominently innervates the hippocampus and amygdala, and facilitates memory functions in both structures. These structures are likely not of critical relevance to AD/HD, but illustrate the general actions of NE in posterior cortical and subcortical areas. The hippocampus is critical for the consolidation of memory, and long term potentiation (LTP) is an electrophysiological measure of increased synaptic strength commonly associated with this process. NE strengthens LTP at mossy fiber synapses in hippocampus through actions at β adrenergic receptors (Hopkins and Johnston, 1984; Hopkins and Johnston, 1988). The consolidation of emotionally relevant information is enhanced by interactions with the amygdala. NE is released in the amygdala during emotional events (including stressors) and is critical to this process (Cahill and McGaugh, 1996). Both β and α1 adrenergic receptor stimulation facilitate memory consolidation in the amygdala (Ferry et al., 1999) while α2 receptor stimulation impairs plasticity (e.g. LTP) in the amygdala (DeBock et al., 2003). Thus, these subcortical structures are modulated in a manner similar to somatosensory cortex, thriving under conditions of high NE release.

NE and the Orchestration of Brain Response

NE may act as a chemical switch to determine which brain regions predominate in the control of behavior under varying environmental conditions. This orchestration of brain response may be accomplished by NE's differing affinities for its receptors: moderate levels of NE release engaging high affinity α2 receptors and a modest number of lower affinity α1 and β receptors under non-stressful conditions, and higher levels of NE release engaging large numbers of α1 and β receptors during stress (reviewed in (Arnsten, 2000a).

The PFC and amygdala both have widespread projections throughout the brain, and are positioned to play the role of "conductor". Both structures are also intimately connected with the LC, and levels of NE release may determine which of the two structures predominates in the control of brain function. There are reciprocal connections between the LC and PFC (Arnsten and Goldman-Rakic, 1984; Jodo et al., 1998), the LC and the amygdala (Cedarbaum and Aghajanian, 1978; Price and Amaral, 1981), and the PFC and amygdala (Ghashghaei and Barbas, 2002). These connections may create a flip-flop switch between 1) PFC regulation of brain and behavior under conditions of normal waking (phasic LC firing, moderate NE release, α2 receptor stimulation predominating, thus favoring PFC function and weakening amygdala), vs. 2) amygdala regulation of brain and behavior under conditions of stress (high tonic LC firing, high levels of NE release, α1 and β receptor stimulation predominating, strengthening amygdala and weakening PFC). While PFC is positioned to either excite or inhibit a variety of structures, including the amygdala, the amygdala may indirectly shut off PFC regulation through its projections to the LC and to the dopamine neurons in midbrain. Biochemical studies have shown that the amygdala initiates high levels of NE and DA release in the PFC during psychological stress (Goldstein et al., 1996), which impair PFC function (Arnsten, 2000b). The amygdala may have a general and powerful excitatory effect on LC via CRF projections which are activated under stressful conditions (Curtis et al., 2002). The PFC is also positioned to regulate LC firing, and may provide one of the few "intelligent" inputs to sculpt appropriate firing to relevant vs. irrelevant environmental stimuli. The PFC projects to the region of the LC (Arnsten and Goldman-Rakic, 1984; Jodo et al., 1998), especially in the dendritic zone medial to the LC cell bodies where there are GABAergic "interneurons" (Aston-Jones et al., 2004). Thus, the PFC is in the position to either excite (Jodo et al., 1998) or inhibit LC responses (Sara and Herve-Minvielle, 1995). This more refined regulation of LC firing may occur during non-stressed waking when the PFC is in its optimal neurochemical state. Inappropriate LC firing patterns could contribute to symptoms of AD/HD (Aston-Jones et al., 2000).

The Role of NE in Medications that Treat AD/HD

It should be evident even from this review that NE mechanisms and thus NE medications would be highly relevant to disorders of attention and behavioral regulation. Biederman and colleagues have long appreciated the importance of NE and NE compounds in AD/HD (Biederman and Spencer, 1999; Biederman and Spencer, 2000). For example, they found that NE reuptake blockers such as desipramine can be highly efficacious in treating AD/HD symptoms, however, cardiac side effects have limited their utility in a pediatric population (Spencer et al., 2002b). The recent success of the safer, NE transporter blocker, atomoxetine (Strattera), in treating AD/HD has refocused the interest of the entire field on the role of NE in this disorder (Spencer et al., 2002a). It is now being appreciated that stimulant medications commonly used to treat AD/HD facilitate NE as well as DA transmission: methylphenidate (Ritalin) blocks both DA and NE transporters, amphetamines (e.g. Adderall) block DA and NE transporters and increase catecholamine release, atomoxetine (Strattera) blocks NE transporters (which take up DA in PFC, thus effectively increasing the concentration of both catecholamines in the synapse and extrasynaptic space (Bymaster et al., 2002)), and guanfacine mimics NE at α2A adrenoceptors. As reviewed above, oral, low dose treatment with stimulants can enhance PFC cognitive function in both normal college students (Mehta et al., 2000) and in AD/HD patients e.g. (Aron et al., 2003). Guanfacine has also been shown to enhance working memory or other PFC tasks (e.g. planning, Stroop interference, CPT), in normal adults (Jakala et al., 1999a) and patients with AD/HD (Scahill et al., 2001; Taylor and Russo, 2001). Neuropsychological assessment of atomoxetine is in progress, and it will be interesting to observe whether this compound also improves performance of PFC tasks.

The important effects of NE in stimulant actions have been relatively neglected, especially as many previous studies in animals have used high doses that have prominent effects on DA. However, recent biochemical evidence from studies in rats indicates that low, oral doses of methylphenidate, that produce plasma levels comparable to those observed in AD/HD patients, have more effect on NE than on DA in subcortical structures (Kuczenski and Segal, 2002). These same low, oral doses *reduce* locomotor activity in rats, highlighting their relevance to AD/HD (ibid). Low doses of stimulant increase NE and DA in PFC, consistent with the greater sensitivity of the PFC than striatal DA systems (Berridge and Stalnaker, 2002). Identification of the appropriate dose regimen for methylphenidate administration in rats has allowed research to be performed of immediate relevance to AD/HD. Our lab has recently found that low, oral doses of methylphenidate improve performance of PFC tasks in rats and mice, and that this improvement results from both α2A adrenoceptor and DA D1 stimulation (Arnsten and Dudley, 2005). Thus, it is highly likely that the therapeutic actions of stimulants such as methylphenidate and amphetamine involve increased NE stimulation of α2A adrenoceptors in PFC, which strengthen PFC executive functions.

Optimizing catecholamine influences in PFC may remediate AD/HD symptomatology irrespective of the cause of AD/HD. It is obvious that such treatments would be helpful if the AD/HD symptomatology was caused by inadequate catecholamine transmission in PFC, as suggested by the Ernst findings (Ernst et al., 1998). However, it is likely to be helpful under other conditions as well- e.g. slowed maturation of PFC circuits, fewer PFC cells (i.e. smaller

PFC volume)- as long as there are normal PFC cells available as a substrate for catecholamine actions.

The finding that high levels of catecholamine release impair PFC function is also informative for the treatment and even diagnosis of AD/HD. For example, high doses of stimulants may impair PFC cognitive abilities and induce perseverative or restricted thinking via excessive catecholamine actions in PFC. We have recently observed this in rats given higher doses of methylphenidate (e.g. 2-3 mg/kg, p.o.) who show impaired spatial working memory performance due to perseverative errors (Arnsten and Dudley, 2005). Exposure to uncontrollable stress (e.g. families going through divorce) may also induce excessive catecholamine release in PFC, impairing PFC function and mimicking AD/HD. In such cases stimulant medications would not be indicated; treatment should focus on remediating the stress and if necessary, use of agents (e.g. prazosin, guanfacine) that can protect PFC from stress in animals (Birnbaum et al., 1999; Birnbaum et al., 2000) and humans (Horrigan, 1996; Raskind et al., 2003).

In summary, the PFC mediates executive abilities such as working memory, attention regulation, behavioral inhibition, planning and organization that are problematic in subjects with AD/HD. Research in animals has shown that NE has vital, beneficial effects on PFC function through actions at post-synaptic α2A adrenoceptors in PFC, strengthening working memory, attention regulation, planning and behavioral inhibition. Many of the symptoms of AD/HD, including impaired working memory, impulsivity and hyperactivity, can be recreated by blocking NE α2A adrenoceptors in the monkey PFC. Conversely, medications that treat AD/HD directly or indirectly stimulate α2A adrenoceptors. Thus, there we are beginning to see a strong correspondence between knowledge of NE mechanisms in PFC and therapeutic drug actions in AD/HD. NE may also be important to attentional processes mediated by posterior cortices, although there has been less basic research in this field. These posterior abilities may be weakened in children with symptoms of inattention, i.e. the inability to allocate attentional processing resources at earlier stages of attention regulation. Our ability to differentiate and treat symptoms of AD/HD will evolve as we develop a more refined understanding of higher cortical mechanisms and their dependence on NE actions.

Acknowledgments

This work was supported by AG06036 and MH066393.

References

Aoki, C., Venkatesan, C., Go, C.-G., Forman, R. and Kurose, H. (1998) Cellular and the subcellular sites for noradrenergic action in the monkey dorsolateral prefrontal cortex as revealed by the immunocytochemical localization of noradrenergic receptors and axons. *Cereb. Cortex,* 8, 269-277.

Arnsten, A.F.T. (2000a) Through the looking glass: Differential noradrenergic modulation of prefrontal cortical function. *Neural Plasticity,* 7, 133-146.

Arnsten, A.F.T. (2000b) Stress impairs PFC function in rats and monkeys: Role of dopamine D1 and norepinephrine alpha-1 receptor mechanisms. *Prog. Brain Res.,* 126, 183-192.

Arnsten, A.F.T. and Goldman-Rakic, P.S. (1984) Selective prefrontal cortical projections to the region of the locus coeruleus and raphe nuclei in the rhesus monkey. *Brain Res.,* 306, 9-18.

Arnsten, A.F.T. and Dudley, A.G. (2005) Methylphenidate improves prefrontal cortical cognitive function through $\alpha 2$ adrenoceptor and dopamine D1 receptor actions: Relevance to therapeutic effects in Attention Deficit Hyperactivity Disorder. *Behav Brain Funct.* 1, 2. <http://www.behavioralandbrainfunctions.com/content/1/1/2>.

Arnsten, A.F.T. and Goldman-Rakic, P.S. (1985) Alpha-2 adrenergic mechanisms in prefrontal cortex associated with cognitive decline in aged nonhuman primates. *Science,* 230, 1273-1276.

Arnsten, A.F.T. and Goldman-Rakic, P.S. (1990) Stress impairs prefrontal cortex cognitive function in monkeys: role of dopamine. *Soc. Neurosci. Abstr.* 16, 164.

Arnsten, A.F.T. and Contant, T.A. (1992) Alpha-2 adrenergic agonists decrease distractibility in aged monkeys performing a delayed response task. *Psychopharmacology,* 108, 159-169.

Arnsten, A.F.T. and Goldman-Rakic, P.S. (1998) Noise stress impairs prefrontal cortical cognitive function in monkeys: Evidence for a hyperdopaminergic mechanism. *Arch. Gen. Psychiatry,* 55, 362-369.

Arnsten, A.F.T., Cai, J.X. and Goldman-Rakic, P.S. (1988) The alpha-2 adrenergic agonist guanfacine improves memory in aged monkeys without sedative or hypotensive side effects. *J. Neurosci.,* 8, 4287-4298.

Arnsten, A.F.T., Steere, J.C. and Hunt, R.D. (1996) The contribution of alpha-2 noradrenergic mechanisms to prefrontal cortical cognitive function: potential significance to Attention Deficit Hyperactivity Disorder. *Arch. Gen. Psychiatry,* 53, 448-455.

Arnsten, A.F.T., Mathew, R., Ubriani, R., Taylor, J.R. and Li, B.-M. (1999) Alpha-1 noradrenergic receptor stimulation impairs prefrontal cortical cognitive function. *Biol. Psychiatry,* 45, 26-31.

Aron, A.R., Robbins, T.W. and Poldrack, R.A. (2004) Inhibition and the right inferior frontal cortex. *Trends Cogn. Sci.,* 8, 170-177.

Aron, A.R., Dowson, J.H., Sahakian, B.J. and Robbins, T.W. (2003) Methylphenidate improves response inhibition in adults with attention-deficit/hyperactivity disorder. *Biol P.ychiatry,* 54, 1465-1468.

Aston-Jones, G., Rajkowski, J. and Cohen, J. (1999) Role of locus coeruleus in attention and behavioral flexibility. *Biol. Psychiatry,* 46, 1309-1320.

Aston-Jones, G., Rajkowski, J. and Cohen, J. (2000) Locus coeruleus and regulation of behavioral flexibility and attention. *Prog. Brain Res.,* 126, 165-182.

Aston-Jones, G., Zhu, Y. and Card, J.P. (2004) Numerous GABAergic afferents to locus ceruleus in the pericerulear dendritic zone: possible interneuronal pool. *J. Neurosci.,* 24, 2313-2321.

Avery, R.A., Franowicz, J.S., Studholme, C., van Dyck, C.H. and Arnsten, A.F.T. (2000) The alpha-2A-adenoceptor agonist, guanfacine, increases regional cerebral blood flow in dorsolateral prefrontal cortex of monkeys performing a spatial working memory task. *Neuropsychopharmacology,* 23, 240-249.

Barbas, H., Medalla, M., Alade, O., Suski, J., Zikopoulos, B. and Lera, P. (2005) Relationship of prefrontal connections to inhibitory systems in superior temporal areas in the rhesus monkey. *Cereb. Cortex,* Jan 5; Epub ahead of print.

Barkley, R.A. (1997) *ADHD and the nature of self-control.* New York: Guilford Press.

Bartus, R.T. and Levere, T.E. (1977) Frontal decortication in rhesus monkeys: A test of the interference hypothesis. *Brain Res.,* 119, 233-248.

Bedard, A.C., Ickowicz, A., Logan, G.D., Hogg-Johnson, S., Schachar, R. and Tannock, R. (2003) Selective inhibition in children with attention-deficit hyperactivity disorder off and on stimulant medication. *J. Abnorm. Child Psychol.,* 31, 315-327.

Berridge, C.W. and España, R.A. (2000) Synergistic actions of b- and a1-noradrenergic receptors in the maintenance of alert waking. *Neurosci.,* 99, 495-505.

Berridge, C.W. and Stalnaker, T.A. (2002) Relationship between low-dose amphetamine-induced arousal and extracellular norepinephrine and dopamine levels within prefrontal cortex. *Synapse,* 46, 140-149.

Berridge, C.W. and Waterhouse, B.D. (2003) The locus coeruleus-noradrenergic system: modulation of behavioral state and state-dependent cognitive processes. *Brain Res Brain Res. Rev.,* 42, 33-84.

Biederman, J. and Spencer, T. (1999) Attention-deficit/hyperactivity disorder (ADHD) as a noradrenergic disorder. *Biol. Psychiatry,* 46, 1234-1242.

Biederman, J. and Spencer, T.J. (2000) Genetics of childhood disorders: XIX. ADHD, Part 3: Is ADHD a noradrenergic disorder? *J. Am. Acad. Child Adolesc. Psychiatry,* 39, 1330-1333.

Birnbaum, S.G., Podell, D.M. and Arnsten, A.F.T. (2000) Noradrenergic alpha-2 receptor agonists reverse working memory deficits induced by the anxiogenic drug, FG7142, in rats. *Pharmacol. Biochem. Behav.,* 67, 397-403.

Birnbaum, S.G., Gobeske, K.T., Auerbach, J., Taylor, J.R. and Arnsten, A.F.T. (1999) A role for norepinephrine in stress-induced cognitive deficits: Alpha-1-adrenoceptor mediation in prefrontal cortex. *Biol. Psychiatry,* 46, 1266-1274.

Birnbaum, S.G., Yuan, P., Bloom, A., Davis, D., Gobeske, K., Sweatt, D., Manji, H.K. and Arnsten, A.F.T. (2004) Protein kinase C overactivity impairs prefrontal cortical regulation of working memory. *Science,* 306, 882-884.

Brozoski, T., Brown, R.M., Rosvold, H.E. and Goldman, P.S. (1979) Cognitive deficit caused by regional depletion of dopamine in prefrontal cortex of rhesus monkey. *Science,* 205, 929-931.

Buzsaki, G., Kennedy, B., Solt, V.B. and Ziegler, M. (1991) Noradrenergic control of thalamic oscillation: The role of alpha-2 receptors. *Eur J. Neurosci.,* 3, 222-229.

Bymaster, F.P., Katner, J.S., Nelson, D.L., Hemrick-Luecke, S.K., Threlkeld, P.G., Heiligenstein, J.H., Morin, S.M., Gehlert, D.R. and Perry, K.W. (2002) Atomoxetine increases extracellular levels of norepinephrine and dopamine in prefrontal cortex of rat: a potential mechanism for efficacy in attention deficit/hyperactivity disorder. *Neuropsychopharmacology,* 27, 699-711.

Cahill, L. and McGaugh, J.L. (1996) Modulation of memory storage. *Curr. Opin. Neurobiol.*, 6, 237-242.

Cai, J.X., Ma, Y., Xu, L. and Hu, X. (1993) Reserpine impairs spatial working memory performance in monkeys: Reversal by the alpha-2 adrenergic agonist clonidine. *Brain Res.*, 614, 191-196.

Casey, B.J., Castellanos, F.X., Giedd, J.N., Marsh, W.L., Hamburger, S.D., Schubert, A.B., Vauss, Y.C., Vaituzis, A.C., Dickstein, D.P., Sarfatti, S.E. and Rapoport, J.L. (1997) Implication of right frontostriatal circuitry in response inhibition and attention-deficit/hyperactivity disorder. *J Am. Acad. Child Adolesc. Psychiatry,* 36, 374-383.

Castellanos, F.X., Giedd, J.N., Marsh, W.L., Hamburger, S.D., Vaituzis, A.C., Dickstein, D.P., Sarfatti, S.E., Vauss, Y.C., Snell, J.W., Lange, N., Kaysen, D., Krain, A.L., Ritchhie, G.F., Rajapakse, J.C. and Rapoport, J.L. (1996) Quantitative brain magnetic resonance imaging in attention deficit/hyperactivity disorder. *Arch. Gen. Psychiatry,* 53, 607-616.

Cedarbaum, J.M. and Aghajanian, G.K. (1978) Afferent projections to the rat locus coeruleus as determined by a retrograde tracing technique. *J. Comp. Neurol.*, 178, 1-16.

Clark, C.R., Geffen, G.M. and Geffen, L.B. (1987) Catecholamines and attention II: Pharmacological studies in normal humans. *Neurosci. Biobehav. Rev.*, 11, 353-364.

Comings, D.E., Gade-Andavolu, R., Gonzalez, N. and MacMurray, J.P. (1999) Additive effect of three noradrenergic genes (ADRA2A, ADRA2C, DBH) on attention-deficit hyperactivity disorder and learning disabilities in Tourette syndrome subjects. *Clin Genet.*, 55, 160-172.

Coull, J.T. and Nobre, A.C. (1998) Where and when to pay attention: The neural systems for directing attention to spatial locations and to time intervals as revealed by both PET and fMRI. *J. Neurosci.*, 18, 7426-7435.

Coull, J.T., Nobre, A.C. and Frith, C.D. (2001) The noradrenergic alpha2 agonist clonidine modulates behavioural and neuroanatomical correlates of human attentional orienting and alerting. *Cereb. Cortex,* 11, 73-84.

Curtis, A.L., Bello, N.T., Connolly, K.R. and Valentino, R.J. (2002) Corticotropin-releasing factor neurones of the central nucleus of the amygdala mediate locus coeruleus activation by cardiovascular stress. *J. Neuroendocrinol.*, 14, 667-682.

Daly, G., Hawi, Z., Fitzgerald, M. and Gill, M. (1999) Mapping susceptibility loci in attention deficit hyperactivity disorder: preferential transmission of parental alleles at DAT1, DBH and DRD5 to affected children. *Mol. Psychiatry,* 4, 192-196.

DeBock, F., Kurz, J., Azad, S.C., Parsons, C.G., Hapfelmeier, G., Zieglgansberger, W. and Rammes, G. (2003) Alpha2-adrenoreceptor activation inhibits LTP and LTD in the basolateral amygdala: involvement of Gi/o-protein-mediated modulation of Ca2+-channels and inwardly rectifying K+-channels in LTD. *Eur. J. Neurosci.*, 17, 1411-1424.

Devilbiss, D.M. and Waterhouse, B.D. (2000) Norepinephrine exhibits two distinct profiles of action on sensory cortical neuron responses to excitatory synaptic stimuli. *Synapse,* 37, 273-282.

Dias, R., Roberts, A. and Robbins, T.W. (1996) Dissociation in prefrontal cortex of affective and attentional shifts. *Nature,* 380, 69-72.

Egan, M.F., Goldberg, T.E., Kolachana, B.S., Callicott, J.H., Mazzanti, C.M., Straub, R.E., Goldman, D. and Weinberger, D.R. (2001) Effect of COMT Val108/158 Met genotype on frontal lobe function and risk for schizophrenia. *Proc. Natl. Acad. Sci. USA,* 98, 6917-6922.

Ernst, M., Zametkin, A.J., Matochik, J.A., Jons, P.H. and Cohen, R.M. (1998) DOPA decarboxylase activity in attention deficit disorder adults. A [fluorine-18]fluorodopa positron emission tomographic study. *J. Neurosci.,* 18, 5901-5907.

Ferry, B., Roozendaal, B. and McGaugh, J.L. (1999) Involvement of alpha-1-adrenoceptors in the basolateral amygdala in modulation of memory storage. *Eur. J. Pharmacol.,* 372, 9-16.

Filipek, P.A., Semrud-Clikeman, M., Steingard, R.J., Renshaw, P.F., Kennedy, D.N. and Biederman, J. (1997) Volumetric MRI analysis comparing subjects having attention-deficit hyperactivity disorder with normal controls. *Neurology,* 48, 589-601.

Foote, S.L., Freedman, F.E. and Oliver, A.P. (1975) Effects of putative neurotransmitters on neuronal activity in monkey auditory cortex. *Brain Res.,* 86, 229-242.

Foote, S.L., Aston-Jones, G. and Bloom, F.E. (1980) Impulse activity of locus coeruleus neurons in awake rats and monkeys is a function of sensory stimulation and arousal. . *Proc. Natl. Acad. Sci. USA,* 77, 3033-3037.

Franowicz, J.S., Kessler, L., Dailey-Borja, C.M., Kobilka, B.K., Limbird, L.E. and Arnsten, A.F.T. (2002) Mutation of the alpha2A-adrenoceptor impairs working memory performance and annuls cognitive enhancement by guanfacine. *J. Neurosci.,* 22, 8771-8777.

French, G.M. (1959) Locomotor effects of regional ablation of frontal cortex in rhesus monkeys. *J. Comp. Physiol. Psychol.,* 52, 18-24.

Funahashi, S., Chafee, M.V. and Goldman-Rakic, P.S. (1993) Prefrontal neuronal activity in rhesus monkeys performing a delayed anti-saccade task. *Nature,* 365, 753-756.

Ghashghaei, H.T. and Barbas, H. (2002) Pathways for emotion: interactions of prefrontal and anterior temporal pathways in the amygdala of the rhesus monkey. *Neurosci.,* 115, 1261-1279.

Giedd, J.N., Blumenthal, J., Molloy, E. and Castellanos, F.X. (2001) Brain imaging of attention deficit/hyperactivity disorder. *Ann. NY Acad. Sci.,* 931, 33-49.

Godefroy, O. and Rousseaux, M. (1996) Divided and focused attention in patients with lesion of the prefrontal cortex. *Brain Cogn.,* 30, 155-174.

Goldman-Rakic, P.S. (1995) Cellular basis of working memory. *Neuron,* 14, 477-485.

Goldstein, L.E., Rasmusson, A.M., Bunney, S.B. and Roth, R.H. (1996) Role of the amygdala in the coordination of behavioral, neuroendocrine and prefrontal cortical monoamine responses to psychological stress in the rat. *J Neurosci,* 16, 4787-4798.

Gross, C.G. (1963) Locomotor activity following lateral frontal lesions in rhesus monkeys. *J. Comp. Physiol. Psychol.,* 56, 232-236.

Gross, C.G. and Weiskrantz, L. (1964) Some changes in behavior produced by lateral frontal lesions in the macaque. In: The frontal granular cortex and behavior (Warren JM and Akert K, eds), pp 74-101. New York: McGraw-Hill Book Co.

Hill, D.E., Yeo, R.A., Campbell, R.A., Hart, B., Vigil, J. and Brooks, W. (2003) Magnetic resonance imaging correlates of attention-deficit/hyperactivity disorder in children. *Neuropsychology,* 17, 496-506.

Hopkins, W.F. and Johnston, D. (1984) Frequency-dependent noradrenergic modulation of long-term potentiation in the hippocampus. *Science,* 226, 350-352.

Hopkins, W.F. and Johnston, D. (1988) Noradrenergic enhancement of long-term potentiation at mossy fiber synapses in the hippocampus. *J. Neurophysiol.,* 59, 667-687.

Horrigan, J.P. (1996) Guanfacine for PTSD nightmares. *J. Am. Acad. Child Adolesc. Psychiatry,* 35, 975-976.

Itami, S. and Uno, H. (2002) Orbitofrontal cortex dysfunction in attention-deficit hyperactivity disorder revealed by reversal and extinction tasks. *Neuroreport,* 13, 2453-2457.

Jakala, P., Riekkinen, M., Sirvio, J., Koivisto, E., Kejonen, K., Vanhanen, M. and Riekkinen, P.J. (1999a) Guanfacine, but not clonidine, improves planning and working memory performance in humans. *Neuropsychopharmacol.,* 20, 460-470.

Jakala, P., Sirvio, J., Riekkinen, M., Koivisto, E., Kejonen, K., Vanhanen, M. and Riekkinen, P.J. (1999b) Guanfacine and clonidine, alpha-2 agonists, improve paired associates learning, but not delayed matching to sample, in humans. *Neuropsychopharmacol.,* 20, 119-130.

Jodo, E., Chiang, C. and Aston-Jones, G. (1998) Potent excitatory influence of prefrontal cortex activity on noradrenergic locus coeruleus neurons. *Neurosci.,* 83, 63-79.

Kates, W.R., Frederikse, M., Mostofsky, S.H., Folley, B.S., Cooper, K., Mazur-Hopkins, P., Kofman, O., Singer, H.S., Denckla, M.B., Pearlson, G.D. and Kaufmann, W.E. (2002) MRI parcellation of the frontal lobe in boys with attention deficit hyperactivity disorder or Tourette syndrome. *Psychiat. Res.,* 116, 63-81.

Kennard, M.A., Spencer, S. and Fountain, G. (1941) Hyperactivity in monkeys following lesions of the frontal lobes. *J. Neurophysiol.,* 4, 512-524.

Kimberg, D.Y., D'Esposito, M. and Farah, M.J. (1997) Effects of bromocriptine on human subjects depend on working memory capacity. *NeuroReport,* 8, 3581-3585.

Knight, R.T., Scabini, D. and Woods, D.L. (1989) Prefrontal cortex gating of auditory transmission in humans. *Brain Res.,* 504, 338-342.

Konishi, S., Nakajima, K., Uchida, I., Kikyo, H., Kameyama, M. and Miyashita, Y. (1999) Common inhibitory mechanism in human inferior prefrontal cortex revealed by event-related functional MRI. *Brain,* 122, 981-991.

Kuczenski, R. and Segal, D.S. (2002) Exposure of adolescent rats to oral methylphenidate: preferential effects on extracellular norepinephrine and absence of sensitization and cross-sensitization to methamphetamine. *J. Neurosci.,* 22, 7264-7271.

Li, B.-M. and Mei, Z.-T. (1994) Delayed response deficit induced by local injection of the alpha-2 adrenergic antagonist yohimbine into the dorsolateral prefrontal cortex in young adult monkeys. *Behav. Neur. Biol.,* 62, 134-139.

Li, B.-M., Mao, Z.-M., Wang, M. and Mei, Z.-T. (1999) Alpha-2 adrenergic modulation of prefrontal cortical neuronal activity related to spatial working memory in monkeys. *Neuropsychopharmacol,* 21, 601-610.

Lidow, M.S., Koh, P.-O. and Arnsten, A.F.T. (2002) D1 dopamine receptors in the mouse prefrontal cortex: Immunocytochemical and cognitive neuropharmacological analyses. *Synapse,* 47, 101-108.

Ma, C.-L., Arnsten, A.F.T. and Li, B.-M. (2005) Locomotor hyperactivity induced by blockade of prefrontal cortical alpha-2-adrenoceptors in monkeys. *Biol. Psychiatry,*57, 192-195.

Ma, C.-L., Qi, X.-L., Peng, J.-Y. and Li, B.-M. (2003) Selective deficit in no-go performance induced by blockade of prefrontal cortical alpha 2-adrenoceptors in monkeys. *NeuroReport,* 14, 1013-1016.

MacDonald, E., Kobilka, B.K. and Scheinin, M. (1997) Gene targeting- Homing in on alpha-2-adrenoceptor subtype function. *Trends Pharmacol. Sci.,* 18, 211-219.

Malmo, R.B. (1942) Interference factors in delayed response in monkeys after removal of frontal lobes. *Neurophysiol.,* 5, 295-308.

Manes, F., Sahakian, B.J., Clark, L., Rogers, R., Antoun, N., Aitken, M. and Robbins, T. (2002) Decision-making processes following damage to the prefrontal cortex. *Brain,* 125, 624-639.

Mao, Z.-M., Arnsten, A.F.T. and Li, B.-M. (1999) Local infusion of alpha-1 adrenergic agonist into the prefrontal cortex impairs spatial working memory performance in monkeys. *Biol. Psychiatry,* 46, 1259-1265.

McCormick, D.A., Pape, H.C. and Williamson, A. (1991) Actions of norepinephrine in the cerebral cortex and thalamus: implications for function of the central noradrenergic system. *Prog. Brain Res.,* 88, 293-305.

McLean, A., Dowson, J., Toone, B., Young, S., Bazanis, E., Robbins, T.W. and Sahakian, B.J. (2004) Characteristic neurocognitive profile associated with adult attention-deficit/hyperactivity disorder. *Psychol. Med.,* 34, 681-692.

Mehta, M.A., Goodyer, I.M. and Sahakian, B.J. (2004) Methylphenidate improves working memory and set-shifting in AD/HD: relationships to baseline memory capacity. *J. Child Psychol. Psychiat.,* 45, 293-305.

Mehta, M.A., Owen, A.M., Sahakian, B.J., Mavaddat, N., Pickard, J.D. and Robbins, T.W. (2000) Methylphenidate enhances working memory by modulating discrete frontal and parietal lobe regions in the human brain. *J. Neurosci.,* 20, RC651-656.

Miller, E.K., Li, L. and Desimone, R. (1993) Activity of neurons in anterior inferior temporal cortex during a short-term memory task. *J. Neurosc.,* 13, 1460-1478.

Moises, H.C., Waterhouse, B.D. and Woodward, D.J. (1981) Locus coeruleus stimulation potentiates Purkinje cell responses to afferent input: the climbing fiber system. *Brain Res.,* 222, 43-64.

Morita, M., Nakahara, K. and Hayashi, T. (2004) A rapid presentation event-related functional magnetic resonance imaging study of response inhibition in macaque monkeys. *Neurosci. Lett.,* 356, 203-206.

Morrison, J.H. and Foote, S.L. (1986) Noradrenergic and serotonergic innervation of cortical, thalamic, and tectal visual structures in Old and New World monkeys. *J. Comp. Neurol.,* 243, 117-138.

Mouradian, R.D., Seller, F.M. and Waterhouse, B.D. (1991) Noradrenergic potentiation of excitatory transmitter action in cerebrocortical slices: evidence of mediation by an alpha1-receptor-linked second messenger pathway. *Brain Res.,* 546, 83-95.

Muir, J.L., Everitt, B.J. and Robbins, T.W. (1996) The cerebral cortex of the rat and visual attentional function: Dissociable effects of mediofrontal, cingulate, anterior dorsolateral, and parietal cortex lesions on a five-choice serial reaction time task. *Cereb. Cortex,* 6, 470-481.

Petrides, M. (1986) The effect of periarcuate lesions in the monkey on the performance of symmetrically and asymmetrically reinforced visual and auditory go, no-go tasks. *J. Neurosci.,* 6, 2054-2063.

Price, J.L. and Amaral, D.G. (1981) An autoradiographic study of the projections of the central nucleus of the monkey amygdala. *J Neurosci.,* 1, 1242-1259.

Quirk, G.J., Likhtik, E., Pelletier, J.G. and Pare, D. (2003) Stimulation of medial prefrontal cortex decreases the responsiveness of central amygdala output neurons. *J. Neurosci.,* 23, 8800-8807.

Rajkowski, J., Kubiak, P., Inanova, S. and Aston-Jones, G. (1998) State-related activity, reactivity of locus coeruleus neurons in behaving monkeys. *Adv. Pharmacol.,* 42, 740-744.

Rajkowski, J., Majczynski, H., Clayton, E. and Aston-Jones, G. (2004) Activation of monkey locus coeruleus neurons varies with difficulty and performance in a target detection task. *J. Neurophysiol.,* 92, 361-371.

Rama, P., Linnankoski, I., Tanila, H., Pertovaara, A. and Carlson, S. (1996) Medetomidine, atipamezole, and guanfacine in delayed response performance of aged monkeys. *Pharmacol. Biochem. Behav.,* 54, 1-7.

Raskind, M.A., Peskind, E.R., Kanter, E.D., Petrie, E.C., Radant, A., Thompson, C., Dobie, D.J., Hoff, D., Rein, R.J., Straits-Troster, K., Thomas, R. and McFall, M.M. (2003) Prazosin reduces nightmares and other PTSD symptoms in combat veterans: A placebo-controlled study. *Am. J. Psychiatry,* 160, 371-373.

Roman, T., Schmitz, M., Polanczyk, G.V., Eizirik, M., Rohde, L.A. and Hutz, M.H. (2002) Further evidence for the association between attention-deficit/hyperactivity disorder and the dopamine-beta-hydroxylase gene. *Am. J. Med. Genet.,* 114, 154-158.

Rubia, K., Smith, A.B., Brammer, M.J. and Taylor, E. (2003) Right inferior prefrontal cortex mediates response inhibition while mesial prefrontal cortex is responsible for error detection. *Neuroimage,* 20, 351-358.

Rubia, K., Overmeyer, S., Taylor, E., Brammer, M., Williams, S.C.R., Simmons, A. and Bullmore, E.T. (1999) Hypofrontality in Attention Deficit Hyperactivity Disorder during higher-order motor control: A study with functional MRI. *Am. J. Psychiatry,* 156, 891-896.

Sara, S.J. and Herve-Minvielle, A. (1995) Inhibitory influence of frontal cortex on locus coeruleus. *Proc. Natl. Acad. Sci. USA,* 92, 6032-6036.

Sawaguchi, T. and Goldman-Rakic, P.S. (1994) The role of D1-dopamine receptors in working memory: local injections of dopamine antagonists into the prefrontal cortex of rhesus monkeys performing an oculomotor delayed response task. *J. Neurophysiol.,* 71, 515-528.

Scahill, L., Chappell, P.B., Kim, Y.S., Schultz, R.T., Katsovich, L., Shepherd, E., Arnsten, A.F.T., Cohen, D.J. and Leckman, J.F. (2001) Guanfacine in the treatment of children with tic disorders and ADHD: A placebo-controlled study. *Am. J. Psychiatry,* 158, 1067-1074.

Segal, M. and Bloom, F.E. (1976) The action of norepinephrine in the rat hippocampus. IV. The effects of locus coeruleus stimulation on evoked hippocampal unit activity. *Brain Res.,* 107, 513-525.

Sowell, E.R., Thompson, P.M., Welcome, S.E., Henkenius, A.L., Toga, A.W. and Peterson, B.S. (2003) Cortical abnormalities in children and adolescents with attention-deficit hyperactivity disorder. *Lancet,* 362, 1699-1707.

Spencer, T., Heiligenstein, J.H., Biederman, J., Faries, D.E., Kratochvil, C.J., Conners, C.K. and Potter, W.Z. (2002a) Results from 2 proof-of-concept, placebo-controlled studies of atomoxetine in children with attention-deficit/hyperactivity disorder. *J. Clin. Psychiatry,* 63, 1140-1147.

Spencer, T., Biederman, J., Coffey, B., Geller, D., Crawford, M., Bearman, S.K., Tarazi, R. and Faraone, S. (2002b) A double-blind comparison of desipramine and placebo in children and adolescents with chronic tic disorder and comorbid attention-deficit/hyperactivity disorder. *Arch. Gen. Psychiatry,* 59, 649-656.

Steere, J.C. and Arnsten, A.F.T. (1997) The alpha-2A noradrenergic agonist, guanfacine, improves visual object discrimination reversal performance in rhesus monkeys. *Behav. Neurosci.,* 111, 1-9.

Swanson, J.M., Posner, M., Potkin, S., Bonforte, S., Youpa, D., Fiore, C., Cantwell, D. and Crinella, F. (1991) Activating tasks for the study of visual-spatial attention in ADHD children: a cognitive anatomic approach. *J. Child Neurol.,* 6, S119-S127.

Tanila, H., Rama, P. and Carlson, S. (1996) The effects of prefrontal intracortical microinjections of an alpha-2 agonist, alpha-2 antagonist and lidocaine on the delayed alternation performance of aged rats. *Brain Res. Bull.,* 40, 117-119.

Tanila, H., Mustonen, K., Sallinen, J., Scheinin, M. and Riekkinen, P. (1999) Role of alpha-2C-adrenoceptor subtype in spatial working memory as revealed by mice with targeted disruption of the alpha-2C-adrenoceptor gene. *Eur J. Neurosci.,* 11, 599-603.

Taylor, F.B. and Russo, J. (2001) Comparing guanfacine and dextroamphetamine for the treatment of adult Attention Deficit-Hyperactivity Disorder. *J. Clin. Psychopharmacol.,* 21, 223-228.

Thompson-Schill, S.L., Jonides, J., Marshuetz, C., Smith, E.E., D'Esposito, M., Kan, I.P., Knight, R.T. and Swick, D. (2002) Effects of frontal lobe damage on interference effects in working memory. *Cogn. Affect Behav. Neurosci.,* 2, 109-120.

Trommer, B., Hoeppner, J. and Zecker, S. (1991) The go-no go test in attention deficit disorder is sensitive to methylphenidate. *J. Child Neurol.,* 6 Suppl., S128-131.

Turner, D.C., Blackwell, A.D., Dowson, J.H., McLean, A. and Sahakian, B.J. (2004) Neurocognitive effects of methylphenidate in adult attention-deficit/hyperactivity disorder. *Psychopharmacol.,* 178, 286-295.

Usher, M., Cohen, J.D., Servan-Schreiber, D., Rajkowski, J. and Aston-Jones, G. (1999) The role of locus coeruleus in the regulation of cognitive performance. *Science,* 283, 549-554.

Vaidya, C.J., Austin, G., Kirkorian, G., Ridlehuber, H.W., Desmond, J.E., Glover, G.H. and Gabrieli, J.D.E. (1998) Selective effects of methylphenidate in attention deficit hyperactivity disorder: A functional magnetic resonance study. *Proc. Natl. Acad. Sci. USA,* 95, 14494-14499.

Van Tol, H.H.M., Bunzow, J.R., Guan, H.-C., Sunahara, R.K., Seeman, P., Niznik, H.B. and Civelli, O. (1991) Cloning of the gene for a human dopamine D4 receptor with high affinity for the antipsychotic clozapine. *Nature,* 350, 610-614.

Wallis, J.D., Anderson, K.C. and Miller, E.K. (2001) Single neurons in prefrontal cortex encode abstract rules. *Nature,* 411, 953-956.

Wang, M., Tang, Z.X. and Li, B.M. (2004a) Enhanced visuomotor associative learning following stimulation of alpha 2A-adrenoceptors in the ventral prefrontal cortex in monkeys. *Brain Res.,* 1024, 176-182.

Wang, M., Ji, J.Z. and Li, B.M. (2004b) The alpha(2A)-adrenergic agonist guanfacine improves visuomotor associative learning in monkeys. *Neuropsychopharmacology,* 29, 86-92.

Watanabe, M. (1986) Prefrontal unit activity during delayed conditional go/no-go discrimination in the monkey I. Relation to the stimulus. *Brain Res. Rev.,* 382, 1-14.

Waterhouse, B.D., Moises, H.C. and Woodward, D.J. (1980) Noradrenergic modulation of somatosensory cortical neuronal responses to iontophoretically applied putative transmitters. *Exp. Neurol.,* 69, 30-49.

Waterhouse, B.D., Moises, H.C. and Woodward, D.J. (1981) Alpha-receptor-mediated facilitation of somatosensory cortical neuronal responses to excitatory synaptic inputs and iontophoretically applied acetylcholine. *Neuropharmacology,* 20, 907-920.

Waterhouse, B.D., Moises, H.C. and Woodward, D.J. (1998) Phasic activation of the locus coeruleus enhances responses of primary sensory cortical neurons to peripheral receptive field stimulation. *Brain Res.,* 790, 33-44.

Wilkins, A.J., Shallice, T. and McCarthy, R. (1987) Frontal lesions and sustained attention. *Neuropsychologia,* 25, 359-365.

Witte, E.A. and Marrocco, R.T. (1997) Alterations of brain noradrenergic activity in rhesus monkeys affects the alerting component of covert orienting. *Psychopharmacology,* 132, 315-323.

Woods, D.L. and Knight, R.T. (1986) Electrophysiological evidence of increased distractability after dorsolateralll prefrontal lesions. *Neurology,* 36, 212-216.

Xu, C., Schachar, R., Tannock, R., Roberts, W., Malone, M., Kennedy, J.L. and Barr, C.L. (2001) Linkage study of the alpha2A adrenergic receptor in attention-deficit hyperactivity disorder families. *Am. J. Med. Genet.,* 105, 159-162.

Yamaguchi, S. and Knight, R.T. (1990) Gating of somatosensory input by human prefrontal cortex. *Brain Res.,* 521, 281-288.

Yeo, R.A., Hill, D., Campbell, R., Vigil, J. and Brooks, W.M. (2000) Developmental instability and working memory ability in children: a magnetic resonance spectroscopy investigation. *Dev. Neuropsychol.,* 17, 143-159.

Zahrt, J., Taylor, J.R., Mathew, R.G. and Arnsten, A.F.T. (1997) Supranormal stimulation of dopamine D1 receptors in the rodent prefrontal cortex impairs spatial working memory performance. *J. Neurosci.,* 17, 8528-8535.

In: Prefrontal Cortex: Roles, Interventions and Traumas ISBN 978-1-60692-415-0
Editors: Lorenzo LoGrasso and Giovanni Morretti

Short Communication A

Prefrontal Cortex: Brodmann and Cajal Revisited

Guy N. Elston[1] and Laurence J. Garey[2]
[1]Centre for Cognitive Neuroscience,
Sunshine Coast, Qld 4562, Australia
[2]Centre for Psychiatric Neuroscience
CH-1008 Lausanne, Switzerland

Abstract

Modern imaging techniques allow the mapping of gross brain structure to an exacting standard; however, these methodologies have been applied inappropriately in recent times to the study of the prefrontal cortex – the structure identified by Brodmann as being central to intelligence. Currently, these methodologies cannot detect prefrontal cortex, nor be used to quantify it. Here we review Brodmann's data on comparative aspects of the gross structure of the cerebral cortex, some of which have been largely ignored in recent times. We believe this still remains the definitive data set for prefrontal cortex. In addition we compare Brodmann's observations with those of his contemporary Santiago Ramon y Cajal. Cajal's studies of the fine structure of the cerebral cortex led him to the conclusion that human intelligence is largely attributable to the complexity of the pyramidal (psychic) cell. These observations are compared and contrasted with modern data on prefrontal cortex, essentially substantiating the conclusions of these two great founding fathers of modern neuroscience.

Introduction

Brodmann on Prefrontal Cortex

Apparently mostly unbeknown to neuroscientists, Korbinian Brodmann published an unprecedented and unsurpassed set of data almost 100 years ago (Brodmann, 1912, 1913;

translated by Elston and Garey, 2004) in which he quantified, among other things, the size of the frontal lobe and "prefrontal cortex" in a variety of primate and non-primate species. Brodmann's definition of prefrontal cortex is clear: granular cortex (that containing an identifiable layer IV) in the frontal lobe. Because this term has become confused in modern studies we use the term granular prefrontal cortex (gPFC) here in accordance with Brodmann's definition. We highlight in italics examples of where the term has been misused. Brodmann's observations of gPFC were derived from his Nissl preparations of the brains of a large number of species, both primate and non-primate (Figure 1). Brodmann's data on the frontal lobe and gPFC (Table 1) reveal several interesting observations which predate modern findings. Moreover, statements made in modern studies are often inconsistent with the Brodmann data. In particular Brodmann's data reveal that the size of the frontal lobe of humans is smaller than that predicted from the non-human primate data (Figure 2A). In addition, his data reveal that the proportion of the frontal lobe occupied by the gPFC varies considerably between species (Figure 2B).

Table 1. Brodmann's (1913) original data on the area of various cortices in the frontal lobe, motor cortex, granular prefrontal cortex, and the total cerebrum in a variety of mammalian species

Species	Frontal	Motor	Prefrontal	Total
Man	49120	9833	39287	135470
Chimpanzee	12108	5389	6719	39572
Gibbon	3490	1651	1839	16301
Mandrill	4362	2194	2168	21321
Baboon (*Papio hamadryas*)	4865	2898	1967	20594
Baboon (*Papio cynocephalus*)	4311	2200	2111	20376
Macaque	3550	1817	1733	15308
Guenon	3601	1976	1625	14641
Capuchin monkey	3082	1822	1260	13682
Marmoset	315	167	148	1649
Black lemur	790	453	337	4054
Dwarf lemur	164	94	70	921
Fruit bat	99	73	26	1097
Dog (fox terrier)	1940	1283	657	9527
Cat	564	412	152	4474
Rabbit	184	148	36	1627
Hedgehog	24	24	0	575
Armadillo	93	93	0	2010
Opossum	51	51	0	804

Notably, the proportion of the frontal lobe occupied by gPFC is considerably higher in human than in all other species studied (Figure 2C). His data also show that the proportion of the cortical mantle occupied by gPFC in man is greater, as a function of either the frontal lobe or the total cortical surface area, than that in all other species studied (Figure 2D).

Because of Brodmann's observations it is widely believed that the disproportionate increase in the size of the gPFC, not the frontal lobe, is related to increasing intelligence during hominine evolution.

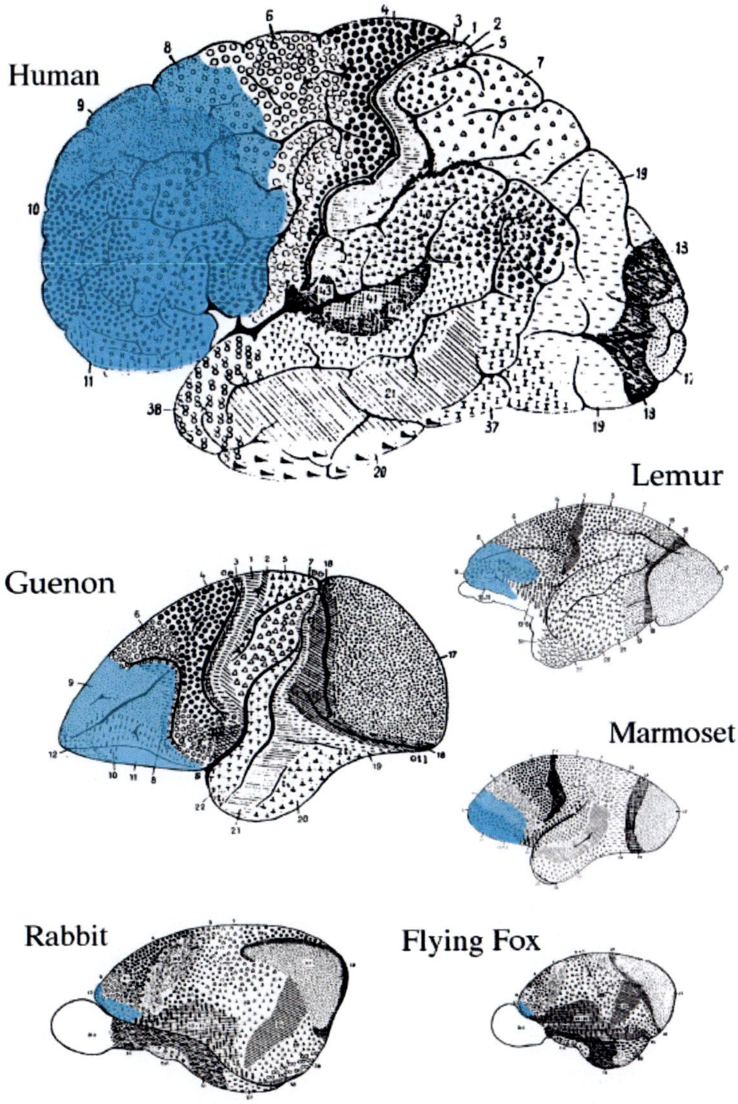

Figure 1. Drawings, based on Brodmann (1909; see Garey, 2006, for a complete translation) illustrating cortical areas identified in the frontal lobe as having a well-developed layer IV ("inner granular layer"). As per Brodmann's definition (1913) these areas (blue) represent the extent of *prefrontal* cortex. Note that the number and size of cortical areas included as granular prefrontal cortex, as well as their topography, differ between species. The most differentiated prefrontal cortex is found in humans, including areas 8, 9, 10, 11, 44, 45, 46 and 47. The number and location of cortical areas in granular prefrontal cortex have since been modified with the advent of new methodologies used to distinguish cortical areas. However, changes to nomenclature do not adversely affect the original Brodmann data (1913) regarding relative differences in the size of the gPFC in different species. Figure modified from Elston, 2003a. Not to scale.

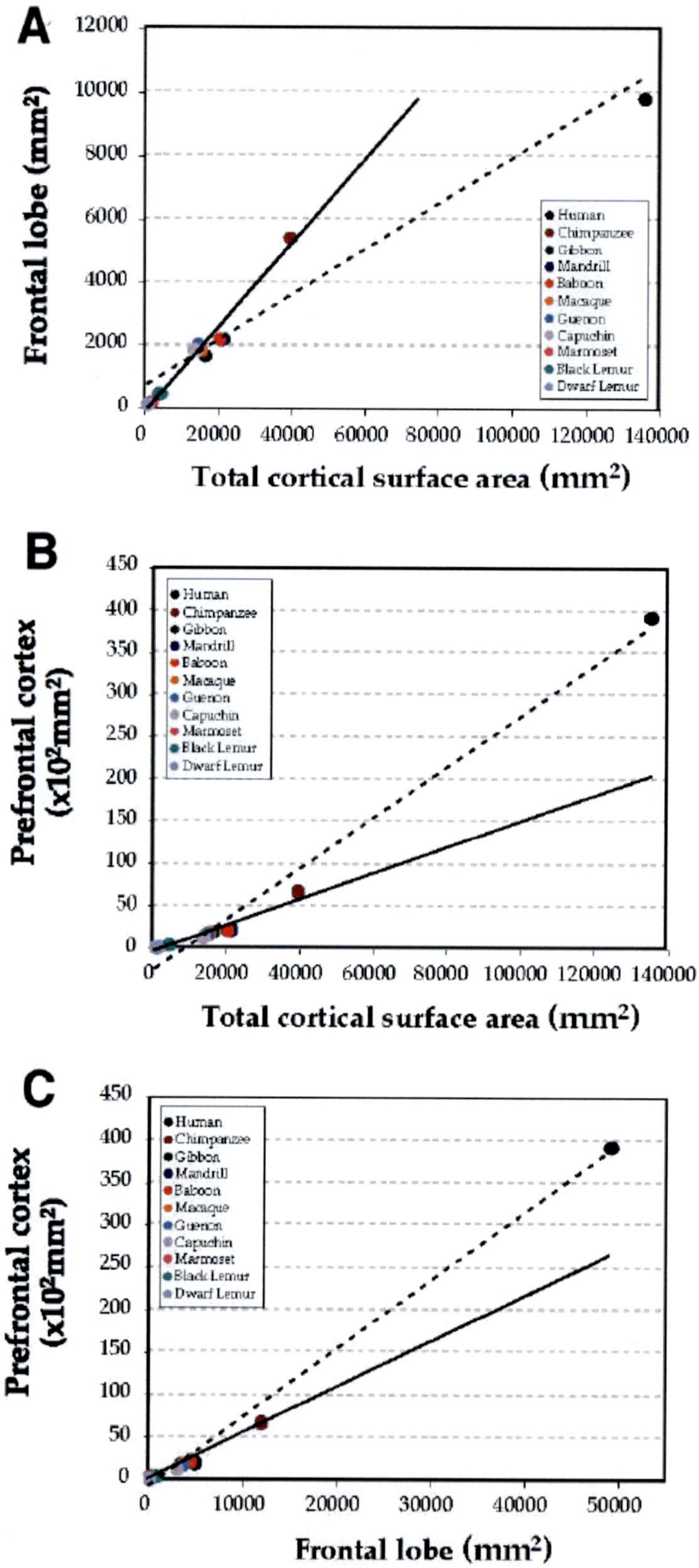
A
Frontal lobe (mm²)
Total cortical surface area (mm²)
B
Prefrontal cortex (x10²mm²)
Total cortical surface area (mm²)
C
Prefrontal cortex (x10²mm²)
Frontal lobe (mm²)
Human
Chimpanzee
Gibbon
Mandrill
Baboon
Macaque
Guenon
Capuchin
Marmoset
Black Lemur
Dwarf Lemur

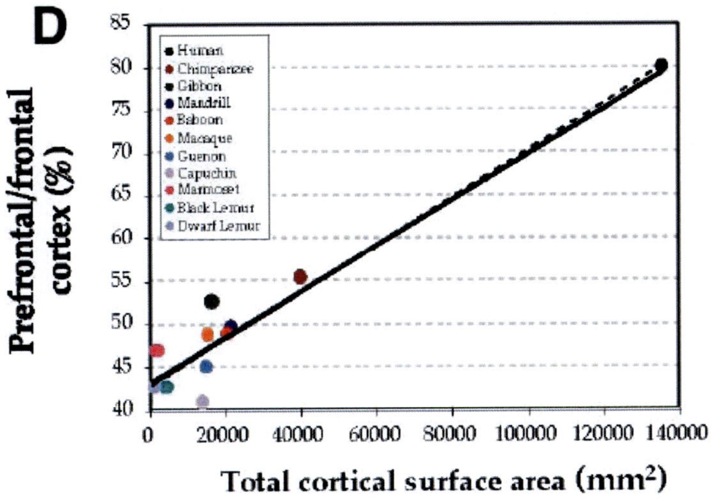

Figure 2. Plots of original data from Brodmann (1913) illustrating (A) the area of the frontal lobe vs. total cortical surface area, (B) area of the granular prefrontal cortex vs. total cortical surface area, (C) area of the granular prefrontal cortex vs. frontal lobe and (D) the proportion of the frontal lobe occupied by granular prefrontal cortex vs. total cortical surface area. Linear regressions of the entire data set are illustrated in dashed black lines; those excluding the human data are illustrated by solid black lines. In A, exclusion of the human data increased the r^2 coefficient. Exclusion of the human data in B-D decreased the r^2 coefficient. Note that according to these data (A) the frontal lobe of the human brain is smaller than that expected from the plot of the non-human primate data. Note also that the proportion of the frontal lobe occupied by granular prefrontal cortex varies quite dramatically between primate species (D). Thus, in some primates, there has been a disproportionate increase in the size of prefrontal cortex during the expansion of the frontal lobe. This is highlighted in C and D; prefrontal cortex occupies a much higher proportion of both the cerebrum and the frontal lobe in humans compared to non-human primates. In addition to these relative values, it should be kept in mind that the absolute size of human prefrontal cortex is considerably larger than that in other species.

Prefrontal Cortex

Modern Imaging Studies

Unfortunately, the field has become confused in recent times as modern imaging technologies have in some cases been applied inappropriately to test Brodmann's conclusion related to the size of the *prefrontal* cortex and intelligence. The confusion arises largely out of a misunderstanding of what *prefrontal cortex* is or because something that is not *prefrontal* cortex has been used to test this relationship. These studies fail to acknowledge the existence of the Brodmann data, which have been reviewed previously (Passingham, 1973). For example, Semendeferi and colleagues (2002) quantified the size of the frontal lobes of great apes and monkeys and concluded that "Human frontal cortices were not disproportionately large in comparison to those of the great apes" (as a function of total cerebral cortical volume). Although this study included a larger number of species than Brodmann's, the conclusion was no different from that made by Brodmann (1913) some 90 years earlier (see

Figure 2A). However, unlike the modern investigators, Brodmann further extended his line of investigation to the gPFC, leading him to conclude that it was this region of the cerebral cortex, not the frontal lobe, that was larger in man than in other species (both absolutely and relatively). Indeed, it is difficult to understand the justification presented by Semendeferi and colleagues (2002) for studying size relationships of the frontal lobe and intelligence. Studying the Brodmann data (1913) reveals that the frontal lobe of humans *and great apes* is considerably smaller than what would be expected in a primate of similar brain size when extrapolating the non-human/non-great ape data. Taking these data together with those of Brodmann (who also studied the chimpanzee), the logical conclusion is that the frontal lobe of humans *and great apes* is considerably smaller than what would be expected in a primate of similar brain size when extrapolating the non-human/non-great ape data. In essence, this is just what Bush and Allman (2004) demonstrated: frontal cortex hyperscaling is greater in lemurs and lorises compared with higher primates. While new and important data have been fleshed out, these modern studies represent no advance over Brodmann's original conclusions (1913): the relative size of the frontal lobe compared to total cortical volume reveals little about cognitive abilities.

As mentioned above, the field has become confused due to a misunderstanding of *what prefrontal cortex is* in estimating its size. Schoenemann and colleagues (2005) concluded that there is a disproportionately larger volume of white matter in human *prefrontal* cortex as compared to that in other primates, and suggested that this reflects a substrate for human cognitive abilities. However, these authors used what they called a "proxy" for the *prefrontal* cortex, which neither reflects granular prefrontal cortex nor is consistent across species. It is likely that white matter in this study was sampled from a different selection of areas in the gPFC of the different species studied due to differences in the size and topography of prefrontal areas (see Brodmann, 1909, translated by Garey, 2006 for pictorial illustration). The study was too ambitious. Moreover, reanalyses of their data led Sherwood and colleagues (2005) to conclude that the white matter volume in the human brain is less that expected from the great ape data. Clearly, there is no agreement among these studies. Moreover, conspicuous in all of these studies is that the methodologies used do not allow identification of the structure in question – gPFC.

Why the Confusion?

Most of the recent confusion arises because inappropriate methodology has been applied to test the relationship between the size of the gPFC and "intelligence". No doubt this last statement will be cause for concern for some, perhaps rightly so. Despite the technological advances available to us today, the only way to quantify prefrontal cortex is to identify granular cortex in the frontal lobe. The only way to identify granular cortex is to employ age-old techniques that generally do not attract funding. Herein lies the conundrum faced by some of today's neuroscientists interested in the study of the gPFC: submit a scientifically sound application that may not attract funding or submit an application based on an "attractive methodology" that will likely get funded. In the latter case, it is necessary to state why the applicant chooses the modern technology over the appropriate technology. In essence, the argument becomes that the modern technique is superior to the old technique and data collected by the old technique are then usually discredited. For these reasons, some discount the Brodmann data: the brains were collected over 100 years ago, methods of preservation may have caused differential shrinkage and it is unclear how many brains were included for study for a given species (see Passingham, 1973 for a review). However, Brodmann published these data at the end of his career after having the benefit of studying the brains of many different species over a period of decades. It is difficult to believe that he was incapable of distinguishing granular from non-granular cortex. In addition, the evidence suggests that Brodmann processed all the brains himself, making it likely that a standard methodology was applied in all studies. Furthermore, at least for the human data, we know that Brodmann studied many brains. Human brain weights were determined from fourteen cases and the size of human granular prefrontal cortex was reported in the brains obtained from two normal and three pathological cases (Brodmann, 1913; Elston and Garey, 2004). While modern imaging techniques allow the sampling of larger numbers of individuals, and reveal important data related to interindividual variation in brain structure (Sherwood et al., 2004), these methodologies still cannot be used to identify and quantify the gPFC - the structure identified by Brodmann as being central to intelligence. This goal remains off-limits to imaging technology until such time as granular cortex can be distinguished from non-granular cortex.

A Glimpse of Circuit Specialisations in Prefrontal Cortex

It is not all bad news. Considerable effort has been focussed on the determination and quantification of patterns of connections between cortical areas in the gPFC - at least, that of the macaque monkey (Felleman and Van Essen, 1991; Young, 1993; Goldman-Rakic, 1996; Hilgetag et al., 1996; Barbas, 2000; Lewis and Van Essen, 2000; Petrides, 2000; Passingham et al., 2002). Moreover, considerable advances have been made in quantifying patterns of intrinsic connections in the gPFC of the macaque (Lund et al., 1993; Melchitzky et al., 1998, 2001; Barbas et al., 1999; González-Burgos et al., 2000; Rempel-Clower and Barbas, 2000; Soloway et al., 2002; Germuska et al., 2006). However, it is remarkable how little has been done to quantify connectivity in the gPFC of other primate species. To the best of our knowledge there exists not a single study in which patterns of connectivity have been quantified systematically in homologous cortical areas of the *granular* prefrontal cortex of primates by a standardised methodology (that allows axon projections to be visualised and quantified). Two studies have addressed this question qualitatively in non-human primates, both from the laboratory of the late Patricia Goldman-Rakic (Bugbee and Goldman-Rakic, 1983; Preuss and Goldman-Rakic, 1991). Petrides and colleagues have utilised patterns of connectivity to determine the internal organisation and homology of cortical areas of the *granular* prefrontal cortex between the macaque monkey and man (Petrides and Pandya, 2001); however, no quantitative comparisons were made between species. This is particularly striking when we consider that methodologies used in these connectional studies were developed over 30 years ago. Perhaps the lack of application of these techniques to comparative analyses results from the fact that these methodologies were developed at a time when it was generally believed that the cortex was uniform in structure. At that time it was widely believed that all functional differences in the cerebral cortex were solely attributed to the origin of inputs (e.g. Szentagothai and Arbib, 1974; Creutzfeldt, 1977; Zeki, 1978). We now know that this very definitely is not the case.

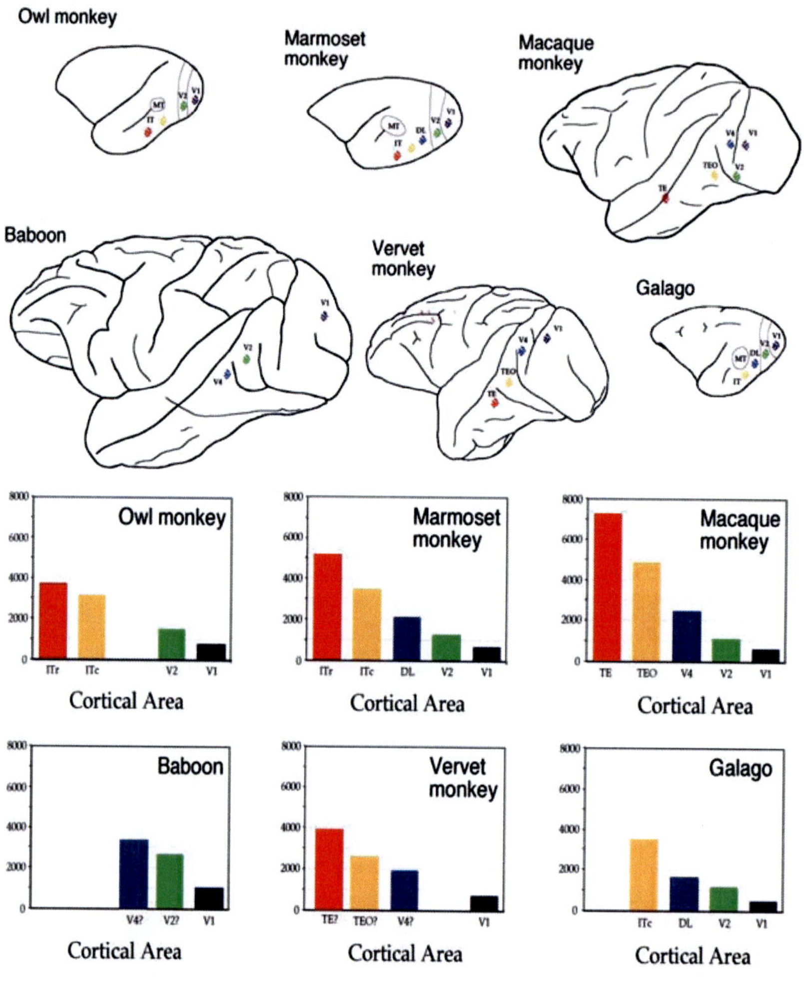

Figure 3. Differences in the number of dendritic spines (sites of excitatory synapses) on the dendritic trees of pyramidal neurons in cortical areas of the ventral visual pathway of the galago, owl monkey, marmoset monkey, macaque monkey, vervet monkey and baboon (dots illustrate regions where neurons were sampled; X-axis = total number of spines in the basal dendritic tree calculated by summing the product of the number of branches by spine density along concentric annuli [25mm] from the cell body and extending to the distal tips). Note there is a clear and consistent trend for neurons to have more spines with anterior progression through cortical areas associated with this pathway. See also Figures 4 and 5. The different brains are not drawn to scale. Modified from Elston (2007).

Cajal's Psychic Cell

Recent studies of the morphology of the pyramidal cell, the archetypal ubiquitous neuron in the cerebral cortex, have revealed extensive phenotypic variation in its structure across the cortical mantle. The dendritic trees of pyramidal cells differ in their size and branching structure between cortical areas. Significant variations have also been demonstrated in the density of spines, the major site for excitatory synaptic input to pyramidal neurons, along the dendrites. Our estimates of the total number of spines in the dendritic trees (calculated by summing the product of the number of branches by spine density along concentric annuli [25mm] from the cell body and extending to the distal tips) reveal systematic differences among cortical areas associated with different cortical pathways (Figures 3-6).

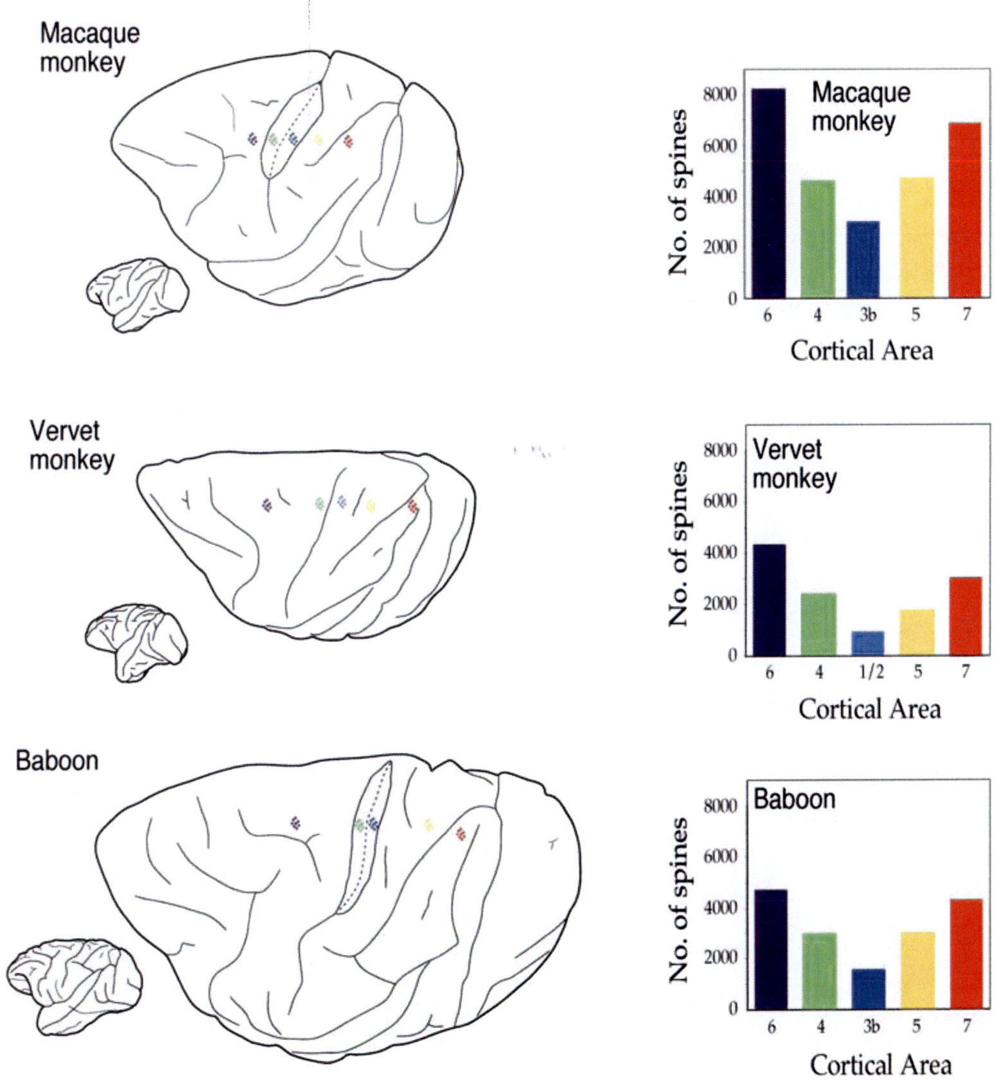

Figure 4. Differences in the number of dendritic spines on pyramidal neurons in cortical areas of the somatosensory-motor cortex of the macaque monkey, vervet monkey and baboon (dots illustrate regions where neurons were sampled; X-axis = total number of spines, calculated as in Figure 3). Note the consistent trend for neurons to have more spines with anterior progression from the primary motor area (area 4) to premotor cortex (area 6) in all three species. Note also the consistent trend for progressively more spinous cells with posterior progression through somatosensory areas from the central sulcus to the angular gyrus. Modified from Elston, 2007.

Moreover, there is a systematic increase in pyramidal cell complexity from primary sensory to sensory association, limbic and granular prefrontal cortex (Lund et al., 1993; Elston et al., 1999a,b, 2001, 2005a-c; Elston, 2000, 2003b; Elston and Rosa, 1998, 2000; Jacobs et al., 2001; Elston and Rockland, 2002). This systematic increase in complexity has a dramatic functional parallel: neurons with simple structure in primary sensory cortex are characterised by phasic discharge, those in sensory association cortex are characterised by tonic discharge that can be interrupted by distractors and those most complex cells in the granular prefrontal cortex are characterised by tonic discharge that is resistant to distractors (see Fuster, 1997; Miller and Cohen, 2001; Elston, 2003a for reviews). Moreover, comparison of pyramidal cell structure in the gPFC of different primates reveals a dramatic variation in the pyramidal cell phenotype among species (Elston et al., 2001, 2007). There is a trend for increasingly more complex pyramidal cells in species with a progressively larger gPFC. Thus, not only is the human *granular* prefrontal cortex larger than that in other species (in absolute terms), but it is composed of neurons of greater functional capacity (see Elston, 2007 for a review).

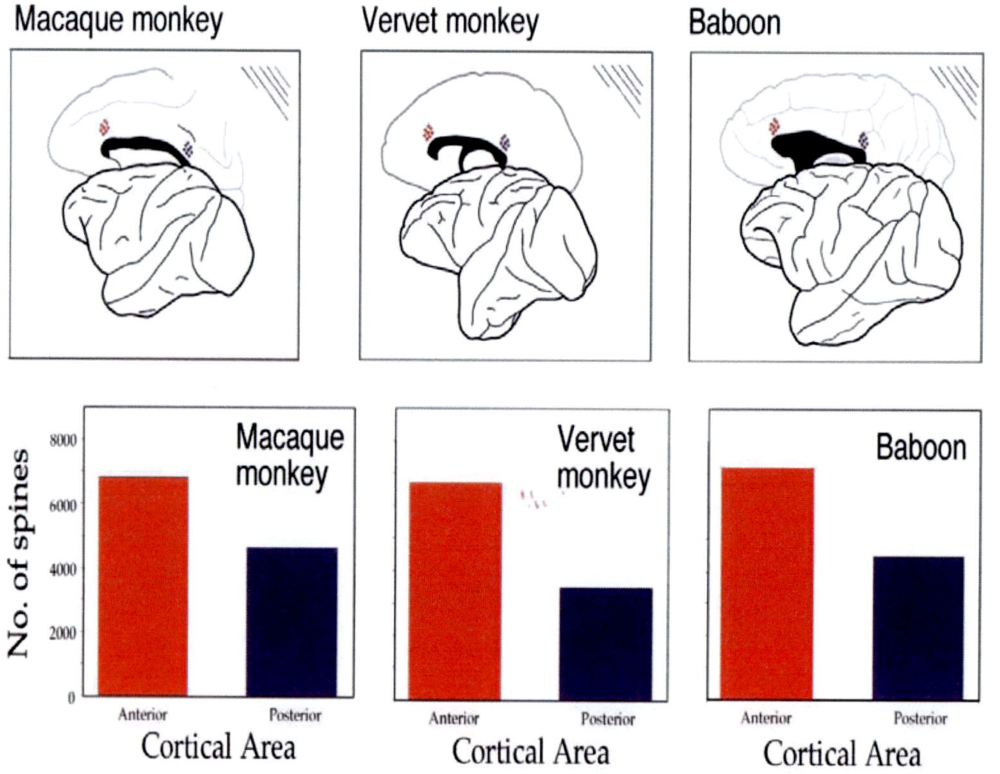

Figure 5. Differences in the number of dendritic spines (sites of excitatory synapses) on the dendritic trees of pyramidal cells in cortical areas of the cingulate gyrus (Brodmann's areas 23 and 24) in macaque monkey, vervet monkey and baboon. (Dots illustrate regions where neurons were sampled; X-axis = total number of spines, calculated as in Figure 3). In all three species there was a consistent trend for pyramidal neurons to have more spines in the anterior cingulate gyrus than in the posterior. The different brains not drawn to scale. Modified from Elston, 2007.

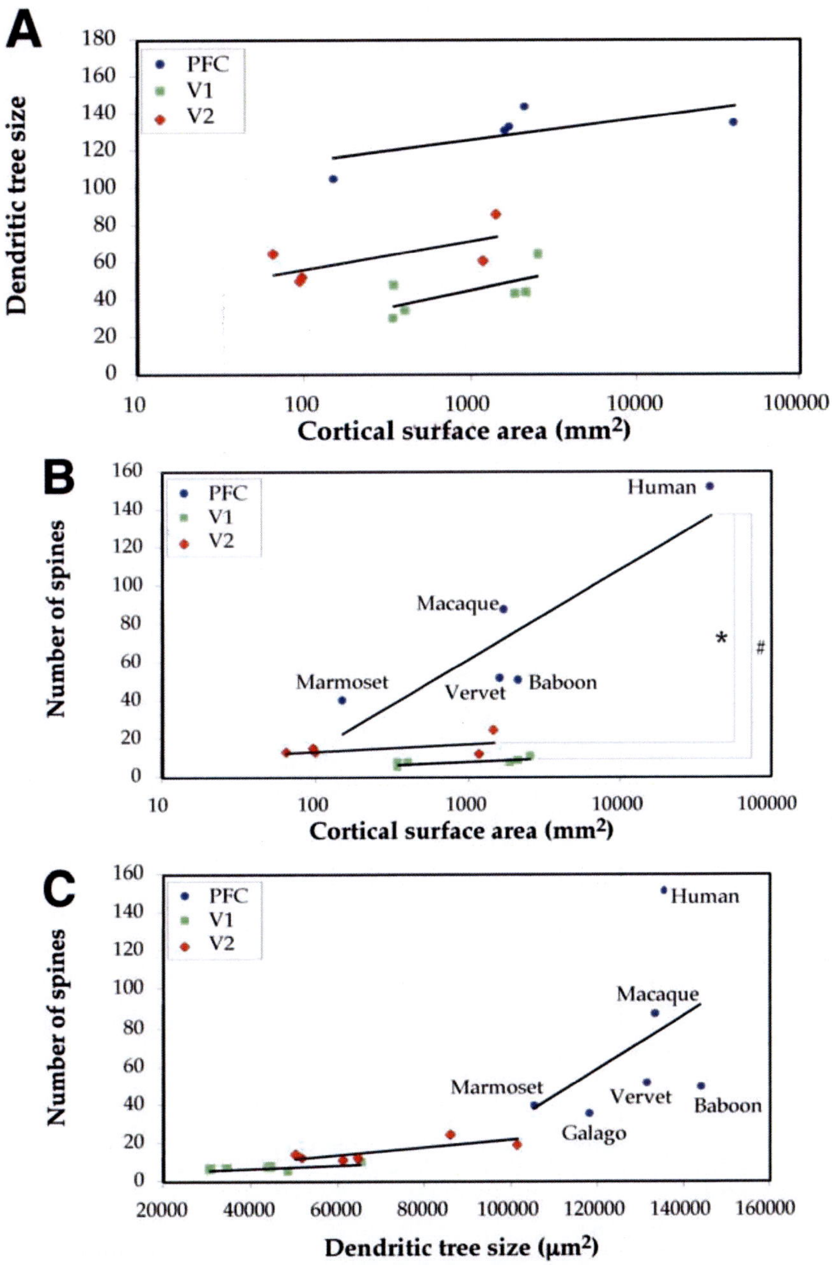

Figure 6. Plots of (A) the area (μm^2 x10^3), and (B) the number of spines (x10^2) on the basal dendritic trees of pyramidal cells in the granular prefrontal cortex (gPFC), primary (V1) and secondary (V2) visual cortex vs. the tangential surface area of each cortical area. (C) Plot of the number of spines (x10^2) vs. the size of the basal dendritic trees of pyramidal cells in the gPFC, primary (V1) and secondary (V2) visual cortex. Moderated multiple regression revealed a significant difference between the slopes of regression lines of gPFC and V2 for comparisons between total number of spines on the dendritic arbors of pyramidal cells vs. cortical surface area (F_{change} (1,6) = 6.19, $p < 0.05$). Significance was approached for the comparison between the total number of spines in the dendritic arbors of pyramidal cells vs. cortical surface area for gPFC and V1 (F_{change} (1,7) = 5.20, $p < 0.057$). Reproduced from Elston et al. 2006.

Conclusion

Brodmann's data reveal that the frontal lobe of modern man is smaller than what might be expected if extrapolating from data obtained from other primate species. However, the size of human granular prefrontal cortex is larger than in other primate species, in both absolute and relative terms. Because of this, it is often stated that the granular prefrontal cortex is associated with intelligence or cognitive ability. Recent studies demonstrate that not only is the human granular prefrontal cortex larger than in other primate species, but it is composed of neurons of more complex structure. The highly complex neuronal structure observed in the gPFC of humans endows a higher degree of connectivity and functional capacity than those in the gPFC of other species. Santiago Ramon y Cajal said it beautifully in 1893: "as one ascends the animal scale the psychic (pyramidal) cell becomes larger and more complex; it is natural to attribute this progressive morphological complexity, in part at least, to its progressive functional state…it can thus be considered probable that the psychic cell performs its activity more amply and usefully the larger the number of somatic and collateral dendrites that it offers".

Just after the one hundredth anniversary of the award of the Nobel Prize to Ramon y Cajal it might be appropriate for modern neuroscientists to embrace this specialisation and further probe the microstructure of intelligence in a series of systematic comparative studies (see also DeFelipe, 2006).

References

Barbas H. Connections underlying the synthesis of cognition, memory, and emotion in primate prefrontal cortices. *Brain Research Bulletin* 2000 52:319-330.

Barbas H, Ghashghaei H, Dombrowski SM, Rempel-Clower NL. Medial prefrontal cortices are unified by common connections with superior temporal cortices and distinguished by input from memory-related areas in the rhesus monkey. *Journal of Comparative Neurology* 1999 410:343-367.

Brodmann K. Vergleichende Lokalisationslehre der Grosshirnrinde in ihren Prinzipien dargestellt auf Grund des Zellenbaues. Barth, Leipzig 1909 (for translation see Garey, 2006, below).

Brodmann K. Neue Ergebnisse über die vergleichende histologische Lokalisation der Grosshirnrinde mit besonderer Berücksichtigung des Stirnhirns. *Anatomischer Anzeiger* 1912 41:157-216.

Brodmann K. Neue Forschungsergebnisse der Grosshirnrindenanatomie mit besonderer Berücksichtigung anthropologischer Fragen. Verhandlungen der Gesellschaft deutscher *Naturforscher und Ärzte* 1913 85:200-240.

Bugbee NM, Goldman-Rakic PS. Columnar organization of corticocortical projections in squirrel and rhesus monkeys: similarity of column width in species differing in cortical volume. *Journal of Comparative Neurology* 1983 220:355-364.

Bush EC, Allman JM. The scaling of frontal cortex in primates and carnivores. *Proceedings of the National Academy of Sciences USA* 2004 101:3962-3966.

Cajal S R y. 1893. Neuvo concepto de la histologia de los centros nerviosos. *Revista de ciencias medicas*, Barcelona 18:21–40.

Creutzfeldt OD. Generality of the functional structure of the neocortex. *Naturwissenschaften* 1977 64:507-517.

DeFelipe J. Brain plasticity and mental processes: Cajal again. *Nature Reviews Neuroscience* 2006 7:811-817.

Elston GN. Pyramidal cells of the frontal lobe: all the more spinous to think with. *Journal of Neuroscience* 2000 20:RC95(1-4).

Elston GN. Cortex, cognition and the cell: new insights into the pyramidal neuron and prefrontal function. *Cerebral Cortex* 2003a 13:1124-1138.

Elston GN. The pyramidal neuron in occipital, temporal and prefrontal cortex of the owl monkey (*Aotus trivirgatus*): regional specialization in cell structure. *European Journal of Neuroscience* 2003b 17:1313-1318.

Elston GN. 2007. Specializations in pyramidal cell structure during primate evolution. In: Kaas JH, Preuss TM (Eds.) *Evolution of Nervous Systems*. Elsevier Oxford. pp 191-242

Elston GN, Benavides-Piccione R, DeFelipe J. The pyramidal cell in cognition: a comparative study in human and monkey. *Journal of Neuroscience* 2001 21:RC163(1-5).

Elston GN, Benavides-Piccione R, Elston A, DeFelipe J, Manger P. Specialization in pyramidal cell structure in the cingulate cortex of the Chacma baboon (*Papio ursinus*): an intracellular injection study of the posterior and anterior cingulate gyrus with comparative notes on the macaque and vervet monkeys. *Neuroscience Letters* 2005a 387:130-135.

Elston GN, Benavides-Piccione R, Elston A, Manger P, DeFelipe J. Specialization in pyramidal cell structure in the sensory-motor cortex of the Chacma baboon (*Papio ursinus*) with comparative notes on macaque and vervet monkeys. *Anatomical Record* 2005b 286A:854-865.

Elston GN, Benavides-Piccione R, Elston A, Zietsch B, DeFelipe J, Manger P, Casagrande V, Kaas JH. Specializations of the granular prefrontal cortex of primates: implications for cognitive processing. *Anatomical Record* 2006 288A:26-35.

Elston GN, Elston A, Casagrande VA, Kaas JH. Pyramidal neurons of granular prefrontal cortex of the galago: complexity in evolution of the psychic cell in primates. *Anatomical Record* 2005c 285A:610-618.

Elston GN, Garey LJ. New research findings on the anatomy of the cerebral cortex of special relevance to anthropological questions. 2004: University of Queensland Printery. Brisbane

Elston GN, Rockland KS. The pyramidal cell of the sensorimotor cortex of the macaque monkey: phenotypic variation. *Cerebral Cortex* 2002 12:1071-1078.

Elston GN, Rosa MG. Morphological variation of layer III pyramidal neurones in the occipitotemporal pathway of the macaque monkey visual cortex. *Cerebral Cortex* 1998 8:278-294.

Elston GN, Rosa MGP. Pyramidal cells, patches, and cortical columns: a comparative study of infragranular neurons in TEO, TE, and the superior temporal polysensory area of the macaque monkey. *Journal of Neuroscience* 2000 20:RC117(1-5).

Elston GN, Tweedale R, Rosa MGP. Cortical integration in the visual system of the macaque monkey: large-scale morphological differences in the pyramidal neurons in the occipital, parietal and temporal lobes. *Proceedings of the Royal Society*, London, Series B 1999a 266:1367-1374.

Elston GN, Tweedale R, Rosa MGP. Cellular heterogeneity in cerebral cortex. A study of the morphology of pyramidal neurones in visual areas of the marmoset monkey. *Journal of Comparative Neurology* 1999b 415:33-51.

Felleman DJ, Van Essen DC. Distributed hierarchical processing in the primate cerebral cortex. *Cerebral Cortex* 1991 1:1-47.

Fuster JM. 1997. *The Prefrontal Cortex: Anatomy, Physiology, and Neuropsychology of the Frontal Lobe.* Lippincott-Raven: Philadelphia.

Garey LJ. 2006. *Brodmann's Localisation in the Cerebral Cortex*. Springer: New York.

Germuska M, Saha S, Fiala J, Barbas H. Synaptic distinction of laminar-specific prefrontal-temporal pathways in primates. *Cerebral Cortex* 2006 16:865-875.

Goldman-Rakic PS. The prefrontal landscape: implications of functional architecture for understanding human mentation and the central executive. Philosophical Transactions of the Royal Society, London, Series B 1996 351:1445-1453.

González-Burgos G, Barrionuevo G, Lewis DA. Horizontal synaptic connections in monkey prefrontal cortex: an in vitro electrophysiological study. *Cerebral Cortex* 2000 10:82-92.

Hilgetag CC, O'Neill MA, Young MP. Indeterminate organization of the visual system. *Science* 1996 271:776-777.

Jacobs B, Schall M, Prather M, Kapler L, Driscoll L, Baca S, Jacobs J, Ford K, Wainwright M, Treml M. Regional dendritic and spine variation in human cerebral cortex: a quantitative study. *Cerebral Cortex* 2001 11:558-571.

Lewis JW, van Essen DC. Corticocortical connections of visual, sensorimotor, and multimodal processing areas in the parietal lobe of the macaque monkey. *Journal of Comparative Neurology* 2000 428:112-137.

Lund JS, Yoshioka T, Levitt JB. Comparison of intrinsic connectivity in different areas of macaque monkey cerebral cortex. *Cerebral Cortex* 1993 3:148-162.

Melchitzky DS, González-Burgos G, Barrionuevo G, Lewis DA. Synaptic targets of the intrinsic axon collaterals of supragranular pyramidal neurons in monkey prefrontal cortex. *Journal of Comparative Neurology* 2001 430:209-221.

Melchitzky DS, Sesack SR, Pucak ML, Lewis DA. Synaptic targets of pyramidal neurons providing intrinsic horizontal connections in monkey prefrontal cortex. *Journal of Comparative Neurology* 1998 390:211-224.

Miller EK, Cohen JD. An integrative theory of prefrontal cortex function. *Annual Reviews of Neuroscience* 2001 24:167-202.

Passingham R. Anatomical differences between the neocortex of man and other primates. *Brain Behavior and Evolution* 1973 7:337-359.

Passingham R, Stephan KE, Kötter R. The anatomical basis of functional localization in the cortex. *Nature Reviews Neuroscience* 2002 3:606-616.

Petrides M. 2000. Mapping prefrontal cortical systems for the control of cognition. In: Toga AW, Mazziotta JC, Frackowiak RS (Eds.) *Brain Mapping: The Systems*. Academic: San Dieg:. pp 159-176.

Petrides M, Pandya DN. Comparative cytoarchitectonic analysis of the human and the macaque ventrolateral prefrontal cortex and corticocortical connection patterns in the monkey. *European Journal of Neuroscience* 2001 16:291-310.

Preuss TM, Goldman-Rakic PS. Ipsilateral cortical connections of granular frontal cortex in the strepsirhine primate Galago, with comparative comments on anthropoid primates. *Journal of Comparative Neurology* 1991 310:507-549.

Rempel-Clower NL, Barbas H. The laminar pattern of connections between prefrontal and anterior temporal cortices in the rhesus monkey is related to cortical structure and function. *Cerebral Cortex* 2000 10:851-865.

Schoenemann PT, Sheehan MJ, Glotzer LD. Prefrontal white matter volume is disproportionately larger in humans than in other primates. *Nature Neuroscience* 2005 8:242-252.

Semendeferi K, Lu A, Schenker N, Damasio H. Humans and great apes share a large frontal cortex. *Nature Neuroscience* 2002 5:272-276.

Sherwood CC, Cranfield MR, Mehlman PT, Lilly AA, Garbe JA, Whittier CA, Nutter FB, Rein TR, Bruner HJ, Holloway RL, Tang CY, Naidich TP, Delman BN, Steklis HD, Erwin JM, Hof PR. Brain structure variation in great apes, with attention to the mountain gorilla (*Gorilla beringei beringei*). *American Journal of Primatology* 2004 63:149-164.

Sherwood CC, Holloway RL, Semendeferi K, Hof PR. Is prefrontal white matter enlargement a human evolutionary specialization? *Nature Neuroscience* 2005 8:537-538.

Soloway AS, Pucak ML, Melchitzky DS, Lewis DA. Dendritic morphology of callosal and ipsilateral projection neurons in monkey prefrontal cortex. *Neuroscience* 2002 109:461-471.

Szentagothai J, Arbib MA. Conceptual models of neural organization. *Neuroscience Research Programme Bulletin* 1974 12:305-510.

Young MP. The organization of neural systems in the primate cerebral cortex. *Proceedings of the Royal Society,* London, Series B 1993 252:13-18.

Zeki SM. Uniformity and diversity of structure and function in rhesus monkey prestriate visual cortex. *Journal of Physiology* (London) 1978 277:273-290.

In: Prefrontal Cortex: Roles, Interventions and Traumas
Editors: Lorenzo LoGrasso and Giovanni Morretti
ISBN 978-1-60692-415-0

Short Communication B

Developmental Characteristics in Category Generation Reflects Differential Prefrontal Cortex Maturation

Julio Cesar Flores Lázaro[1, 2] and Feggy Ostrosky-Solís[1*]
[1]Universidad Nacional Autónoma de México, Psychology Faculty,
Laboratory of Neuropsychology and Psychophysiology México, D.F.
[2]Universidad Juárez Autónoma de Tabasco,
división académica de ciencias de la salud,
Villahermosa Tabasco, México

Abstract

The developmental characteristics of semantic category generation were studied in a sample of 200 neurologically intact subjects from 6 to 30 years old. Results indicate that diverse brain areas support different the category criteria used: subjects in the 6-8 age range used a concrete criteria (posterior brain areas), in the 9-11 age range a functional criteria is dominant (dorsolateral prefrontal cortex), while abstract criteria becomes dominant in the 12-14 age-range (anterior prefrontal cortex) and continuous to develop in the 16 to 30 age range. It is proposed that different prefrontal areas participate during development, shaping cognitive approach to categorisation during childhood and adolescence.

Keywords: categorisation, prefrontal cortex, development

* Correspondence: Feggy Ostrosky-Solís, Universidad Nacional Autónoma de México, facultad de Psicología, Laboratorio de Neuropsicología y Psicofisiología. Rivera de Cupia 110-71. Lomas de Reforma. México D.F. C.P. 11900. E-mail address: feggy@servidor.unam.mx.

Introduction

The ability to categorize is fundamental for cognitive development. The evolution from concrete to abstract thinking goes trough different developmental stages that shape cognitive performance in children (Gelaes and Thibaut, 2006).

Young children frequently compare and categorize objects using perceptual features, like for example the shape of an object. Progressively when children learn new words that represent semantic labels, they prefer to use the category such as "animals" or "furniture", rather than a perceptual criteria (Gentner and Namy, 2000). While performing comparisons between objects, children systematically introduce cognitive changes and variations in their semantic representations. These changes allow the transformation and construction of experiences into categories, achieved by continuously delineating each category's characteristics and its boundaries, thus creating a conceptual structure for each representation (Borodistky, 2007).

The processes of comparison are mainly based on similarity, a basic component of cognition. As Markman and Gentner (1996) point out, humans tend to categorize objects based mainly on similarities. Similar objects are grouped into the same categories and serve to support inductive inferences between each other. These categories also form a structure to further acquire and learn new information.

The development of categorization transforms experience into well-defined categories by constructing conceptual structures that goes beyond concrete experience (Boroditsky 2007).

When young children have to include objects within categories they prefer to use perceptual features (Gelaes and Thibaut, 2006). Children continuously compare objects, and integrate them into categories formed by structurally related items. Throughout children's development, perceptual comparison leads to the continuously dynamic identification of similarities and differences, but most importantly to conceptual category development that progressively evolves from concrete to abstract features (Gelaes and Thibaut, 2006).

It has already been found that children are able to know and differentiate a significant number of complex categories showed by adults. However, this can only happen when these categories are shown by the adult, and not necessarily when children have generate them spontaneously (Gentner and Namy, 2000).

Frontal Lobes and Categorization

The capacity to generate abstract classification criteria and to maintain an attitude for an adequate abstract thinking is a very important property of the frontal lobes (Lezak, 2004; Luria, 1986). Normal adults (with average education) tend to analyze information in an abstract form, even if instructed not to do so (Noppeney et al., 2005). This phenomenon has been named *abstract attitude* (Lezak, 2004).

It is a common characteristic that damage to the frontal lobes frequently alters the capacity to identify abstract classification criteria in both spontaneous and active form (Delis et al., 1992; Kertesz, 1994; Luria, 1986). Often patients with frontal lobe damage don't lose the ability for abstract processing, but prefer to analyze objects, events and situations in a concrete form. This phenomenon has been named *concretism* (Lezak, 2004). A severe bilateral frontal lobe damage affects the ability for abstract processing in a significant way (Kertsez, 1994; Luria, 1989).

Recent neuroimaging studies have found that during abstract categorization in adults, the prefrontal cortex and mainly the anterior prefrontal cortex (APFC) are significantly activated (Green et al., 2006). This can be seen particularly during visual object categorization that requires a dynamic scan of elements and an active features comparison, where the right prefrontal cortex, mainly areas 10 and 47, are the most active (Bright, Most and Tyler, 2004; Pernet et al., 2004; Reber et al., 1998). In contrast, the comparison and retrieval of concrete and perceptual object features activates mainly the posterior cortex (occipito-temporal cortex) (Rossion et al., 2000).

Within neuropsychology, there is a conceptual division between semantic representations and their active utilization, where semantic representation activates posterior-cortical areas (Rossion et al., 2000), while the active processing occurs mainly in the prefrontal cortex (Delis et al., 1992). This dissociation represents the neural basis for the division between knowledge and its adequate use, named *know/do* (Bright et al., 2004; Noppeney et al., 2005 Peranni et al., 1999).

As a result of diverse neuroimaging studies, a functional division between the anterior prefrontal cortex (APFC) and the dorsolateral prefrontal cortex (DLPFC) has been found, in which the latter region participates during executive categorization: updating specific information and directs element feature comparison (Rossion et al., 2000). In contrast, the APFC participates during semantic comparison (Cools, Clark and Robbins, 2004; Kroger et al., 2002; Noppeney et al., 2002; Ricci et al., 1999).

Classification tests regularly used in neuropsychological evaluations depend on the capacity to generate abstract classification criteria, and normal performance in these tests requires prefrontal cortex participation

In neuropsychological testing as well as in most developmental studies, evaluators or researchers ask the child to intentionally produce a specific category or they provide a prompt-cue to influence the subject to generate this category, however in this testing situation the examiner is given the structure thus is acting as the "child's frontal lobes". Here, the question of whether the child possesses the conceptual level of knowledge for the category or if he can recognize it is answered, however, the question regarding what type of category the child chooses spontaneously can't be answered by these evaluation procedures. Therefore, the main objective was to study the developmental characteristics for the capacity of self-regulated category generation in subjects between 6 and 30 years old. Specific questions were 1) How do children spontaneously use their semantic knowledge in a production category task? 2) At what moment during development is present the "abstract attitude present" and finally 3) at what age does abstract category generation reach maximum performance?

By adopting a cognitive neuropsychological perspective, we tried to answer each one of these different questions by using a particular evaluation form that is sensitive to different brain network involvement during development, mainly anterior vs. posterior network divisions and their functional dissociations.

Method

A transversal and comparative study was performed, using the self-regulated category generation test, extracted from the *Executive Functions Battery* (Flores Lázaro and Ostrosky-Solis, 2005). This battery contains several tests that evaluate diverse executive functions, which depend on different prefrontal cortical areas. The sample included 200 normal subjects between 6 to 30 years of age. All subjects were free from neurological, neuropsychological or psychiatric background. All had average school performance. The sample was divided into five age groups: 6-8, 9-11,12-14, 15-17 and 18-30 years old.

Material: The instrument is a category-generation test based on one A4 size foil including 25 animal figures extracted from Snodgrass and Vandertwart´s (1980). Each of these animals can be classified into several semantic categories, such as mammals, aquatic animals, etc. It also gives the opportunity to generate other types of classification, named *concrete*: size, shape, feathers, and other physical attributes; *functional:* they fly; they are fast, etc. (see figure 1).

Procedure: subjects were given the following instruction: you must generate as many categories as you can, in a maximum time of five minutes. For children between ages 6-8, instructions were: you must make as many animals groups as you can, I'll give you five minutes to do so. Test application was individual, and it was part of a larger research on the development of executive functions.

Statistical Analysis: Results were registered in a database with SPSS 11. Statistical analysis included one way ANOVA. Contrast analysis was made considering the age range as the independent variable and curvilinear estimation was made considering year by year as a lineal as the independent variable.

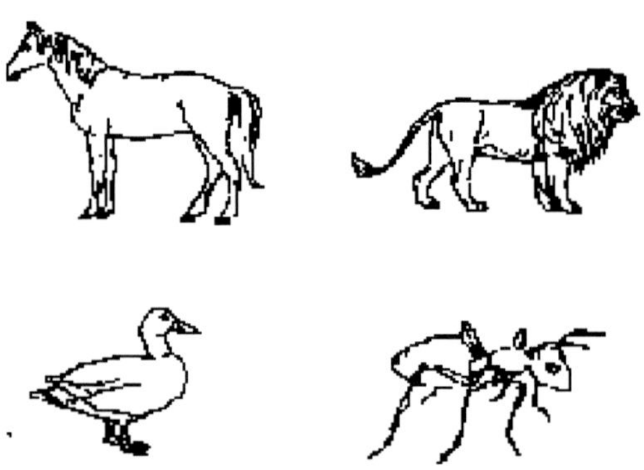

Figure 1. Examples of animals included in the test.

Results

Results are divided by age ranges and presented by category type. Table 1 shows the category type percentages (in round numbers). It can be noticed (outlined in bold) that *concrete* category type is the preferred classification criteria for children between 6-8 years of age; functional characteristics are the preferred classification criteria for 9-11 year old children, abstract criteria is the preferred classification criteria for the 12-14 year old subject group, in the 15-17 and 18-30 year old groups, abstract categories represent the dominant semantic criteria for category generation. Category type averages are shown in table 2. It can be seen that abstract category average increases as a function of age, whereas concrete category average decreases, although it never completely disappears (not even in university students). Number of functional categories increases between ages 6-8 and 9-11, but later decreases.

Table 1. Category type percentage according to age range groups

AGE RANGE GROUPS	CONCRETE	FUNCTIONAL	ABSTRACT
1 (6-8)	58 %	34 %	8 %
2 (9-11)	20 %	47 %	33 %
3 (12-14)	11 %	26 %	63 %
4 (15-17)	10 %	19 %	71 %
5 (18-30)	8 %	16 %	76 %

Table 2. Category type average produced by age range groups

AGE RANGE GROUPS	CONCRETE	FUNCTIONAL	ABSTRACT
1 (6-8)	3.84	2.23	0.61
2 (9-11)	1.38	3.18	2.22
3 (12-14)	0.67	1.76	4.24
4 (15-17)	0.73	1.33	5.03
5 (18-30)	0.63	1.33	6.36

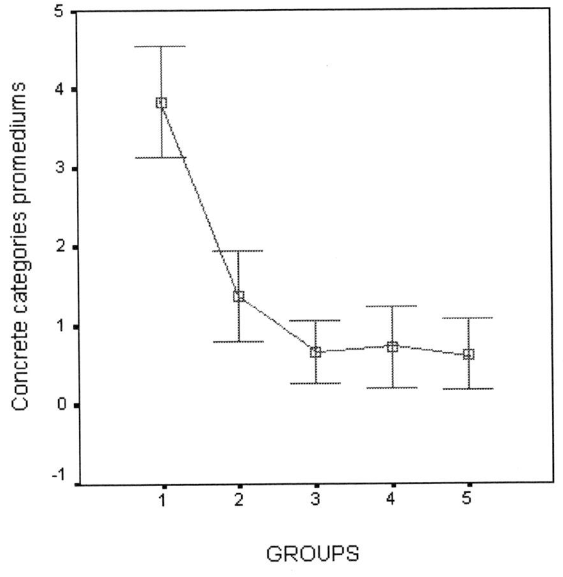

Figure 2. Average of concrete categories by age range . Contrast analysis values present a significant inverse relationship (F= 75.587 p= .000). Curvilinear analysis detects a main inverse lineal effect (R^2= .407, F= 117.92 p=. 000) Age range of group 1=(6-8), 2=(9-11) 3= (12-14), 4=(15-17).

Figure 2 presents a graphical representation of the data, where it can be observed that concrete categories fall dramatically between 6-8 and 9-11, presenting statistical significance among these age ranges (table 3). After this, decrement is very slow and it is not statistically significant among any group, from the 9-11 age range and later age groups. Contrast analysis reveals a main linear relationship, while linear analysis reveals an inverse effect (see figure 2).

Table 3. Statistical differences between averages in number of Concrete categories, produced by age range

Age Range Groups	9-11	12-14	15-17	18-30
1 (6-8)	2.46 (p= .000)	3.17 (p= .000)	3.11 (p= .000)	3.21 (p= .000)
2 (9-11)		0.71 (p= .239)	0.65 (p= .430)	0.75 (p= .240)
3 (12-14)			- 0.06 (p= 1.000)	0.03 (p=1 .000)
4 (15-17)				0.09 (p=. 999)

One-way ANOVA between groups showing mean differences and statistical significance (F(4,181)= 27.739 p= .000).

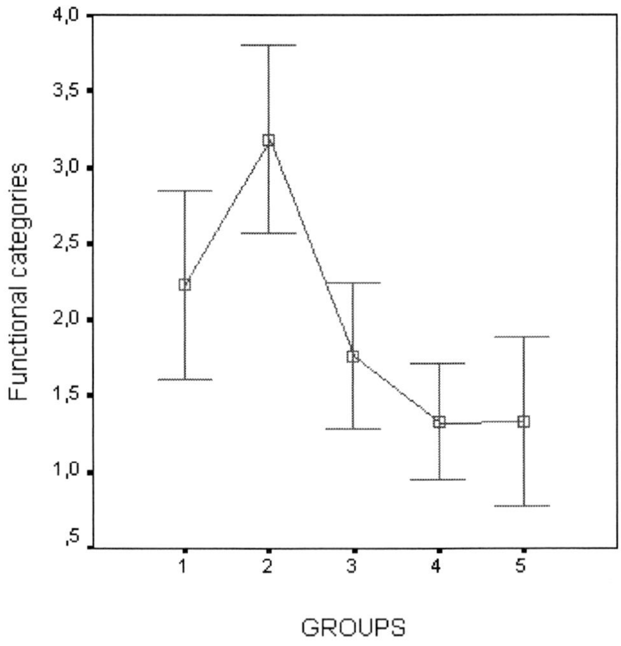

Figure 3. Average of functional categories by age range. Contrast analysis presents a significant lineal relationship (F= 15.833 p= .000). Curvilinear analysis detects a main discreet lineal effect (F=14.34 p=. 000); although quadratic model was significant, its value was inferior to lineal (F= 8.18 p= .000). Age range of group 1=(6-8), 2=(9-11) 3= (12-14), 4=(15-17).

The generation of functional categories presents the most interesting behavior during development (see figure 3), increasing between 6-8 and 9-11 years of age and decrementing through the 12-14 age range (see figure 2). Statistical significance is presented between 9-11 year old group and the subsequent groups. No statistical differences are presented between 6-

8 and 9-11 year old group. Abstract category production presents a linear type of behavior during development. All groups were statistically different except group 12-14 and 15-17 (see table 5 and figure 4).

Table 4. Statistical differences between averages in number of Functional categories, produced by age range

Age Range Groups	9-11	12-14	15-17	18-30
1 (6-8)	-0.96 (p= .187)	0.47 (p= .752)	0.89 (p= .106)	0.89 (p= .199)
2 (9-11)		1.42 (p= .004)	1.85 (p= .000)	1.86 (p= .000)
3 (12-14)			0.43 (p= .622)	0.43 (p= .760)
4 (15-17)				0.00 (p= 1.000)

One-way ANOVA between groups showing mean differences and statistical significance (F(4,182)= 7.677 p= .000).

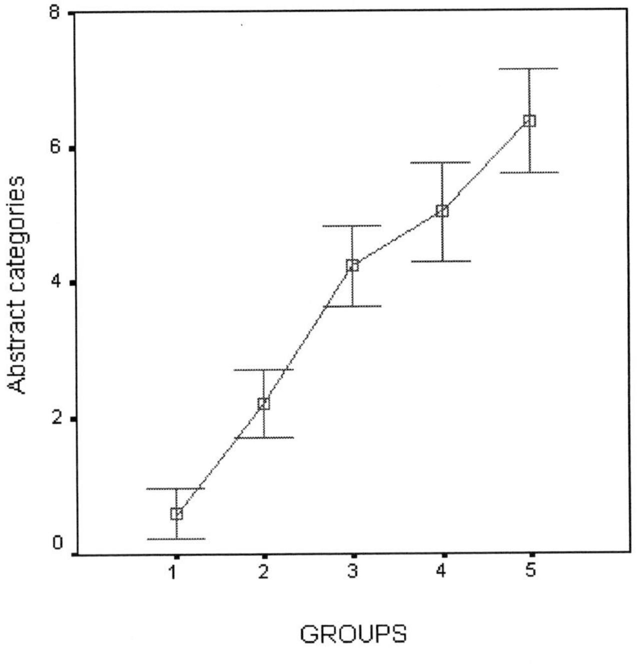

Figure 4. Average of abstract categories by age range . Contrast analysis values present a significant lineal relationship (F=238.946 p= .000). Curvilinear analysis detects a main inverse lineal effect (R2= .592, F=271.31 p=. 000). Age range of group 1=(6-8), 2=(9-11) 3= (12-14), 4=(15-17).

Considering that although some category types are the main preferred category, a second category is also present, shaping cognitive development in a more complex form. In table 6 it can be seen that in the 6-8 age group, concrete categories represent the dominant cognitive approach, accompanied by the functional features. An inverse relation occurs in the next age range (9-11). In the 12-14 age range, abstract classification is the dominant cognitive approach accompanied by the functional criteria. The 15-17 age range it can be noticed that abstract classification is the dominant cognitive criteria for spontaneous semantic classification (see table 6).

Table 5. Statistical differences in average number of Abstract categories, produced by age range

Age Range Groups	9-11	Comparison 12-14	15-17	18-30
1 (6-8)	-1.61 (p= .000)	- 3.63 (p= .000)	- 4.42 (p= .000)	- 5.75 (p= .000)
2 (9-11)		- 2.02 (p= .000)	- 2.81 (p= .000)	- 4.14 (p= .000)
3 (12-14)			0.79 (p= .437)	- 2.12 (p= .000)
4 (15-17)				-1.33 (p= .089)

One-way ANOVA between groups showing mean differences and statistical significance ($F_{(4,184)}$= 60.973 p= .000).

Table 6. Category combination reflecting spontaneous cognitive approach to classification

Age Range Groups	Category's Combination	Percentage relationship
1 (6-8)	Concrete-functional	58-34 %
2 (9-11)	Functional-abstract	47-33 %
3 (12-14)	Abstract-Functional	63-26 %
4 (15-17)	Abstract	71 %
5 (18-30)	Abstract	77 %

Discussion

If we consider that concrete classification criteria depend mainly on posterior cortical networks (or the lack of involvement of APFC) (Noppeney et al., 2002), that functional classification criteria depend mainly on prefrontal cortex -fronto-parietal network- (Piatt et al., 1999; Wood et al., 2004) and that abstract classification criteria depend mainly on APFC (Cools, Clark and Robbins, 2004; Reber et al., 1998), then results show different prefrontal cortex development stages and their influence on cognitive development processes, like categorization.

During the 6-8 age range, concrete features are the preferred criteria for spontaneous classification of objects, indicating that until these ages, children do not present a sufficiently active (or dominant) APFC-network. For this reason, they prefer to spontaneously categorize objects by concrete features (posterior cortical mode of processing). Recent neuroimaging studies have found that the anterior temporal lobe participates in the perceptual analysis of concrete objects' features (Noppeney et al., 2002). The combination of classification criteria reflects that DLPFC is already active and also present during spontaneous classification in this age range. A concrete-functional form of processing indicates a dominant posterior network, combined with an emergent and secondary DLPFC network (fronto-parietal) participation.

In the 9-11 age range, functional features are the dominant criteria for spontaneous classification; this may reflect a very important shift from posterior cortical to prefrontal processing. Action naming is closely related to dorsolateral prefrontal cortex functioning in adults and children (Holland et al., 2001; Piatt et al., 1999; Weiss et al., 2003; Wood et al., 2004). These results show that from ages 9-11, the dominant networks for spontaneous classification depend mainly on DLPFC. Other studies have outlined the acceleration in cognitive performance in tests that depend on DLPFC during this same period, suggesting that these brain regions present the most important growth during late childhood (Diamond, 2002). A secondary abstract criterion is already present and shapes categorization during this phase. These results indicate that DLPFC (fronto-parietal) is the dominant network and that APFC begins to appear as a secondary cortical network during this age range.

During the 12-14 age range the abstract categorization criteria becomes dominant and the functional criteria becomes secondary, reflecting an interesting within-frontal network shifting stage from DLPFC to APFC networks. The last phase occurs from 15-17 years old in which a clear dominant abstract criteria for categorization is present, with a slow but linear increment in the next age range (18-30).

According to our results, four developmental stages have been determined during spontaneous classification: Stage 1 (6-8 years old): concrete-functional. Stage 2 (9-11years old): functional-abstract. Stage 3 (12-14 years old): abstract-functional, Stage 4 (15-17 and 18-30 years old): abstract.

Contrast and curvilinear analysis show different lineal age-effects for each categorization criteria: an inverse effect for concrete criteria, a lineal and discrete quadratic effect for functional criteria, and a clear lineal effect for abstract criteria. The cognitive resources (indeed prefrontal cortex networks) slowly but linearly increase spontaneous attention to abstract processing, while rapidly decreasing the concrete form. Spontaneously functional analysis presents an increment in a very specific age-range (9-11), to later decrease slowly but continuously.

Results suggest that during cognitive development, the prefrontal cortex provide the active use of abstract processing, transforming concrete and functional cognition into abstract spontaneous processing. The development of the prefrontal cortex restructures cognition from concrete to functional, and later on to abstract. Results also suggest a developmental functional dissociation within the prefrontal cortex for the 9-11 age range dorsolateral prefrontal cortex may be the particular dominant prefrontal cortex network, while anterior prefrontal cortex networks are already dominant at the beginning of adolescence, reaching almost exclusively cognitive dominance at the end of adolescence. Regarding these findings, we consider that abstract categorization is more closely related to AFPC than DLPFC, and is clearly present at the beginning of adolescence. Therefore, the operational phase described by Piaget seem to depend not on "the prefrontal cortex" as a whole but mainly on APFC development.

In conclusion, the ability to spontaneously categorize into semantic fields passes through several cognitive stages that in turn depend on developmental characteristics of the prefrontal cortex. Gradual transition occurs from concrete categorization in early childhood to functional criteria utilization in late childhood. At the beginning of adolescence, abstract features become the main preferred criteria for categorization, whereas inn later age ranges including young adulthood, abstract criteria (indeed abstract attitude) develops further and becomes the more dominant cognitive analysis mode. A posterior to frontal cortical network shift occurs during childhood. During adolescence a shift occurs from DLPFC (functional categorization criteria) to APFC (abstract categorization criteria) within the prefrontal cortex. Results indicate how prefrontal cortex development shapes cognitive development from childhood to youthood.

References

Borodistky, L. (2007). Comparison and the development of knowledge. *Cognition,* 102, 118-128.

Bright, P., Most, H., and Tyler, L.K. (2004). Unitary vs multiple semantics: PET studies of word and picture processing. *Brain and Language,* 89, 17-32.

Cools, R., Clark L., and Robbins, T.W. (2004). Differential responses in human striatum and prefrontal cortex to changes in object and rule relevance. *Journal of Neuroscience*, 4, 1129-35.

Delis, D.C., Squire, L.R., Bihrle, A., and Massman, P. (1992). Componential analysis of problem-solving ability: performance of patients with frontal lobe damage and amnesic patients on a new sorting test. *Neuropsychologia*, 30, 683-97.

Diamond, A. (2002) Normal development of prefrontal cortex from birth to young adulthood, cognitive functions, anatony and biochemistry. In D. T. Stuss and R. T. Knight, (Eds.), *Principles of frontal lobes function* (pp. 466-503). New York: Oxford University Press.

Flores Lázaro, J. C., and Ostrosky-Solís, F. (2005). Batería de funciones ejecutivas. *Instituto nacional de derechos de Autor.* Registro: 03-2005-03141105400-01. México, D. F.

Gelaes, S., and Thibaut, J.P. (2006). The role of the structure of parts and of the overall object shape in children's generalization of novel object names. *Cognitive development,* 21, 369-376.

Gentner, D., and Namy, L.L. (2000). Comparison in the development of categories. *Cognitive development*, 14,487-513.

Green, A.E., Fugelsang, J.A., Kraemer, D.J., Shamosh, N.A., Dunbar, K.N. (2006). Frontopolar cortex mediates abstract integration in analogy. *Brain Research*. 22,125-37.

Holland, S.K., Plante, E,, Byars, W.B. (2001). Normal fMRI brain activation patterns in children performing a verb generation task. *Neuroimage*, 14 837-843.

Kertesz, A. (1994). *Localization and Neuroimaging in Neuropsychology*. San Diego: Academic Press.

Kroger, J.K., Sabb, F.W., Fales, C.L., Bookheimer, S.Y., Cohen, S., and Holyoak, K.J. (2002). Recruitment of anterior dorsolateral prefrontal cortex in human reasoning: a parametric study of relational complexity.*Cerebral Cortex*. 12 (5), 477-85.

Lezak, M.D. (2004). *Neuropsychological Evaluation*. 4th Edition. New York: Oxford University Press.

Luria, A.R. (1986). *Las Funciones Corticales Superiores del Hombre*. México: Fontamara.

Luria, A.R. (1989). *El Cerebro en Acción*. España: Roca.

Markman, A.B. and Gentner, D., (1996) Commonalities and differences in similarity comparisons. *Memory and Cognition*. 24, 235-49.

Noppeney, U., Price, C.J., Penny, W.D., and Friston, K.J. (2005). Two Distinct Neural Mechanisms for Category-selective Responses. *Cerebral Cortex*. 16(3), 437-45.

Perani, D., Schnur, T., Tettamanti, M., Gorno-Tempini, M., Cappa, S.F., and Fazio, F. (1999). Word and picture matching: a PET study of semantic category effects. *Neuropsychologia*. 37(3), 293-306.

Pernet, C,, Franceries, X,, Basan, S., Cassol, E., Demonet, J.F., and Celsis, P. (2004). Anatomy and time course of discrimination and categorization processes in vision: an fMRI study. *Neuroimage,* 22 (4), 1563-77.

Piatt, A., Fields, J., Paolo, A.M., Troster, A.I. (1999). Action (verb naming) fluency as an executive function measure: convergent and divergent evidence of validity. *Neuropsychologia*, 37, 1499-1503.

Reber, P.J., Stark, C.E., and Squire, L.R. (1998). Cortical areas supporting category learning identified using functional MRI. *Proceedings of the National Academy of Science U. S. A*. 20 (2), 747-50.

Ricci, P.T., Zelkowicz, B.J., Nebes, R.D., Meltzer, C.C., Mintun, M.A., Becker, J.T. (1999). Functional neuroanatomy of semantic memory: recognition of semantic associations. *Neuroimage*, 9, 88-96.

Rossion, B., Bodart, J.M., Pourtois, G., Thioux, M., Bol, A., Cosnard, G., Benoit, G., Michel, C., and De Volder, A. (2000). Functional imaging of visual semantic processing in the human brain. *Cortex*. 36(4), 579-91.

Snodgrass, J. G., and Vanderwart, M. (1980). A standardized set of 260 pictures: Norms for name agreement, familiarity and visual complexity. *Journal of Experimental Psychology: Human Learning and Memory*, 6, 174-215.

Weiss, E.M., Siedentopf, C., Hofer, A., and Deisenhammer, E.A. (2003). Brain activation patterns during a verbal fluency test in healthy male and female volunteers: a functional magnetic imaging study, *Neuroscience letters*, 352,191-194.

Wood, A.G., Harvey, A.S., Wellard, R.M., Abbott, D.F., Anderson, V., Kean, M., Saling, M.M., and Jackson, G.D. (2004). Language cortex activation in normal children. *Neurology*. 28, (6), 1035-44.

Index

A

B

C

E

G

H

I

N

O

T